TOPICS IN OSTEOPOROSIS

Edited by **Margarita Valdés-Flores**

Topics in Osteoporosis
http://dx.doi.org/10.5772/50259
Edited by Margarita Valdés-Flores

Contributors
Emilio González Jiménez, Luiz Eugenio Garcez Leme, Maria do Carmo Sitta, Margarita Valdés-Flores, Rafael Velázquez Cruz, Lorena Orozco, Alma Parra-Torres, Mehreen Lateef, Mukhtiar Baig, Abid Azhar, Olga Cvijanovic, Zeljka Crncevic Orlic, Sandra Pavicic Zezelj, Nenad Bicanic, Robert Domitrovic, Dragica Bobinac, Silvija Lukanovic, Tulay Okman-Kilic, Cengiz Sagiroglu, Lucas Emmanuel Teixeira, Joelma Magalhães, Stella Peccin, Kelson Silva, Tiago Jose De Paiva Teixeira, Aline Mizusaki Imoto, Virginia Trevisani, Yan Zhang, Yoseph Asmelash Gebru, Shiqi Peng, Ming Zhao, Satoshi Iwase, Leticia Rao, Venketeshwer Rao

Published by InTech
Janeza Trdine 9, 51000 Rijeka, Croatia

Publishing Process Manager Iva Simcic
Technical Editor InTech DTP team
Cover InTech Design team

Additional hard copies can be obtained from orders@intechopen.com

Topics in Osteoporosis, Edited by Margarita Valdés-Flores
p. cm.
ISBN 978-953-51-1066-8

For EU product safety concerns :
IN TECH d.o.o., Prolaz Marije Krucifikse Kozulić 3, 51000 Rijeka, Croatia,
info@intechopen.com or visit our website at intechopen.com.

Meet the editor

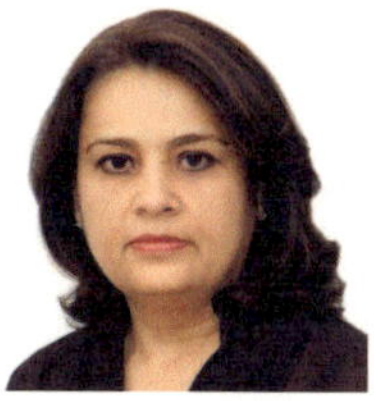

Dr. Margarita Valdés Flores received M.D. at Autonomous University of Coahuila in 1989, title of Genetic specialist in 1995 and Ph.D in 2002, at the National Autonomous University of Mexico. From 1998, Dr. Valdés Flores is working at National Rehabilitation Institute as Genetics specialist and Researcher. She supervises the Masters and Doctorate in Medical Sciences Program and in the Genetics Specialty of Medicine, at National Autonomous University of Mexico. Currently, Dr. Valdés Flores is member of the National System of Researchers, the Mexican Academy of Sciences and Mexican Academy of Surgery. Between her research lines, highlights the investigation of the genetic component of Mexican population in relation to osteoporosis. Most of her published articles are related with these investigations.

Contents

Preface

In the last decades the world has faced several epidemic health problems; among them are osteoporosis, osteoarthritis, diabetes mellitus, obesity and cardiovascular diseases. All these diseases share characteristics as their multifactorial and polygenic origin and the extensive involvement of the environment in their etiology strongly associated with the actual lifestyle (bad dietary habits, sedentary life and eating disorders, among others). At present, the above mentioned diseases do not exclusively affect elderly people and are currently afflicting young adults and even children, obligating us to intensify our efforts to prevent them.

The progressive loss of bone mineral density and bone microarchitecture deterioration in osteoporosis, promote the occurrence of fractures which can develop complications and disabilities and imply high costs to the healthcare services. There is no doubt that the efforts should focus on prevention and on strengthening of programs directed toward protecting and improving the bone health to induce bone mass gain in early stages of life and to limit the potential risks related with the onset of the disease. Actually a great number of investigations throughout the world continuously contribute with information about functioning of bone tissue and the physiopathology of osteoporosis which enable researchers to explore new therapeutic possibilities in bone resorption disorders.

Dr. Margarita Valdés-Flores
Genetics Unit, National Institute of Rehabilitation,
Health Secretary (Secretaria de Salud),
Faculty of Medicine, Universidad Nacional Autónoma Mexico
Mexico D.F.

Chapter 1

Molecular Aspects of Bone Remodeling

Alma Y. Parra-Torres, Margarita Valdés-Flores,
Lorena Orozco and Rafael Velázquez-Cruz

Additional information is available at the end of the chapter

http://dx.doi.org/10.5772/54905

1. Introduction

Bone is a dynamic tissue in constant change; maintenance of bone mass throughout life relies on the bone remodeling process, which continually replaces old and damaged bone with new bone. This remodeling is necessary to maintain the structural integrity of the skeleton and allows the maintenance of bone volume, the repair of tissue damage and homeostasis of calcium and phosphorous metabolism. This process allows the renewal of 5% of cortical bone and trabecular 20% in a year, and although the cortical portion makes up most of the bone (75%), the metabolic activity is ten times greater in the trabecular since the relationship between surface and volume is greater in this, which is achieved by an annual renewal of 5-10% of bone volume and although this remodeling takes place throughout life, your balance is positive only during the first three decades. The skeleton is particularly dependent on mechanical information to guide the resident cell population towards adaptation, maintenance and repair; a wide range of cell types depend on mechanically induced signals to enable appropriate physiological responses. The bone remodeling has two main phases: a resorption phase, consisting of the removal of old bone by osteoclasts, and a later phase of formation of new bone by osteoblasts that replaces the tissue previously resorbed. While osteoclasts are derived from hematopoietic precursor cells and degrade the bone matrix, osteoblasts originate from mesenchymal stem cells, they deposit a collagenous bone matrix and orchestrate its mineralization. While the interaction of bone cells with their mechanical environment is complex, an understanding of mechanical regulation of bone signaling is crucial to understanding bone physiology, the etiology of bone diseases such as osteoporosis, and to the development of interventions to improve bone strength. The clinical importance of bone formation has stimulated a lot of research aimed at understanding its mechanism. Much knowledge has been gained in the recent years, especially in relation with the signaling pathways controlling osteoblast differentiation. The purpose of this chapter is to review current knowledge on biochemical and physiological mechanisms of remodeling bone, with particular attention to the role in the cell involved, the process, regulation signals into the control and pathophysiology of bone remodeling (diseases).

2. Cells involved in bone remodeling

Two bone cell lineages have been identified: cells of the osteoblast lineage (osteoblasts, osteocytes and bone-lining cells) and bone resorbing cells (osteoclasts) that together with their precursor cells and associated cells (e.g. endothelial cells, nerve cells) are organized in specialized units called bone multi cellular units (BMU). The main function of the BMU is to mediate a bone "rejuvenation" mechanism called "bone remodeling". Bone remodeling maintains the integrity of the skeleton by removing old bone of high mineral density and high prevalence of fatigue micro-fractures through repetitive cycles of bone resorption and bone formation [1]. This is a direct and crucial interaction that has been well established in vivo. Once osteoblasts and osteoclasts are fully differentiated, there is a less direct relationship [2]. Despite the know close physiological interactions of the two main cellular systems in bone, there are effectively separate and distinct origins of osteoblast (hematopoietic cell origin) and stromal/osteoblast linages from the developing fetus onward in mammalian development; circulating osteogenic precursor cells are blood-borne cells that express a variety of osteoblastic markers and are able to form bone in vivo. Strong evidence suggests that cells are derived from bone marrow and are of hematopoietic origin [3].

2.1. Osteoblast

Osteoblasts derive from mesenchymal precursor cells, which also originate, chondrocytes (cartilage), adipocytes (bone marrow stroma), fibroblasts (periosteum), and adventitial reticular cells (bone marrow stroma). Although the claim that bone marrow stromal cell can also give raise chondrocytes, myoblasts, adipocytes and tendon cells, depending on the transcription factors that regulate the pathway [4]. There are four stages that have been identified in osteoblast differentiation: the preosteoblast, osteoblast, osteocyte and bone-lining cell that histologically these cells stain positively for alkaline phosphatase, however, only mature osteoblasts have the ability to produce mineralized tissue [5], and can be identified by their cuboidal morphology and strong alkaline phosphatase positivity. The master gene that encodes for a protein involved in the osteogenic differentiation process from mesenchymal precursors is the nuclear transcriptional factor Runx-2 (Runt related transcription factor 2, cbfa-1) (Figure 1) [6].

The osteoblast resides along the bone surface at sites of active bone formation. They secrete type 1 collagen, the basic building block of bone; non-collagenous proteins including osteocalcin and alkaline phosphatase, which is essential for mineral deposition [7]. The principal function of the osteoblast is bone formation and these occur via two distinct mechanisms: the intramembranous ossification (flat bones of the skull and most of the clavicle) and the endochondral ossification, which produces most bones, involves the transformation of mesenchyme

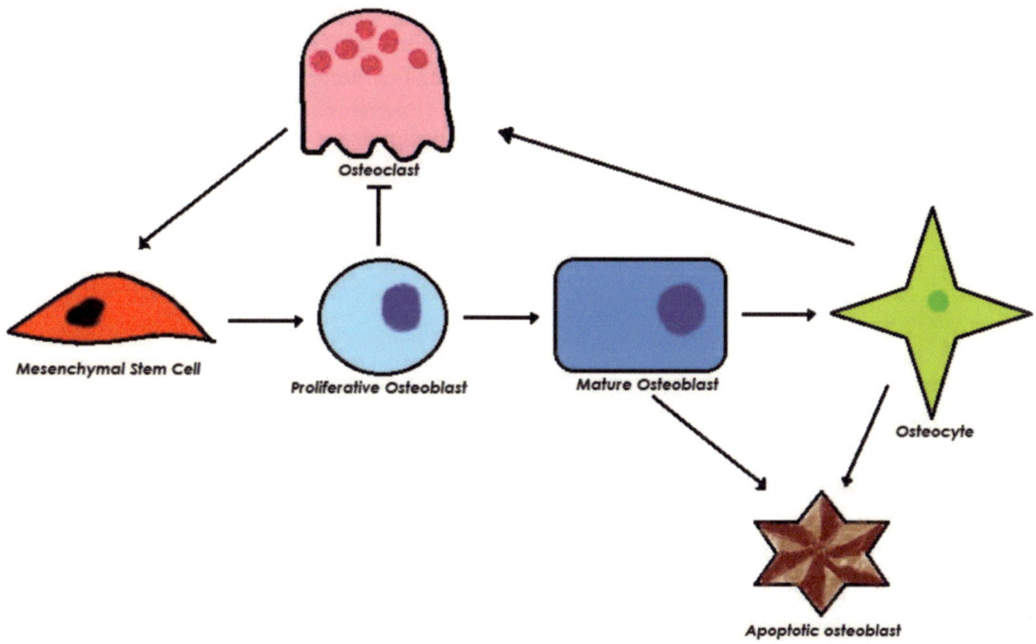

Figure 1. Osteoblasts derive from Mesenchymal Stem Cells. Osteoclasts derive from by the fusion of mononuclear progenitors of the monocyte/macrophage family, and Osteocytes are non-proliferative differentiated cells of the osteoblast lineage.

into a cartilage model that resembles the shape of the bone [8]. They are also responsible for the mineralization, although the exact mechanism by which mineralization occurs remains unclear [9]. Mature osteoblasts have one of three fates: they undergo apoptosis, differentiate further into osteocytes or become quiescent lining cells. Approximately 50 to 70% of osteoblasts undergo apoptosis [10].

2.2. Osteocyte

Osteocytes are non-proliferative, terminally differentiated cells of the osteoblast lineage, how osteoblasts transform into osteocytes is dependent on the mode of ossification (Figure 1). They reside both in the mineralized bone matrix and in newly formed osteoid, locked inside small lacuna spaces in the hard substance of bone are smaller than osteoblasts and have lost many of their cytoplasmic organelles [11-13]. They compose over 90–95% of all bone cells in the adult skeleton and are thought to respond to mechanical strain to send signals of resorption or formation, due to their distribution throughout the bone matrix and extensive interconnectivity, osteocytes are thought to be one if not the major bone cell type responsible for sensing mechanical strain and orchestrating signals of resorption and formation. Evidence suggests that the primary function of the osteocyte relates to the determination and maintenance of bone structure. Osteocytes are mechanosensors capable of transducing musculoskeletal derived mechanical input into biological output [14], the osteocyte appears to be capable of relating the intensity of strain signals and the distribution of the strain throughout the whole bone into signals to regulate [15]. Microdamage in the bone matrix has been shown to initiate bone remodeling, the osteocytes located near these sites undergo apoptosis correlated with increased bone remodeling due to enhanced RANKL production and an increase in osteoclast formation [16], and the osteocytes may be the major source of RANKL during bone remodeling [17-19]. For some time it has been estimated that the average life of this cell would be 25 years. The percentage of dead osteocytes increases with age senescence, being from 1% to 75% rise in the eighth decade [20,21].

2.3. Osteoclast

Osteoclasts, which are the only cells capable of resorbing bone, are multinucleated giant cells formed from by the fusion of mononuclear progenitors of the monocyte/macrophage family in a process termed osteoclastogenesis (Figure 1) [22], they are located on endosteal surfaces within the Haversian system and on the periosteal surface beneath the periosteum, in the bone has only two to three per μm^3 [23]. Osteoclasts are terminally differentiated myeloid cells that are uniquely adapted to remove mineralized bone matrix. These cells have distinct morphological and phenotypic characteristics that are routinely used to identify them, including multinuclearity and expression of tartrate-resistant acid phosphatase and the calcitonin receptor. Osteoclast differentiation is supported by cells of the osteoblast lineage that express membrane-bound receptor activator (RANK) of RANKL (NF-kB ligand) and macrophage-colony stimulating factor (M-CSF) [22]; this process is also regulated by a secreted decoy receptor of RANKL, osteoprotegerin (OPG), which functions as a paracrine inhibitor of osteoclast formation [24]. The balance between OPG and RANKL regulates bone resorption and formation and one imbalance of the RANKL/OPG system have been implicated in the pathogenesis of various primary and secondary bone malignancies [25]. In the motile state the osteoclast migrate from the bone marrow to their resorptive site and in the resorptive phase they exert their bone resorbing function, in each state the osteoclast display morphological differences [26], the motile osteoclasts are flattened, non-polarised cells and they are characterised by the presence of membrane protrusions (lamellipodia), and podosome. Upon reaching the resorptive site, osteoclasts become polarised through cytoskeletal reorganization, results in the formation of a ruffled border, sealing zone, functional secretory domain and basolateral membrane. The sealing zone is an osteoclast specific structure, which separates the acidic resorptive environment from the rest of the cell, forming an organelle free area [27].

2.4. Bone-lining cells

The bone lining cells constitute a subpopulation of the osteoblast family. Bone lining cells were characterized by their long, slender, and flattened appearance; and their association with the bone surface at sites where a thin no mineralized collagen layer was present [28]. Although not being osteoblasts in the sense that they produce an osteoid layer, belong to the same lineage as osteoblasts for the following reasons: they are alkaline phosphatase positive, respond to PTH, and are associated with the bone surface. The bone lining cells contained a low level of labeled osteocalcin, and they have electron-dense vacuoles containing crossbanded collagen fibrils in the cytoplasm [28]. It has been proposed that bone lining cells play a role in bone remodeling by preventing the inappropriate interaction of osteoclast precursors with the bone surface. It is thought that the signals that initiate osteoclast formation may stimulate the bone lining cells to prepare for bone resorption, through the actions of collagenase which digests a thin layer of non-mineralized bone, revealing the mineralized matrix underneath [29,30]. The bone lining cells migrate to form a canopy over the remodeling area, particularly at sites adjacent to osteoclasts, creating a microenvironment (in phagocytosis of collagen at the bone surface) for the coupling required during bone remodeling. It has been proposed that the bone lining cells are responsible for the cell to cell interactions between RANKL and RANK receptor on osteoclast precursors [31].

3. Bone remodeling: The process

The normal bone remodeling is a process that couples bone resorption and bone formation, it occurs in discrete locations and involves a group of different kinds of cells and takes 2 to 5 years for an area on the bone surface to complete one bone remodeling cycle [32]. The bone tissue is morphologically and physiologically separated from the marrow by bone lining cell; the process of cancellous bone remodeling occurs on the surface of trabeculae at the boundary between bone and marrow. In normal bone length of the remodeling is about 200 days, with the majority of that time (approx. 150 days) devoted to bone formation [33]. The bone remodeling takes place in the BMU and the skeleton contains millions which comprises the next: osteoclasts that resorbing the bone, the osteoblasts that replacing the bone, the osteocytes within the bone matrix, the bone lining cells that covering the bone surface and the capillary blood supply. All BMU are in different stages, and the life span of individual cells in a BMU is much shorter than that of a BMU [31,35,36]. Mechanical stress in the bone can be sensed by osteocytes that can signal giving to lining cells to form a new BMU at cortical or cancellous surfaces and estimates that the duration is 2-8 months [12]. The bone remodeling follows coordination of distinct and sequential phases of this process, (Figure 2):

Activation Phase- The first stage of bone remodeling involves detection of an initiating remodeling signal, the activation is a continuing process that occurs at the cutting edge of the BMU, and this signal can take several forms as a direct mechanical strain on the bone that results in structural damage or hormone (e.g. estrogen or PTH) action on bone cells in response to more systemic changes in homeostasis [32]. Conceivably, osteocyte apoptosis and possible release of osteotropic growth factors and cytokines could be attractants for blood vessels, which would then subsequently initiate the formation of a resorptive of the bone remodeling compartment which are a prerequisite for osteogenesis, including bone development, fracture healing, and cortical bone remodeling that support recruitment of osteoblast progenitors to bone remodeling sites, thus highlight a link between activation of bone remodeling on the cancellous bone surfaces and activation of neighbouring bone marrow events [12,34,36,37]. The mechanical environment to which bone cells are exposed is a dynamic milieu of biophysical stimuli that includes strain, stress, shear, pressure, fluid flow, streaming potentials and acceleration. While ultimately it may not be possible to separate specific effects of each of these factors, it is clear that several of these parameters independently have the ability to regulate cellular responses and influence remodeling events within bone. Furthermore, components of these specific factors (such as magnitude, frequency, and strain rate) also affect the cellular response [38].

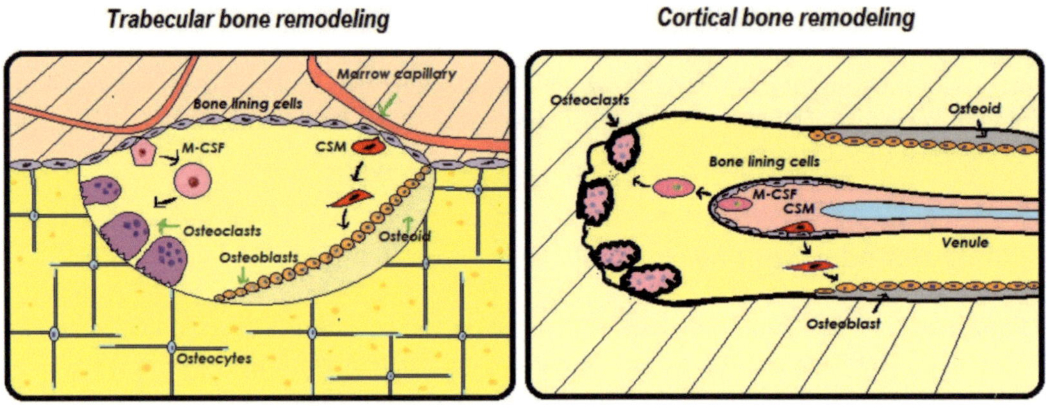

Figure 2. Schematic presentation of trabecular and cortical bone remodeling by BMU. In trabecular, the osteoclast create Howship´s lacunas that are refilled by osteoblast, and in the cortical bone, the osteoclast erode bone tissue and are followed by osteoblast that refill the gap with new bone.

The osteocyte, which is uniquely situated in cortical bone to sense mechanical strain and load generated factors (e.g., fluid flow, streaming and pressure) through a connected network of sister cells contributes to the perception of and response to loading and unloading [12], this canalicular network responds to unloading, or a decrease in mechanical signals, with upregulation of the proteins sclerostin and RANKL that control bone remodeling at multiple levels. The long osteocytic processes are able to pass information between cells separated by hard tissue [16,19]. Osteoblast linage cells and bone marrow stromal cells (BMSCs) are thought to be the major cell types that express RANKL in support of osteoclastogenesis [39,40]; however the actual major source of RANKL in vivo is the osteocyte [12].

Resorption Phase- In this phase, the formation and activity of osteoclasts is controlled by cells of the osteoblast lineage that recruit osteoclast precursors to the remodeling site with the expression of the master osteoclastogenesis cytokines, CSF-1, RANKL, and OPG, is also modulated in response to PTH [32,45,46]. Remodeling is initiated by osteoclastic resorption, which erodes a resorption lacuna, they attach to the bone surface, sealing a resorbing compartment that they acidify by secreting H^+ ions, facilitating dissolution of the bone mineral and thereby exposing the organic matrix to proteolytic enzymes that degrade it, during resorption the bone matrix and bone mineral is digested. Some fragments can be used as biochemical markers for overall bone resorption [43]. The depth of which varies between 60-40 μm in young and older individuals, and the resorption period has a median duration of 30–40 days [45]. In cortical bone, the BMUs proceed by osteonal tunnelling, during which osteoclasts excavate a canal that is refilled by osteoblasts, the so-formed Haversian systems are 100–200 μm wide and may become as long as 10 mm; their orientation is along the main loading direction trabecular, by contrast, are eroded as grooves along the bone surface with a depth of 60–70 μm (Figure 2), [36].

Reversal Phase- This phase lasts ~9 days, occurs after the maximum eroded depth has been achieved. In the reversal period the osteoclasts undergo apoptosis whilst osteoblasts are recruited and begin to differentiate [44], therefore the reversal phase is a transition from osteoclast to osteoblast activity [35]. After withdrawal of the osteoclast from the resorption pit, bone-lining cells enter the lacuna and clean its bottom from bone matrix leftovers. This cleaning proves to be a prerequisite for the subsequent deposition of a first layer of proteins (collagenous) in the resorption pits and form a cement line (glycoprotein) that helps in attaching osteoblasts (Figure 2), [28,41].

Formation Phase- The bone formation by the osteoblasts lasts the longest, and is slower than bone resorption, involves new bone formation and mineralization. It was proposed that the coupling molecules were stored in the bone matrix and liberated during bone resorption. TGF-β appears to be a key signal for recruitment of mesenchymal stem cells to sites of bone resorption and osteoclasts produce the coupling factors [32,45], once mesenchymal stem cells or early osteoblast progenitors have returned to the resorption lacunae, they differentiate [28, 34,46] and the proliferating osteoblasts forming multilayers of cells. Several genes associated with formation of the extracellular matrix (Type I collagen, fibronectin, and TGF-β) are actively expressed and then gradually decline being maintained at a low basal level during subsequent stages of osteoblast differentiation. Collagen type I is the primary organic component of bone and accumulation contributes, in part, to the cessation of cell growth. When proliferation ceases, proteins associated with bone cell phenotype are detected, e.g. alkaline phosphatase enzyme, osteocalcin [7,47]. Bone matrix is built up of type I collagen (88%) and the remaining 10% is composed of a large number of non-collagenous proteins (e.g. osteocalcin, osteonectin, bone sialoprotein and various proteoglycans) and lipids and glycosaminoglycans represent 1–2% [48]. For bone to assume its final form, hydroxylapatite is incorporated into this newly deposited osteoid [47,49]. The extracellular matrix undergoes a series of modifications in composition and organization that renders it competent for mineralization that begins ~15 days after osteoid has been formed, and non-collagenous proteins participate in the process of matrix maturation, mineralization and may regulate the functional activity of bone cells. With the onset of mineralization, several other bone expressed genes are induced to maximal levels (bone sialoprotein, osteopontin and osteocalcin) [32,47]. The composition of bone is approximately 10% cells, 60% mineral crystals (crystalline hydroxyapatite), and 30% organic matrix [48]. When an equal quantity of resorbed bone has been replaced, the remodeling cycle concludes (Figure 2).

Termination Phase- The termination signals are largely unknown, and include the terminal differentiation of the osteoblast. The role of osteocytes is emerging [12,32]. The cells then gradually flatten as they slow production, and finally they become quiescent lining cells. Some of the osteoblast differentiate into osteocytes and remain in the matrix [12]. The osteocytes may secrete inhibitory factors that slow the rate of bone formation as the resorbed cavity is nearly filled. Bone remodeling is mediated by a balance of osteoblast and osteoclast cell activity, which together, maintain bone mass and mineral homeostasis. Both decreased bone formation and increased bone resorption may result in bone loss. Therefore, the stimulation of bone formation may be another important factor for the prevention and treatment of bone loss (Figure 2).

4. Regulation signals into the control of bone remodeling

4.1. Systemic regulation of bone remodeling

The process of bone remodeling is essential for adult bone homeostasis. This control involves a complex mechanism compound by numerous local and systemic factors, and their expression and release is controlled finely. The main factor that affects normal bone remodeling is the regulation of osteoblasts and osteoclasts. Local and systemic factors can affect bone remodeling by directly or indirectly targeting mature cells and their respective progenitor cells. The metabolic functions of the bone are mediated by two major calcium-regulating hormones, parathyroid hormone (PTH) and 1,25-dihydroxy vitamin D (Table 1) [50].

	Bone reabsorption (osteoclast activity)	**Bone Formation (osteoblast activity)**
Parathyroid hormone (PTH)	↑	↑*
1,25(OH)2 Vitamin D	↑	↑*
Calcitonin	↓	?
Estrogen	↓	↓#
Growth hormone/IGF	↑	↑
Thyroid hormone	↑	↑

? = Effects are not Known

* PTH and vitamin D decrease collagen synthesis in high doses.

Estrogen decreases bone formation by decreasing remodeling, but formation is decreased less than resorption and bone mass increases.

Data and modified from Raisz, L. G. (1999). Physiology and pathophysiology of bone remodeling. Clinical chemistry, 45 (8B): 1353-1358.

Table 1. Local and systemic regulation of bone remodeling.

PTH is a stimulator of bone resorption and 1,25-Dihydroxy vitamin D has its greatest effect on intestinal calcium and phosphate absorption, but it may also have direct effects on bone and other tissues. It is probably critical for the differentiation of both osteoblasts and osteoclasts and can stimulate bone resorption and formation under some experimental conditions. A third hormone, calcitonin (Table 1), in contrast to PTH and 1,25(OH)2 D3, both of which increase calcium release from the mineralized matrix, calcitonin is an inhibitor of osteoclast activity. It is a potent inhibitor of bone resorption and is used clinically in the treatment of bone diseases. Other systemic hormones are keys in regulating bone remodeling, such as: Growth hormone acting through both systemic and local insulin-like growth factor (IGF) production, can stimulate bone formation and resorption. Glucocorticoids are necessary for bone cell differentiation during development. Indirect effects of glucocorticoids on calcium absorption and sex hormone production may, however, increase bone resorption (Table 1). O the other hand, probably the most important systemic hormone in maintaining normal bone turnover is estrogen. Estrogen deficiency leads to an increase in bone remodeling in which resorption overcome formation and bone mass decreases (Table 1). The increase in bone remodeling and in bone resorption in the estrogen deficient state is associated with an increase in bone formation at the tissue level [51]. Therefore, sex steroid deficiency is associated with a defect in bone formation. Based on the available evidence, there are currently at least three key mechanisms by which estrogen deficiency may lead to a relative deficit in bone formation through direct effects on osteoblasts: increased apoptosis, increased oxidative stress, and an increase in NF-kB activity (Figure 3). In addition, estrogen inhibits the activation of bone remodeling, and this effect is most likely mediated via the osteocyte [52].

4.2. Parathyroid hormone (TH) and PTHrP signals

The parathyroid hormone (PTH) increases bone formation in bone diseases. The anabolic effects of PTH on bone formation are mediated through the PTH/PTH-related peptide (PTHrP) receptor-dependent mechanisms that generate multiple G protein-dependent signals (Table 1). PTH mediated cyclic AMP/protein kinase phosphorylates the osteoblast transcription factor Runx2, which in turn upregulates the expression of osteoblast genes. Intermittent PTH also activates ERK1/2-mitogen-activated protein kinase (MAPK) Erk1/2 and phosphatidylinositol phosphate (PI3K) signaling, resulting in increased osteoblastogenesis and osteoblast survival (Figure 3) [53]. PTH induces the synthesis of IGF-I that works with PTH in osteoblasts to stimulate osteoblast proliferation and differentiation as well as indirectly regulates osteoclast activity [54,55]. Also, PTH was inferred to interact with various local signaling molecules, including insulin-like growth factors and Wnt antagonist sclerostin (SOST) [55-57]. It was recently shown that, in addition to reducing SOST, PTH reduces Dkk1 expression and thereby increases Wnt signaling, which contributes to the anabolic effect of PTH in bone [58]. This does not exclude the possibility that PTH receptor signaling may increase bone mass and bone remodeling by affecting Wnt signaling in other cell types. Recent data indicate that the activation of the PTH receptor in T lymphocytes plays a role in PTH-induced bone formation and bone mass by promoting the production of Wnt10b by these cells [59]. These observations and the finding that PTH signaling also acts by phosphorylating the Wnt coreceptor LRP6 and β-catenin indicate that direct and indirect crosstalks between PTH and Wnt signaling are important mechanisms regulating bone formation.

4.3. Wnt and Wnt antagonists

Genetic studies in human and animal models suggest that the canonical Wnt/β-catenin pathway (Table 2), together with BMP signaling and key transcription factor RUNX2(CBFA1/AML3), has an key role in skeletal development, osteoblast differentiation and bone formation [60,61]. Wnt/β-catenin signaling plays a significant role in promoting mesenchymal commitment to the osteoblastic lineage during the embryonic bone development. The canonical Wnt/β-catenin signaling activity is promoted in the forming osteoblast, and this activity promotes osteoblast differentiation during endochondral bone formation, and the skeletal development is affected and the osteoblast differentiation is reduced when Wnt/β-catenin signaling is interrupted in the mesenchyme (Figure 3) [62]. The *in vivo* stimulation of the Wnt10b signaling cascade in the FABP4 promoter-Wnt10b transgenic mice led to a significantly higher bone mass because of the stimulation of osteoblastogenesis and the inhibition of adipogenesis. In addition, the Wnt10b–/–mice had decreased trabecular bone and serum osteocalcin [63]. Recent advances have been made in our understanding of the role of Wnt proteins in bone cell biology. It was found that, in addition to Wnt10b [63], several other Wnt proteins (Wnt6a, Wn10a) influence the differentiation of mesenchymal precursors into osteoblasts or adipocytes, and thereby control bone mass [64]. The Wnt signal is modulated by various antagonists, including secreted factors, transmembrane modulators, and intracellular signals. Dickkopf family members (Dkk1 and Dkk2) and secreted frizzled related proteins (Sfrps) are families of extracellular proteins that negatively modulate canonical Wnt signalling [60].

4.4. Transforming growth factor-β

The transforming growth factor-β (TGF-β) signaling pathway, is known to control bone remodeling and maintenance. However, TGF-β exerts both positive and negative effects on bone cells, causing bone loss or bone gain in mice. There are three isoforms of TGF-β, namely, TGF-β1, TGF-β2, and TGF-β3. TGF-β1, known as the most abundant TGF-β isoform in the bone tissue, has been intensively studied during bone remodeling [65]. A study on the mechanism of TGF-β for osteoblast regulation has indicated that TGF-β1 stimulates bone matrix apposition and osteoblast proliferation in vitro. Additional research revealed that although TGF-β1 stimulates the early differentiation of osteoblast cells, this factor suppresses the late stage of osteoblast differentiation. These signals are transduced together by the activation of R-smads and Cosmads as well as through the mitogen-activated protein kinase (MAPK) pathway (Table 2). A cross talk exists between the TGF-β signal and the parathyroid hormone (PTH) in the regulation of osteoblastogenesis [66]. PTH stimulates the production of TGF-β1 and TGF-β2 in the osteoblast. In addition to regulating the osteoblastic bone formation, TGF-β1 has a key role in regulating bone remodeling by connecting bone formation and bone resorption (Figure 3). TGF-β proteins are present in their latent form in the bone matrix, and osteoclasts can release, as well as activate, TGF-β from the bone matrix via osteoclastic bone resorption. The released TGF-β may in turn stimulate the osteoblastic bone formation [45].

4.5. Bone morphogenetic proteins

Bone morphogenetic proteins (BMPs), they are so named for their osteoinductive properties, and regulate differentiation of mesenchymal cells into components of bone, cartilage or adipose tissue. TGF-β/BMP ligand signal is mediated by serine/threonine protein kinases (receptor types 1 and 2) and a family of receptor substrates (the Smad proteins) that move into the nucleus. BMP signaling is important for skeletal development and maintenance of bone mass through activation of BMP type 1A (BMPR1A) and type 1B receptors that control osteoblast function and bone remodeling (Table 2) [67]. Notably, BMPR1A in osteoblasts negatively regulates bone mass and Wnt/β-catenin signaling through upregulation of the Wnt inhibitors Sost and Dkk1 in mice [68]. Also, BMPs promote osteoblastogenesis through the Smad and MAPK pathways, which upregulates the expression of *Runx2* and *Osx*, and thus stimulate the bone formation (Figure 3). BMP signaling is modulated by multiple agonists and antagonists acting at the extracellular level, which are also important for bone remodeling and may be potential therapeutic targets [69]. It was found that the Wnt-induced secreted protein 1 (WISP-1/CCN4) enhances BMP2-induced signaling (Smad-1/5/8 phosphorylation and activation), resulting in increased osteogenic differentiation and bone mass in mice.

Ligand	Receptors	Activated pathways	Target Cells
PTH	PTH/PTHrP	cAMP/PCA, PKC, PI3K/Akt, Wnt	Osteoblasts
Wnt3a	LRP5/LRP6/Frizzled	Wnt, PI3K/Akt	Osteoblasts
TGFB	TGF-B type II	cAMP/PCA, PKC, PI3K/Akt, Wnt	Osteoblats/osteoclasts
BMP	BMPR1A	Wnt	Osteoblasts/osteoclasts
Ephrins	Eph	c-Fos-NFATc1	Osteoblasts/osteoclasts
EGFR	ERBB1-4	Ras-Raf-Map-Kinase	
FGF2	FGFR1/2	Erk1/2, PKCa, Wnt	Osteoblasts
IGF-1/IGFBP2	IGFR	Akt, Wnt	Osteoblats
Brain derived serotonin (BDS)	Htr2c	Wnt	Osteoblasts
Wnt5a	Ror2	JNK	Osteoblasts/osteoclasts
Semaphorin 4D	Plexin-B1	RhoA/IGF1	Osteoblasts/osteoclasts

Table 2. Signaling pathways affecting bone cells and bone remodeling.

4.6. Eph and Ephrin interactions

The interactions between Eph and Ephrin play important roles in bone cell differentiation and patterning by exerting effects on osteoblast and osteoclast differentiation, resulting in the

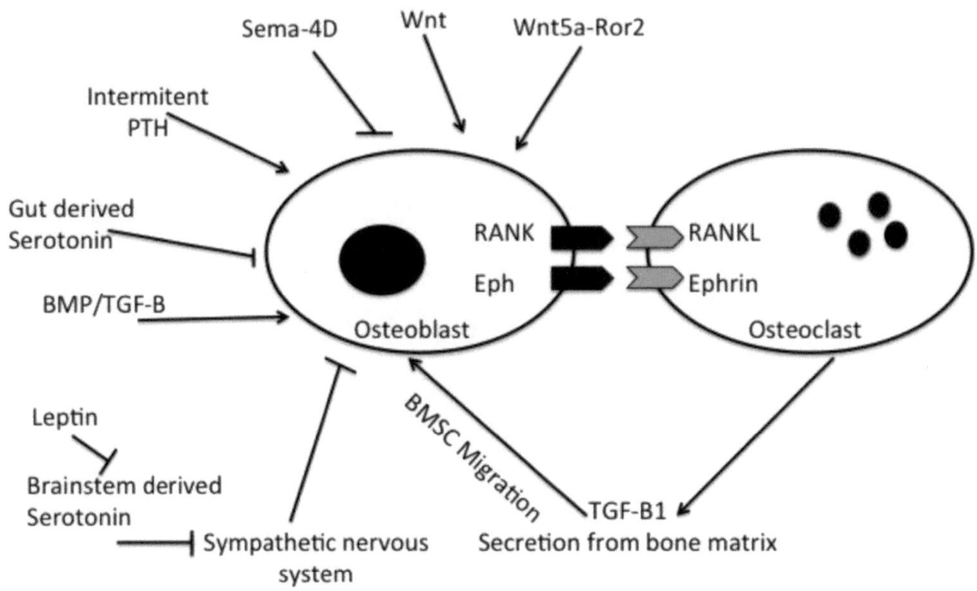

Figure 3. Key signaling pathways for regulating osteoblastogenesis in bone remodeling. BMPs/TGF-β, Wnt, intermittent PTH and Wnt5a-Ror2 stimulate osteoblast differentiation. Eph–Ephrin and RANKL-RANK signal mediate osteoblast–osteoclast interaction. TGF-β1 secretion mediated by osteoclastic bone resorption induces BMSC migration and bone formation. Leptin–brainstem-derived serotonin-sympathetic nervous system and Sema4D pathway suppresses osteoblast proliferation, whereas gut-derived serotonin inhibits osteoblast proliferation.

coupling of bone resorption and bone formation. Eph receptors are tyrosine kinase receptors activated by ligands called ephrins (Eph receptor interacting proteins). Both Ephs and ephrins are divided into two A and B groups [70]. To date, ephrinB2, a transmembrane protein expressed on osteoclasts, and its engagement with its receptor, EphB4, on osteoblasts, lead to bi-directional signaling between these cells; this is one of the cell-cell contact mechanisms that mediate crosstalk between these cells. EphrinB2 (as reverse signaling), located on the surface of osteoclast precursors, suppresses osteoclast precursor differentiation by inhibiting the osteoclastogenic c-Fos-NFATc1 cascade (Table 2) [71]. In addition, the signaling mediated by EphB4 (as forward signaling) located on the surface of osteoblast enhances the osteogenic differentiation. Ephrin B1 induces osteoblast differentiation by transactivating the nuclear location of transcriptional coactivator with PDZ-binding motif (TAZ), a co-activating protein of Runx2. TAZ, together with Runx2, induces osteoblast-related gene expression [72]. The functional role of the EphrinA2–EphA2 complex differs significantly in its interactions compared with the EphrinB2– EphB4 complex. Both the reversed signaling EphrinA2 and forward signaling EphA2 stimulate osteoclast differentiation, but EphA2 has a negative role in bone formation by inhibiting osteoblast differentiation through the regulation of RhoA activity (Figure 3) [71].

4.7. Epidermal growth factor receptor (EGFR)

The epidermal growth factor receptor (EGFR) is a glycoprotein on the cell surface of a variety of cell types and is characterized by its ligand-dependent tyrosine kinase activity. After ligand binding to the extracellular domain, the EGFRs are activated by homo- or heterodimerization with auto- and transphosphorylation on tyrosine residues at the intracellular domain, and then a variety of signaling pathways, such as Ras-Raf-MAP-kinase and PI-3- kinase-Akt, are activated to influence cell behaviors, such as proliferation, differentiation, apoptosis, and migration (Table 2) [73]. In recent years, several experiments indicate that the epidermal growth factor receptor (EGFR) system plays important roles in skeletal biology and pathology. This network, including a family of seven growth factors – the EGFR ligands – and the related tyrosine kinase receptors EGFR (ERBB1), ERBB2, ERBB3 and ERBB4, regulates aspects such as proliferation and differentiation of osteoblasts, chondrocytes and osteoclasts, parathyroid hormone-mediated bone formation and cancer metastases in bone (Figure 3) [74]. In addition, EGFR signaling affects osteoclasts, albeit this could be an indirect effect mediated by inhibition of OPG expression and increased RANKL expression by osteoblasts [74]. It was recently found that decreasing EGFR expression in pre-osteoblasts and osteoblasts in mice results in decreased trabecular and cortical bone mass as a consequence of reduced osteoblastogenesis and increased bone resorption [48].

4.8. Fibroblast Growth Factors (FGFs)

Signaling induced by Fibroblast Growth Factors (FGFs) regulate osteoblastogenesis and bone formation. Multiple signaling pathways activated by FGF receptors 1 and 2 control osteoblast proliferation, differentiation, and survival (Table 2). FGFs bind to high affinity FGF receptors (FGFR), leading to FGFR dimerization, phosphorylation of intrinsic tyrosine residues and activation of several signal transduction pathways [75]. Recent studies provided some insights into specific signaling pathways induced by FGF/FGFR signaling that control osteoblasts. Activation of ERK1/2 signaling by FGF was found to be essential for promoting cell proliferation in osteoblast precursor cells [76]. In addition, activation of ERK1/2 is involved in FGFR2-mediated osteoblast differentiation. Activation of ERK-MAP kinase by activating FGFR2 mutations results in increased transcriptional activity of Runx2, an essential transcription factor involved in osteoblastogenesis, and increased osteogenic marker gene expression (Figure 3) [77]. Recent data indicate that FGF2 stimulates osteoblast differentiation and bone formation in part by activating Wnt signaling suggesting that Wnt signaling may mediate, at least in part, the positive effect of FGF/FGFR signaling on bone formation in mice [78]. Besides Wnt signaling, FGF/FGFR signaling interacts with other pathways. One interaction involves a negative regulation of the BMP antagonist Noggin by FGF2 during skull development [79]. Another interaction involves the upregulation of the BMP2 gene by endogenous FGF/FGFR signaling in calvarial osteoblasts. In vivo, FGF2 treatment of developing bone fronts promotes BMP2 gene expression through the modulation of Runx2 expression [80]. These studies support a positive role of FGF and BMP signaling crosstalks on bone formation.

4.9. Insulin-like growth factor-I

The Insulin-like growth factor-I (IGF-I) signaling through its type 1 receptor generates a complex signaling pathway that stimulates cell proliferation, function, and survival in osteoblasts (Table 2) [81]. Accordingly, mice lacking functional IGF-I exhibit severe deficiency in bone formation and a 60% deficit in peak bone mineral density (BMD) [82]. IGF-I can act in an endocrine, paracrine or autocrine manner and is regulated by a family of six IGF binding proteins (IGFBPs). The IGFBPs, have received considerable attention as regulators of IGF actions. The IGFBPs have been reported to have stimulatory or inhibitory actions on the IGFs in bone, and recent experiments have provided evidence that some of IGFBPs function independently of IGF to increase parameters of bone formation. The IGFBPs are often found bound to IGF-I in the circulation or complexed with IGF-I in osteoblasts. IGFBP-3 and -5 are known stimulators of IGF-I actions, whereas IGFBP-1, -2, -4 and -6 are known inhibitors of IGF-I action in bone. Once IGF-I binds to its receptor (type 1 IGF receptor) it initiates a complex signaling pathway including the phosphoinositol 3-kinase (PI3-K)/3-PI-dependent kinase (PDK)-1/Akt pathway and the Ras/Raf/mitogen-activated protein (MAP) kinase pathway which stimulate cell function and/or survival (Figure 3) [83]. Recent findings indicate that many of the IGFBPs and specific proteins in the IGF-I signaling pathways are also potent anabolic factors in regulating osteoblast function and may serve as potential targets to stimulate osteoblast function and bone formation locally.

4.10. Leptin–serotonin system pathway regulation of bone formation through gut-derived serotonin

A new regulation mode of osteoblastic bone formation controlled by leptin-serotonin (BDS)-sympathetic nervous system pathway has emerged in recent years. Leptin is a hormone produced by adipocytes that, besides its function in regulating body weight and gonadal function, can also act as an inhibitor of bone formation (Figure 3) [84]. Latest data indicates that these leptin functions require brainstem-derived serotonin [85]. Serotonin is a bioamine produced by neurons of the brainstem (brainstem-derived serotonin, BDS) and enterochromaffin cells of the duodenum (gut-derived serotonin, GDS). BDS acts as a neurotransmitter, while GDS as an autocrine/paracrine signal that regulates mammary gland biogenesis, liver regeneration, and gastrointestinal tract motility [86]. There are two Tph genes that catalyze the rate-limiting step in serotonin biosynthesis: Tph1 expressed mostly, but not only, in enterochromaffin cells of the gut and is responsable for the production of peripheral serotonin [86]. Tph2 is expressed exclusively in raphe neurons of the brainstem and is responsible for the production of serotonin in the brain [87]. Leptin inhibits BDS synthesis by decreasing the expression of Tph2, a major enzyme involved in serotonin synthesis in brain [85]. In addition, other data indicate, the key role of GDS in regulating bone formation as well as the relationship between GDS, Lrp5, and bone remodeling. Lrp5 controls bone formation by inhibiting GDS synthesis in the duodenum, and GDS directly acts on the osteoblast cells to inhibit osteoblast proliferation and suppress bone formation (Table 2) [88]. However, recent data to argue that Lrp5 affect bone mass mainly through local Wnt signaling pathway, and that the experiments did not support the Lrp5-GDS-osteoblast model because they found that there was no relevance between GDS and bone mass in their mouse model system [89].

4.11. New signals in bone remodeling

More recently, other signaling pathways that link regulation of the osteoclasts and osteoblasts have been identified. Osteoblast-lineage cells expressed Wnt5a, whereas osteoclast precursors expressed Ror2. Connection between these two cells leads to Wnt5a-Ror2 signaling between osteoblast-lineage cells and osteoclast precursors enhanced osteoclastogenesis, through increased RANK expression mediated by JNK signaling. A soluble form of Ror2 acted as a decoy receptor of Wnt5a and abrogated bone destruction in the mouse model, suggesting that the Wnt5a-Ror2 pathway is crucial for osteoclastogenesis in physiological and pathological environments and may represent a therapeutic target for bone diseases (Figure 3) [90]. Finally, a recent study reported that semaphorin 4D (Sema4D), previously shown to be an axon guidance molecule, expressed by osteoclasts and which potently inhibits bone formation [91]. Several studies have suggested that axon-guidance molecules, such as the semaphorins and ephrins, are involved in the cell-cell communication that occurs between osteoclasts and osteoblasts. The Binding of Sema4D to its receptor Plexin-B1 in osteoblasts resulted in the activation of the small GTPase RhoA, which inhibits bone formation by suppressing insulin-like growth factor-1 IGF-1 signaling and by modulating osteoblast motility. Notably, the suppression of Sema4D using a specific antibody was found to markedly prevent bone loss in a model of postmenopausal osteoporosis (Table 2) [91]. This finding identifies a new link between osteoclasts and osteoblast signaling, and suggests that suppression of the Sema4D-Plexin-B1-RhoA signaling axis may provide a new therapeutic target for reducing bone loss and development of bone-increasing drugs.

5. Pathophysiology of bone remodeling (diseases)

Several lines of evidence have established that the cells that remodel the skeleton under physiological conditions are the same cells that mediate these processes in pathologic states. Mature bone consists of: an organic matrix (osteoid) composed mainly of type 1 collagen formed by osteoblasts; a mineral phase which contains the bulk of the body's reserve of calcium and phosphorus in crystalline form (hydroxyapatite) and deposited in close relation to the collagen fibers; bone cells; and a blood supply with sufficient levels of calcium and phosphate to mineralize the osteoid matrix. Bone turnover and remodeling occurs throughout life and involves the two-coupled processes of bone formation by osteoblasts and bone resorption by osteoclasts and perhaps osteolytic osteocytes. Abnormalities of bone remodeling can produce a variety of skeletal disorders (Table 3). The metabolic bone diseases may reflect disturbances in the organic matrix, the mineral phase, the cellular processes of remodeling, and the endocrine, nutritional, and other factors that regulate skeletal and mineral homeostasis. These disorders may be hereditary or acquired and usually affect the entire bony skeleton. The acquired metabolic bone diseases are the more common and include: osteoporosis, osteomalacia, the skeletal changes of hyperparathyroidism and chronic renal failure (renal osteodystrophy), and Paget's disease [48,50].

5.1. Osteoporosis

Osteoporosis is a common disease of bone remodeling characterized by low bone mass and defects in the microarchitecture of bone tissue; it causes bone fragility and an increased vulnerability to fractures. The loss of bone mass and strength can be contributed to by (a) failure to reach an optimal peak bone mass as a young adult, (b) excessive resorption of bone after peak mass has been achieved, or (c) an impaired bone formation response during remodeling. Osteoporosis, is traditionally classified into primary and secondary types. Primary osteoporosis is the most common metabolic disorder of the skeleton and has been divided into two subtypes: type I osteoporosis and type II osteoporosis, on the basis of possible differences in etiology. Type I osteoporosis or postmenopausal osteoporosis is a common bone disorder in postmenopausal women and is caused primarily by estrogen deficiency resulting from menopause, whereas type II osteoporosis or age-related osteoporosis is associated primarily with aging in both women and men (Table 3). In contrast, secondary osteoporosis refers to bone disorders that are secondary complications of various other medical conditions, consequences of changes in physical activity, or adverse results of therapeutic interventions for certain disorders [92].

Osteoporosis
Primary
Menopause Associated
Age related
Secondary
Glucocorticoid induced
Immobilization induced
Renal osteodystrophy
Paget's disease
Osteopetrosis

Table 3. Diseases of bone remodeling.

5.2. Postmenopausal osteoporosis

Postmenopausal osteoporosis is a common disease with a spectrum ranging from asymptomatic bone loss to disabling hip fracture (Table 3). The pathogenesis of postmenopausal osteoporosis is caused primarily by the decline in estrogen levels associated with menopause [93]. Since the establishment of a central role for estrogen deficiency in the pathogenesis of postmenopausal osteoporosis, enormous effort has been focused on elucidating the mechanisms by which estrogens exert their bone-sparing effects. Since the discovery of the RANKL/RANK/OPG axis, it has become clear that estrogen also exerts bone-sparing effects by targeting this regulatory axis. Specifically, estrogen stimulates the expression of OPG in mouse osteoblasts and stromal cells [94]. Moreover, the expression of RANKL was elevated on the surface of bone marrow cells, such as osteoblasts and lymphocytes, from postmenopausal women with osteoporosis compared with cells from premenopausal controls [94]; this finding indicates that RANKL plays an important role in the pathogenesis of postmenopausal osteoporosis.

5.3. Age-related osteoporosis

As the global population ages, the prevalence of age-related osteoporosis (e.g., postmenopausal osteoporosis, male osteoporosis) and related fractures is likely to increase considerably (Table 3). Recent studies indicate that significant trabecular bone loss begins as early as the twenties in men and women long before any major hormonal changes [95]. In women, however, bone loss accelerates for 5 to 10 years after menopause due to the rapid decline in estrogen levels; after this phase, bone loss continues at approximately the same rate as in elderly males. Thus, the pathogenesis of osteoporosis in women involves primarily osteoclasts (bone resorption) and results from changes in estrogen and FSH levels at menopause and age related, is centered on osteoblasts (bone formation), and engages a number of distinct factors associated with the aging process in both men and women. Thus, age-related changes in the activity of either cell type may lead to bone loss [96]. Age-related osteoporosis in men also has a multifactorial etiology. The decreased bone formation caused by changes in ROS, IGF-1, and PTH levels associated with aging plays a predominant role in the pathogenesis of age-related osteoporosis in men. However, age-related changes in the levels of sex steroids, including both estrogen and androgen, also contribute to the pathogenesis of age-related osteoporosis in men [97].

5.4. Glucocorticoid-induced osteoporosis

Glucocorticoids (GCs) are potent immunomodulatory drugs that are commonly used to treat a variety of inflammatory conditions and autoimmune disorders. GCs increase bone resorption and reduce bone formation (Table 3) [98]. Pharmacological doses of GCs induce osteoporosis primarily by altering normal bone remodeling. GCs exert deleterious effects on the differentiation, function, and survival of multiple cell types involved in the remodeling process. GCs have profound effects on osteoblast differentiation and function. As in other target tissues, glucocorticoids exert their effects on gene expression via cytoplasmic glucocorticoid type 2 receptors. In adult bone, functional glucocorticoid receptors are found in pre-osteoblast/stromal cells, osteoblasts (the cells that produce bone matrix), but not in osteoclasts [99]. Instead, glucocorticoids stimulate osteoclast proliferation by suppressing synthesis of osteoprotegerin, an inhibitor of osteoclast differentiation from hematopoietic cells of the macrophage lineage, and by stimulating production of the receptor activator of nuclear factor kappa-B (RANK), which is required for osteoclastogenesis. High glucocorticoid levels also stimulate RANKL synthesis by pre-osteoblast/stromal cells, supporting osteoclast differentiation and net bone resorption [100].

5.5. Immobilization-induced osteoporosis

One of the major functions of bone remodeling is to adapt bone material and structural properties to the mechanical demands that are placed on the skeleton, including mechanical loading and weight bearing (Table 3). The importance of the mechanical balance of bone has been more recently stressed by the research on the effect of weightlessness on bone, and by the introduction of the concept of "mechanostat" in the pathogenesis of osteoporotic conditions. Immobilization osteoporosis has clinical (fractures, sometimes hypercalcemia, urinary lithiasis) and radiological features. Immobilization has an effect on bone modeling and remodeling, through an increased activation of remodeling loci, and a decrease of the osteoblastic stimulus. For ordinary individuals, the skeleton is developed in childhood and then constantly remodeled throughout adulthood to maintain mechanical strength that can sufficiently support normal weight bearing and routine physical activities. However, for individuals such as athletes, the mechanical needs increase for certain regions of the skeleton; consequently, bone modeling results in the formation of stronger bone to replace old bone that could not adequately meet the increased mechanical demands [101].

5.6. Renal osteodystrophy

Renal osteodystrophy the term used to describe a heterogeneous group of metabolic bone diseases that accompany chronic kidney disease, is a multifactorial disorder of bone remodeling (Table 3). The bone disorders in renal osteodystrophy include: osteomalacia of adults and rickets of children (so-called "renal rickets"); osteitis fibrosa and other bone changes of secondary hyperparathyroidism; osteopenia; and osteosclerosis. Renal osteodystrophy is an alteration of bone morphology in patients with CKD (Chronic Kidney Disease). The pathophysiology of renal osteodystrophy is complex and clearly reflects the importance of PTH and vitamin D on bone turnover and related pathological abnormalities. The bone changes are brought about by the abnormal metabolism of vitamin D, the overproduction of parathyroid hormone (PTH), and chronic metabolic acidosis. The diminished renal mass leads to a decreased renal conversion of 25-hydroxyvitamin D into 1,25-dihydroxyvitamin D, the active metabolite of vitamin D, resulting in diminished intestinal absorption of calcium, hypocalcemia, and defective bone mineralization characterized by the presence of wide osteoid seams, osteomalacia in adults, and rickets in children [102].

5.7. Paget's disease

Paget's disease is known as a bone remodeling disorder and that involves abnormal bone destruction and regrowth, which results in deformity. In Paget's disease, the bone remodeling process is disregulated (Table 3). New bone is placed where it is not needed, and old bone is removed where it is needed. This disregulation can distort the normal skeletal architecture [103]. Paget's disease is most commonly diagnosed in the sixth decade, and increases in prevalence as age increases. Paget's disease is very uncommon in individuals under 40 years of age. The most common bones affected by Paget's disease are the pelvis, femur, spine, skull, and tibia. Paget's disease is believed to be a primary disorder of increased osteoclast bone resorption with a secondary marked increase in osteoblast activity and new bone formation.

http://dx.doi.org/10.5772/54905

The cause of Paget's disease is not entirely known, but it is thought to be caused in part from a childhood virus. A virus particle, known as a paramyxovirus nucleocapsid, has been identified within the bone cells of individuals with Paget's disease. This virus particle is not found in normal bone. Genetics plays a role, several genes have been implicated; however, the most commonly described mutation is a gene that encodes an ubiquitin-binding protein that plays a role in NF-κB signaling [104].

5.8. Osteopetrosis

There are several syndromes of osteopetrosis or osteosclerosis in which bone resorption is defective because of impaired formation of osteoclasts or loss of osteoclast function (Table 3). In these disorders, bone modeling as well as remodeling are impaired, and the architecture of the skeleton can be quite abnormal [105]. Osteopetrosis is a congenital disease that interferes with the formation of the bone marrow, and causes abnormal bone development, blindness, rickets, abnormal tooth development and fragile bones. It results from a defect in cells called osteoclasts, which are necessary for the formation of the bone marrow. In patients with osteopetrosis, osteoclasts not function properly, and no cavity is formed to the bone marrow [106]. The subclassification of these disorders is based upon the mode of inheritance, age of onset, severity, and clinical symptoms [107]. The pathophysiology of osteopetrosis involves mutations that affect osteoclast function. The three most important mutations are: carbonic anhydrase II, proton pump, and chloride channel [48].

6. Conclusions

Bone is a specialized and dynamic tissue, in constant change. It has a complex structure and undergoes constant remodeling. The basic multicellular unit of bone, which comprises osteocytes, osteoclasts and osteoblasts, conducts the remodeling process. In the last years, more knowledge in bone cell biology and genetic studies, have been helped in our understanding of the essential signaling pathways that control bone remodeling and bone mass. They act in a coordinated manner to form or resorb bone. Recent advances in molecular biology and a thorough understanding of the remodeling process bone, many molecules have been discovered that have important roles in bone biology and novel signaling pathways regulating bone remodeling have also been identified. Now understand how PTH, Wnt signaling, and growth factors may trigger anabolic effects in bone. The explosion of this knowledge may serve as a basis for the development of novel therapeutic approaches targeted on the identified signaling molecules enable us to define the abnormalities in cells of the osteoblastic and osteoclastic lineages that lead to bone disease with the hope to the diagnosis and treatment of bone remodeling disorders. With this knowledge, can expect the development of even more therapies to evolve from a better understanding of the complex molecular aspects of bone remodeling.

Author details

Alma Y. Parra-Torres[1,2], Margarita Valdés-Flores[3], Lorena Orozco[4] and Rafael Velázquez-Cruz[2*]

*Address all correspondence to: rvelazquez@inmegen.gob.mx

1 Program in Biomedical Sciences-UNAM, Mexico

2 Genomics of Bone Metabolism Laboratory, National Institute of Genomic Medicine, Mexico City, Mexico

3 Department of Genetics, National Rehabilitation Institute, Mexico City, Mexico

4 Immunogenomics and Metabolic Diseases Laboratory, National Institute of Genomic Medicine, Mexico City, Mexico

References

[1] Kassem M, Abdallah BM, Saeed H. Osteoblastic cells: Differentiation and transdifferentiation. Arch Biochem Biophys. 2008;473(2):183–187.

[2] Pignolo RJ, Shore EM. Circulating osteogenic precursor cells. Crit Rev Eukaryot Gene Expr. 2010;20(2):171-180.

[3] Schmitt JM, Hwang K, Winn SR, Hollinger JO. Bone morphogenetic proteins: an update on basic biology and clinical relevance. J Orthop Res. 1999;17(2):269-278.

[4] Bianco P, Gehron RP, Simmons PJ. Mesenchymal Stem Cells: Revisiting History, Concepts, and Assays. Cell Stem Cell. 2008;2(4):313–319.

[5] Aubin JE, Liu F. The osteoblast lineage. In: Bilezikian J, Raisz L, Rodan G, editors. Principles of bone biology. San Diego: Academic Press; 1996:51–68.

[6] Carbonare LD, Innamorati G, Valenti M. Transcription Factor Runx2 and its Application to Bone Tissue Engineering. Stem Cell Rev and Rep. 2012;8(3):891–897.

[7] Clarke B. Normal bone anatomy and physiology. Clin J Am Soc Nephrol. 2008;3:S131–139.

[8] Westendorf JJ, Kahler RA, Schroeder TM. Wnt signaling in osteoblasts and bone diseases. Gene. 2004;341:19–39.

[9] Anderson H. Matrix vesicles and calcification. Curr Rheumatol Rep. 2003;5(3):222–226.

[10] Lynch MP, Capparelli C, Stein JL, Stein GS, Lian JB. Apoptosis during bone-like tissue development in vitro. J Cell Biochem. 1998;68:31–49.

[11] Noble BS. The osteocyte lineage. B.S. Arch Biochem Biophys. 2008;473:106–111.

[12] Bonewald LF. The Amazing Osteocyte. J Bone Miner Res. 2011;26(2):229–238.

[13] Franz-Odendaal TA, Hall BK, Witten EP. Buried Alive: How Osteoblasts Become Osteocytes. Dev Dyn. 2006;235:176–190.

[14] Cowin SC, Moss-Salentijn L, Moss ML. Candidates for the mechanosensory system in bone. J Biomech Eng. 1991;113:191–197.

[15] Lanyon LE. Osteocytes, strain detection, bone modeling and remodeling. Calcif Tissue Int. 1993;53:S102–S106; discussion S106-7.

[16] Tatsumi S, Ishii K, Amizuka N, Li M, Kobayashi T, Kohno K, et al. Targeted ablation of osteocytes induces osteoporosis with defective mechanotransduction. Cell Metab. 2007;5:464–475.

[17] Nakashima T, Hayashi M, Fukunaga T, Kurata K, Oh-hora M, Feng JQ, et al. Evidence for osteocyte regulation of bone homeostasis through rankl expression. Nat Med. 2011;17:1231–1234.

[18] O'Brien CA, Nakashima T, Takayanagi H. Osteocyte control of osteoclastogenesis. Bone. 2012. http://dx.doi.org/10.1016/j.bone.2012.08.121 (accessed September 2012).

[19] Xiong J, Onal M, Jilka RL, Weinstein RS, Manolagas SC, O'Brien CA. Matrix-embedded cells control osteoclast formation. Nat Med. 2012;17(10):1235–1241.

[20] Tate MK. Whither flows the fluid in bone? An osteocyte´s perspective. J Biomech. 2003;36:1409-1424.

[21] Tomkinson A, Reeve J, Shaw RW, Noble BS. The death of osteocytes via apoptosis accompanies estrogen withdrawal in human bone. J Clin Endocrinol Metab. 1997;82:3128-3135.

[22] Teitelbaum SL. Bone resorption by osteoclasts. Science. 2000;289(5484):1504–1508.

[23] Hill P. Bone remodelling. Br J Orthod. 1998;25:101–107.

[24] Yasuda H, Shima N, Nakagawa N, Yamaguchi K, Kinosaki M, Mochizuki SI, et al. Osteoclast differentiation factor is a ligand for osteoprotegeriny osteoclastogenesis inhibitory factor and is identical to RANCE/RANKL. Proc Natl Acad Sci U S A. 1998;95(7):3597-3602.

[25] Hofbauer LC, Neubauer A, Heufelder AE. Receptor activator of nuclear factor-Kb ligand and osteoprotegerin: potential implications for the pathogenesis and treatment of malignant bone diseases. Cancer. 2001;92(3):460–470.

[26] Li Z, Kong K, Qi W. Osteoclast and its roles in calcium metabolism and bone development and remodeling. Biochem Biophys Res Commun. 2006;343:345–350.

[27] Vaananen HK, Horton M. The osteoclast clear zone is a specialized cell-extracellular matrix adhesion structure. J Cell Sci. 1995;108:2729–2732.

[28] Everts V, Delaisse JM, Korper W, Jansen DC, Tigchelaar-Gutter W, Saftig P, et al. The Bone Lining Cell: Its Role in Cleaning Howship's Lacunae and Initiating Bone Formation. J Bone Miner Res. 2002;17(1):77-90.

[29] Chambers T, Darby J, Fuller K. Mammalian collagenase predisposes bone surfaces to osteoclastic resorption. Cell Tissue Res. 1985;241:671–675.

[30] Chambers TJ, Fuller K. Bone cells predispose bone surfaces to resorption by exposure of mineral to osteoclastic contact. J Cell Sci. 1985;76:155–165.

[31] Hauge EM, Qvesel D, Eriksen EF, Mosekilde L, Melsen F. Cancellous bone remodeling occurs in specialized compartments lined by cells expressing osteoblastic markers. J Bone Miner Res. 2001;16:1575–1582.

[32] Raggatt LJ, Partridge NC. Cellular and Molecular Mechanisms of Bone Remodeling. J Biol Chem. 2010;285(33):25103–25108.

[33] Hernandez CJ, Hazelwood SJ, Martin RB. The Relationship Between Basic Multicellular Unit Activation and Origination in Cancellous Bone. Bone. 1999; 25(5):585–587.

[34] Eriksen EF. Cellular mechanisms of bone remodeling. Rev Endocr Metab Disord. 2010;11:219–227.

[35] Kular J, Tickner J, Chim SM, Xu J. An overview of the regulation of bone remodelling at the cellular level. Clin Biochem. 2012;45:863–873.

[36] Smit TH, Burger EH. Is BMU-Coupling a Strain-Regulated Phenomenon? A Finite Element Analysis. J Bone Miner Res. 2000;15(2):301-307.

[37] Kristensen HB, Andersen TL, Marcussen N, Rolighed L, Delaisse JM. Increased presence of capillaries next to remodeling sites in adult human cancellous bone. J Bone Miner Res. 2012. doi: [10.1002/jbmr.1760].

[38] MacKelvie KJ, Khan KM, Petit MA, Janssen PA, McKay HA. A School-Based Exercise Intervention Elicits Substantial Bone Health Benefits: A 2-Year Randomized Controlled Trial in Girls. Pediatrics. 2003;112(6):e447-e452.

[39] Suda T, Takahashi N, Udagawa N, Jimi E, Gillespie MT, Martin TJ. Modulation of Osteoclast Differentiation and Function by the New Members of the Tumor Necrosis Factor Receptor and Ligand Families. Endocr Rev. 1999;20(3):345–357.

[40] Takayanagi H. Osteoimmunology and the effects of the immune system on bone. Nat Rev Rheumatol. 2009;5(12):667-676.

[41] Gallagher JC, Sai AJ. Molecular biology of bone remodeling: implications for new therapeutic targets for osteoporosis. Maturitas. 2010;65(4):301–307.

[42] Baron R, Neff L, Van PT, Nefussi JR, Vignery A. Kinetic and Cytochemical Identfication of Osteoclast Precursors and Their Differentiation Into Multinucleated Osteoclasts. Am J Pathol. 1986;122(2):363-378.

[43] Martin TJ, Sims NA. Osteoclast-derived activity in the coupling of bone formation to resorption. Trends Mol Med. 2005;11(2):76-81.

[44] Matsuo K, Irie N. Osteoclast–osteoblast communication. Arch Biochem Biophys. 2008;473:201–209.

[45] Tang Y, Wu X, Lei W, Pang L, Wan C, Shi Z, et al. TGF-β1-induced Migration of Bone Mesenchymal Stem Cells Couples Bone Resorption and Formation. Nat Med. 2009;15(7):757–765.

[46] Teti A. Bone Development: Overview of Bone Cells and Signaling. Curr Osteoporos Rep. 2011;9:264–273.

[47] Lian JB, Stein GS. Development of the osteoblast phenotype: molecular mechanisms mediating osteoblast growth and differentiation. Iowa Orthop J. 1995;15:118-140.

[48] Feng X, McDonald JM. Disorders of Bone Remodeling. Annu Rev Pathol. 2011;6:121-145.

[49] Confavreux CB. Bone: from a reservoir of minerals to a regulator of energy metabolism. Kidney Int Suppl. 2011;(121):S14-19.

[50] Raisz LG. Physiology and pathophysiology of bone remodeling. Clin Chem. 1999;45(8 Pt 2):1353-1358. Review. Erratum in: Clin Chem 1999;45(10):1885.

[51] Weitzmann MN, Pacifici R. Estrogen deficiency and bone loss: an inflammatory tale. J Clin Invest. 2006;116(5):1186-1194.

[52] Khosla S. Update on estrogens and the skeleton. J Clin Endocrinol Metab. 2010;95(8): 3569-3577.

[53] Jilka RL. Molecular and cellular mechanisms of the anabolic effect of intermittent PTH. Bone. 2007;40:1434–1446.

[54] Bikle DD, Sakata T, Leary C, Elalieh H, Ginzinger D, Rosen CJ, et al. Insulin-like growth factor I is required for the anabolic actions of parathyroid hormone on mouse bone. J Bone Miner Res. 2002;17:1570–1578.

[55] Wang Y, Nishida S, Boudignon BM, Burghardt A, Elalieh HZ, Hamilton MM, et al. IGF-I receptor is required for the anabolic actions of parathyroid hormone on bone. J Bone Miner Res. 2007;22:1329–1337.

[56] Keller H, Kneissel M. SOST is a target gene for PTH in bone. Bone. 2005;37:148–158.

[57] Kramer I, Loots GG, Studer A, Keller H, Kneissel M. Parathyroid hormone (PTH)-induced bone gain is blunted in SOST overexpressing and deficient mice. J Bone Miner Res. 2010;25:178–189.

[58] Guo J, Liu M, Yang D, Bouxsein ML, Saito H, Galvin RJ, et al. Suppression of Wnt signaling by Dkk1 attenuates PTH-mediated stromal cell response and new bone formation. Cell Metab. 2010;11:161–171.

[59] Bedi B, Li JY, Tawfeek H, Baek KH, Adams J, Vangara SS, et al. Silencing of parathyroid hormone (PTH) receptor 1 in T cells blunts the bone anabolic activity of PTH. Proc Natl Acad Sci USA. 2012;109:E725–733.

[60] Krishnan V, Bryant HU, Macdougald OA. Regulation of bone mass by Wnt signaling. J Clin Invest. 2006;116:1202–1209.

[61] Monroe DG, McGee-Lawrence ME, Oursler MJ, Westendorf JJ. Update on Wnt signaling in bone cell biology and bone disease. Gene. 2012;492(1):1-18.

[62] Hill TP, Spater D, Taketo MM, Birchmeier W, Hartmann C. Canonical Wnt/beta-catenin signaling prevents osteoblasts from differentiating into chondrocytes. Dev Cell. 2005;8(5):727–738.

[63] Bennett CN, Longo KA, Wright WS, Suva LJ, Lane TF, Hankenson KD, et al Regulation of osteoblastogenesis and bone mass by Wnt10b. Proc Natl Acad Sci USA. 2005;102:3324–3329.

[64] Cawthorn WP, Bree AJ, Yao Y, Du B, Hemati N, Martinez- Santibanez G, et al. Wnt6, Wnt10a and Wnt10b inhibit adipogenesis and stimulate osteoblastogenesis through a beta-catenin dependent mechanism. Bone. 2012;50:477–489.

[65] Janssens K, ten Dijke P, Janssens S, Van Hul W. Transforming growth factor-beta1 to the bone. Endocr Rev. 2005;26:743–774.

[66] Qiu T, Wu X, Zhang F, Clemens TL, Wan M, Cao X. TGF beta type II receptor phosphorylates PTH receptor to integrate bone remodeling signaling. Nat Cell Biol. 2010;12:224–234.

[67] Lowery JW, Pazin D, Intini G, Kokabu S, Chappuis V, Capelo LP, et al. The role of BMP2 signaling in the skeleton. Crit Rev Eukaryot Gene Expr. 2011;21:177–185.

[68] Kamiya N, Kobayashi T, Mochida Y, Yu PB, Yamauchi M, Kronenberg HM, et al. Wnt inhibitors Dkk1 and Sost are downstream targets of BMP signaling through the type IA receptor (BMPRIA) in osteoblasts. J Bone Miner Res. 2010;25:200–210.

[69] Gazzerro E, Canalis E. Bone morphogenetic proteins and their antagonists. Rev Endocr Metab Disord. 2006;7:51–65.

[70] Matsuo K. Eph and ephrin interactions in bone. Adv Exp Med Biol. 2010;658:95–103.

[71] Matsuo K, Otaki N. Bone cell interactions through Eph/ephrin: Bone modeling, remodeling and associated diseases. Cell Adh Migr. 2012;6(2):148-156.

[72] Xing W, Kim J, Wergedal J, Chen ST, Mohan S. Ephrin B1 regulates bone marrow stromal cell differentiation and bone formation by influencing TAZ transactivation via complex formation with NHERF1. Mol Cell Biol. 2010;30:711–721.

[73] Zhang X, Tamasi J, Lu X, Zhu J, Chen H, Tian X, et al. Epidermal growth factor receptor plays an anabolic role in bone metabolism in vivo. J Bone Miner Res. 2011;26(5): 1022-1034.

[74] Schneider MR, Sibilia M, Erben RG. The EGFR network in bone biology and pathology. Trends Endocrinol Metab. 2009;20:517–524.

[75] Marie PJ, Miraoui H, Severe N. FGF/FGFR signaling in bone formation: progress and perspectives. Growth Factors. 2012;30(2):117–123.

[76] Choi SC, Kim SJ, Choi JH, Park CY, Shim WJ, Lim DS. Fibroblast growth factor-2 and -4 promote the proliferation of bone marrow mesenchymal stem cells by the activation of the PI3K-Akt and ERK1/2 signaling pathways. Stem Cells Dev. 2008;17:725–736.

[77] Park J, Park OJ, Yoon WJ, Kim HJ, Choi KY, Cho TJ, et al. Functional characterization of a novel FGFR2 mutation, E731K, in craniosynostosis. J. Cell. Biochem. 2012;113:457–464.

[78] Fei Y, Xiao L, Doetschman T, Coffin DJ, Hurley MM. Fibroblast growth factor 2 stimulation of osteoblast differentiation and bone formation is mediated by modulation of the wnt signaling pathway. J. Biol. Chem. 2011;286:40575–40583.

[79] Warren SM, Brunet LJ, Harland RM, Economides AN, Longaker MT. The BMP antagonist noggin regulates cranial suture fusion. Nature. 2003;422:625–629.

[80] Choi KY, et al. Runx2 regulates FGF2-induced Bmp2 expression during cranial bone development. Dev. Dyn. 2005;233:115–121.

[81] Govoni KE. Insulin-like growth factor-I molecular pathways in osteoblasts: potential targets for pharmacological manipulation. Curr Mol Pharmacol. 2012;5(2):143-152.

[82] Mohan S, Richman C, Guo R, Amaar Y, Donahue LR, Wergedal J, et al. Insulin-like growth factor regulates peak bone mineral density in mice by both growth hormone-dependent and -independent mechanisms. Endocrinology. 2003;144(3):929-936.

[83] Miraoui H, Marie PJ. Fibroblast growth factor receptor signaling crosstalk in skeletogenesis. Sci Signal. 2010;3(146):re9.

[84] Ducy P, Amling M, Takeda S, Priemel M, Schilling AF, Beil FT, et al. Leptin inhibits bone formation through a hypothalamic relay: a central control of bone mass. Cell. 2000;100:197–207.

[85] Yadav VK, Oury F, Suda N, et al. A serotonin-dependent mechanism explains the leptin regulation of bone mass, appetite, and energy expenditure. Cell. 2009;138:976–989.

[86] Gershon MD, Tack J. The serotonin signaling system: from basic understanding to drug development for functional GI disorders. Gastroenterology. 2007;132:397-414.

[87] Walther DJ, Peter JU, Bashammakh S, Hörtnagl H, Voits M, Fink H, Bader M. Synthesis of serotonin by a second tryptophan hydroxylase isoform. Science. 2003;299(5603):76.

[88] Yadav VK, Ryu JH, Suda N, et al. Lrp5 controls bone formation by inhibiting serotonin synthesis in the duodenum. Cell. 2008;135:825–837.

[89] Cui Y, Niziolek PJ, MacDonald BT, et al. Lrp5 functions in bone to regulate bone mass. Nat Med. 2011;17:684–691.

[90] Maeda K, Kobayashi Y, Udagawa N, Uehara S, Ishihara A, Mizoguchi T, et al. Wnt5a-Ror2 signaling between osteoblast lineage cells and osteoclast precursors enhances osteoclastogenesis. Nat Med. 2012;18:405–412.

[91] Negishi-Koga T, Shinohara M, Komatsu N, Bito H, Kodama T, Friedel RH, et al. Suppression of bone formation by osteoclastic expression of semaphorin 4D. Nat Med. 2011;17:1473–1480.

[92] Marcus R, Bouxsein M. 2008. The nature of osteoporosis. In Osteoporosis, ed. R Marcus, D Feldman, DA Nelson, CJ Rosen, pp. 27–36. San Diego: Academic.

[93] Saika M, Inoue D, Kido S, Matsumoto T. 17β-estradiol stimulates expression of osteoprotegerin by a mouse stromal cell line, ST-2, via estrogen receptor α. Endocrinology. 2001;142:2205–2212.

[94] Eghbali-Fatourechi G, Khosla S, Sanyal A, Boyle WJ, Lacey DL, Riggs BL. Role of RANK ligand in mediating increased bone resorption in early postmenopausal women. J. Clin. Investig. 2003;111:1221–1230.

[95] Raisz LG. Pathogenesis of osteoporosis: concepts, conflicts, and prospects. J. Clin. Investig. 2005;115:3318–3325.

[96] Khosla S, Riggs BL. Pathophysiology of age-related bone loss and osteoporosis. Endocrinol.Metab. Clin. N. Am. 2005;34:1015–1030.

[97] Hoppé E, Morel G, Biver E, Borg S, Chopin F, Legrand E. Male osteoporosis: do sex steroids really benefit bone health in men? Joint Bone Spine. 2011;78 Suppl 2:S191-196.

[98] Weinstein RS. Glucocorticoid-induced osteoporosis and osteonecrosis. Endocrinol Metab Clin North Am. 2012;41(3):595-611.

[99] Weinstein RS, Jilka RL, Parfitt AM, Manolagas SC. Inhibition of osteoblastogenesis and promotion of apoptosis of osteoblasts and osteocytes by glucocorticoids. Potential mechanisms of their deleterious effects on bone. J. Clin. Invest. 1998;102(2):274–282.

[100] Hofbauer LC, Gori F, Riggs BL, Lacey DL, Dunstan CR, et al. Stimulation of osteoprotegerin ligand and inhibition of osteoprotegerin production by glucocorticoids in

human osteoblastic lineage cells: potential paracrine mechanisms of glucocorticoid-induced osteoporosis. Endocrinol. 1999;140:4382–4389.

[101] Gaudio A, Pennisi P, Bratengeier C, Torrisi V, Lindner B, Mangiafico RA, et al. Increased sclerostin serum levels associated with bone formation and resorption markers in patients with immobilization-induced bone loss. J Clin Endocrinol Metab. 2010;95(5): 2248-2253.

[102] Block GA, Cunningham J. Morbidity and mortality associated with abnormalities in bone and mineral metabolism in CKD. In Clinical Guide to the Basics of Bone and Mineral Metabolism in CKD, ed. K Olgaard, 2006. p77–92. New York: Natl. Kidney Found.

[103] Ralston SH, Layfield R. Pathogenesis of Paget disease of bone. Calcif Tissue Int. 2012;91(2):97-113.

[104] Britton C, Walsh J. Paget disease of bone - an update. Aust Fam Physician. 2012;41(3): 100-103.

[105] Tolar J, Teitelbaum SL, Orchard PJ. Osteopetrosis. N. Engl. J. Med. 2004;351:2839–2849.

[106] Stark Z, Savarirayan R. Osteopetrosis. Orphanet J Rare Dis. 2009;4:5.

[107] McCarthy EF. Genetic diseases of bones and joints. Semin Diagn Pathol. 2011;28(1): 26-36.

Chapter 2

Genetic Diseases Related with Osteoporosis

Margarita Valdés-Flores, Leonora Casas-Avila and
Valeria Ponce de León-Suárez

Additional information is available at the end of the chapter

http://dx.doi.org/10.5772/55546

1. Introduction

Osteoporosis is a disease entity characterized by the progressive loss of bone mineral density (BMD) and the deterioration of bone microarchitecture, leading to the development of fractures. Its classification encompasses two large groups, primary and secondary osteoporosis [1].

Primary osteoporosis is the disease's most common form and results from the progressive loss of bone mass related to aging and unassociated with other illness, a natural process in adult life; its etiology is considered multifactorial and polygenic. This form currently represents a growing worldwide health problem due in part, to the contemporary environmental conditions of modern civilization. Risk factors that are considered as "modifiable" also play an important role and include physical activity, dietary habits and eating disorders. Furthermore, there is another group of associated risk factors that are considered "non-modifiable", including gender, age, race, a personal and/or family history of fractures that in turn, indirectly reflect the degree of genetic susceptibility to this disease [2-4]. Secondary osteoporosis encompasses a large heterogeneous group of primary conditions favoring osteoporosis development. Table 1 summarizes some of the disease entities associated to primary and secondary osteoporosis.

1.1. Genetic aspects of primary osteoporosis

This form of osteoporosis results from the interaction of several environmental and genetic factors, leading to difficulties in its study. It is not easy to define the magnitude of the effect of genetic susceptibility since it is a trait determined by multiple genes whose products affect the bone phenotype; moreover, the environmental factors compromising bone mineral density are also difficult to analyze. However, in spite of these barriers, research suggests that inherited factors affect BMD in ranges between 40 – 70% in the spine, 70 – 85% in the hip and 50 – 60%

Type of osteoporosis	Causes
Primary	Multifactorial, polygenic. Senile/Involutional
Secondary	Drugs compromising bone quality: anticonvulsants, antidepressants, anticoagulants, antacids with aluminum, aromatase inhibitors, barbiturates, cimetidine, corticosteroids, glucocorticoids, birth control pills, cancer drugs, gonadotropin releasing hormone (GnRH), loop diuretics, methotrexate, phenobarbital, phenothiazines, among others.
	Other entities: nephropathies, malabsorption syndromes, neoplasias, rheumatoid arthritis, ankylosing spondylitis, multiple sclerosis, any process leading to decreased mobility or prolonged immobility.
	Metabolic diseases: diabetes, hyperthyroidism, hyperparathyroidism.
	Hypogonadism: Turner and Klinefelter syndromes.
	Behavioral disorders: anorexia nervosa, depression, prolonged physical inactivity, malnutrition, high caffeine intake, smoking and/or chronic alcoholism.
	Monogenic diseases: osteogenesis imperfecta, glioma syndrome, osteoporosis.

Table 1. Osteoporosis classification.

in the wrist. Bone density studies in monozygotic (MZ) and dizygotic (DZ) twins suggest that spinal and femoral neck BMD concordance is higher (6-8:1) in MZ versus DZ twins. Other studies have estimated that fracture predisposition heritability per se ranges between 25 – 35% and up to 40% of patients with osteoporotic fractures have a positive family history of fractures, thus reflecting the great influence of genetic factors in this disease. On the other hand, the geometry and length of the femoral neck, the bone's properties on ultrasound, growth speed and bone remodeling variations are also dependent on genetic factors. The genes associated with the bone phenotype are distributed throughout the human genome and located in practically all chromosomes; their products fulfill specific functions and contribute in different manners to the genetic control of the bone tissue phenotype [5-12]. Some of these genes and their products are presented in Table 2 [13-23].

It is important to mention that the mechanisms conditioning the hereditary susceptibility to osteoporosis are determined, among other factors, by the presence of mutations or genetic polymorphisms (natural genomic variations) in one or several genes involved in bone phenotype genetic control. These polymorphisms follow a well-defined inheritance pattern and their distribution is different among racial groups and populations. There are several reports in the world literature, of associations between specific genetic variants and

http://dx.doi.org/10.5772/55546

osteoporosis development or the risk of fractures; these risks may vary according to the fractures' anatomic location [3, 4, 24-30]

Product Function	Genes
Matrix components	COL1A1, COL1A2, OPN
Hormones and their receptors	ESR1, ESR2, AR, VDR, PTHR1, CASR, PTH, CYP1A1, PRL, LEP, LEPR, INS, INSR
Participants in osteoblastogenic proccesses	ALOX12, ALOX15, BMP4, BMP7, IGF-1 LRP5, LRP6, SOST
Participants in osteoclastogenic proccesses	P53, RANK, RANK-L
Citokines and their receptors	IL1α, IL1β, IL6, TNF, TNFR2
Other	MTHFR, APOE

Table 2. Genes involved in bone metabolism.

2. Mendelian diseases and osteoporosis

The description in the literature of some genetic diseases of monogenic inheritance and whose phenotype includes the loss or increase in bone mineral density and even fractures, has suggested and even proved that bone phenotype has an important genetic component. These diseases include idiopathic osteoporosis, osteogenesis imperfecta in all its variants, osteopetrosis, pycnodysostosis and the osteoporosis syndrome associated to pseudoglioma, among others. In some cases of severe osteoporosis, mutations in the estrogen and even the androgen receptor genes have been detected.

2.1. Idiopathic juvenile osteoporosis

This is an unusual variety of osteoporosis whose frequency has not been precisely determined. This disease may develop in females and males, usually around 7 – 10 years of age; children present difficulty in gait, pain in the lower extremities, ankles, knees, occasionally in the hip and fractures tend to develop particularly in long bones. Radiologically, it is characterized by diffuse osteopenia, metaphyseal fractures – especially of the femur -, and vertebral collapse that may lead to severe kyphoscoliosis or collapse of the thoracic cage. This disease is considered potentially reversible whereby in most cases, there is almost complete recovery of the bone tissue; growth, however, may be compromised.

In these patients, it is important to exclude other disease entities or conditions manifesting secondarily as osteoporosis. A differential diagnosis must be made with other genetic diseases, particularly the different variants of osteogenesis imperfecta; this is relatively easy due to its clinical characteristics, lacking in idiopathic osteoporosis. The genetic basis of this disease has of yet, not been established but it is possible that genetic mutations with preferential tissue expression in bone and with great impact on the tissue's phenotype, may explain some of these cases [31, 32].

2.2. Osteogenesis imperfecta

Osteogenesis imperfecta, also known as "brittle bone disease", has an estimated incidence of approximately 1 in 20 000 births. It has great phenotypic variability, different patterns of inheritance and a wide clinical spectrum ranging from very mild forms of the disease to severe cases with an unfavorable prognosis. It is caused by the defective synthesis of one of the two alpha chains of type I collagen (COL1A1 and COL1A2), leading to anomalies in these protein's structure; it is normally constituted by 3 coiled sub-units, two $\alpha 1$ chains and one $\alpha 2$ chain. This type of collagen is considered the most abundant component of structural protein in bone as well as in ligaments, tendons, sclerae and skin. Quantitative or qualitative defects in this protein lead to bone fragility and hence, to an increased risk of fractures.

The genes encoding the $\alpha 1$ and $\alpha 2$ chains are located in the 17q21.31-q22 and 7q22.1 chromosomes, respectively. Aside from brittle bones, these patients may also present long bones with no curvatures, severe deformities preventing appropriate gait and even standing, conductive deafness due to malformations of the auditory canal, dentinogenesis imperfecta, joint hyperlaxity and intervertebral disc herniation. Patients with severe forms of the disease have a long history of fractures on mild impact and variable bone deformities. The most severe variants may even lead to fractures in utero and pre or perinatal death. Tables 3 and 4 shows different forms of the disease [33-35].

2.3. Osteoporosis – Pseudoglioma Syndrome (OPPG)

This syndrome is an autosomal recessive disease characterized by bone and visual abnormalities including short stature, osteoporosis development during infancy, spontaneous fractures, scoliosis, platyspondyly and long bone deformities. A crucial associated finding is the presence of pseudoglioma that may be associated to microcephaly, blindness during childhood, cataracts and iris atrophy. Occasionally, some patients present interventricular septal defects and mental retardation. This disease is conditioned by mutations of the LRP5 gene, located on chromosome 11q13.4 and that encodes the low-density lipoprotein receptor-related protein 5 (LRP5). It was initially believed that this entity was another variant of osteogenesis imperfecta (OI) but the study of collagen in patients with OPPG established that this protein was normal and the hypothesis was discarded; however, this is still the most relevant differential diagnosis [36-41].

2.4. Neuromuscular disorders

Muscular dystrophies, peripheral neuropathies and muscle atrophies of hereditary origin, represent broad groups of diseases that aside from their characteristic clinical stigmata, can be associated with osteoporosis as one of their complications. As the disease progresses in these patients, there is increased difficulty and limitation in walking and periods of immobility become progressively more prolonged leading to the gradual loss of the mechanical stimuli that bone needs to maintain its strength and hence, favoring the development of osteoporosis. As all Mendelian diseases, these neuromuscular abnormalities follow different inheritance patterns and present phenotypic variability [42-44].

2.5. Inborn errors of metabolism

This group of genetic diseases encompasses a great number of inborn defects with repercussions in several aspects of carbohydrate, amino acid, protein, vitamin, mineral, complex molecule, neurotransmitter and energy metabolism. The genetic basis of most of these entities hinges on gene mutations encoding proteins, particularly enzymes, leading to partial or complete blockade of one or several metabolic processes. In these diseases, symptoms arise for different reasons, including: a deficit of the products generated by the compromised enzymatic reaction, accumulation of the precursor immediate to the defect, an increase in alternative products due to increased activation of alternate metabolic pathways or inhibition of these alternate pathways due to the accumulated substrate. In most cases, inheritance of these diseases is autosomal recessive and less frequently, X-linked recessive.

In cases of metabolic errors, osteoporosis tends to develop for different reasons: in some cases, it is secondary to nutritional deficiencies, progressive neurologic or muscular impairment or as a consequence of the therapeutic measures taken in the management of the primary disease: their secondary effects directly compromise bone quality (steroids, antiseizure drugs, etc.). The number of monogenic diseases whose phenotype may include osteoporosis is large and are shown in Tables 3-5, according to their Mendelian inheritance pattern [45-56].

Disease	Gene	Product	Genomic Location	Reference
Hutchinson-Gilford progeria syndrome; HGPS	LMNA	Prelamin-A/C precursor (LMNA)	1q22	57, 58
Osteogenesis imperfecta, Type I; OI1	COL1A1	Collagen, type I, alpha 1 (COL1A1)	17q21.33	33, 34
Osteogenesis imperfecta, Type II; OI2	COL1A1	Collagen, type I, alpha 1 (COL1A1)	17q21.33	33, 59
	COL1A2	Collagen, type I, alpha 2 (COL1A2)	7q21.3	
Osteogenesis imperfecta, Type III; OI3	COL1A1	Collagen, type I, alpha 1 (COL1A1)	17q21.33	33, 60
	COL1A2	Collagen, type I, alpha 2 (COL1A2)	7q21.3	
Marfan syndrome; MFS	FBN1	Fibrillin 1 (FBN1)	15q21.1	61, 62

Disease	**Gene**	**Product**	**Genomic Location**	**Reference**
Loeys-Dietz syndrome, Type 1A; LDS1A	TGFBR1	Transforming growth factor-beta receptor, Type I (TGFBR1)	9q22.33	63, 64
Loeys-Dietz syndrome, Type 1B; LDS1B	TGFBR2	Transforming growth factor-beta receptor, Type II (TGFBR2)	3p24.1	65, 66
Loeys-Dietz syndrome, Type 2B; LDS2B	TGFBR2	Transforming growth factor-beta receptor, Type II (TGFBR2)	3p24.1	63, 65
Loeys-Dietz syndrome, Type 3; LDS3	MADH3/ SMAD3	Mothers against decapentaplegic homolog 3 (Drosophila) (SMAD3)	15q22.33	67, 68
Ehlers-Danlos syndrome, Type I	COL5A2	Collagen, type V, alpha 2 (COL5A2)	2q32.2	69, 70
	COL5A1	Collagen, type V, alpha 1 (COL5A1)	9q34.3	
	COL1A1	Collagen, type I, alpha 1 (COL1A1)	17q21.33	
Ehlers-Danlos syndrome, Type II	COL5A1	Collagen, type V, alpha 1 (COL5A1)	9q34.3	70, 71
	COL5A2	Collagen, type V, alpha 2 (COL5A2)	2q32.2	
Pseudohypoparathyroidism, Type IA; PHP1A	GNAS	GNAS complex locus (GNAS) [Gs, alpha subunit, included]	20q13.32	72, 73
Pseudohypoparathyroidism, Type IC; PHP1C	GNAS	GNAS complex locus (GNAS) [Gs, alpha subunit, included]	20q13.32	73, 74
Pseudopseudohypopara-thyroidism; PPHP	GNAS	GNAS complex locus (GNAS) [Gs, alpha subunit, included]	20q13.32	73, 75
Epiphyseal dysplasia, multiple, 1; EDM1	COMP	Cartilage oligomeric matrix protein (COMP)	19p13.11	76, 77

Disease	Gene	Product	Genomic Location	Reference
Prader-Willi syndrome; PWS	NDN SNRPN /PWCR	Necdin homolog (mouse) (NDN) Small nuclear ribonucleoprotein-associated protein N (SNRPN/PWCR)	15q11.2 15q11.2	78, 79
Hajdu-Cheney syndrome; HJCYS	NOTCH2	Neurogenic locus Notch homolog protein 2 (NOTCH2)	1p12-p11	80, 81
Nephrolithiasis/osteoporosis, hypophosphatemic, 1; NPHLOP1	SLC34A1	Sodium-dependent phosphate transport protein 2A (SLC34A1/ .NPT2A)	5q35.3	82, 83
Nephrolithiasis/osteoporosis, hypophosphatemic, 2; NPHLOP2	SLC9A3R1/ NHERF	Na(+)/H(+) exchange regulatory cofactor NHE-RF1 (SLC9A3R1/ NHERF)	17q25.1	84-86
Cardiomyopathy, dilated, with hypergonadotropic hypogonadism	LMNA	Prelamin-A/C precursor (LMNA)	1q22	87, 88
Dyskeratosis congenita, autosomal dominant, 1; DKCA1	TERC	Telomerase RNA component (TERC) (RNA)	3q26.2	87, 88
Dyskeratosis congenita, autosomal dominant, 2; DKCA2	TERT	Telomerase reverse transcriptase (TERT)	5p15.33	89, 90
Dyskeratosis congenita, autosomal dominant, 3; DKCA3	TINF2	TERF1-interacting nuclear factor 2 (TINF2)	14q12	91, 92
Pigmented nodular adrenocortical disease, primary, 1; PPNAD1	PRKAR1A	cAMP-dependent protein kinase type I-alpha regulatory subunit (PRKAR1A/ TSE1)	17q24.2	93, 94
Pigmented nodular adrenocortical disease, primary, 2; PPNAD2	PDE11A	Dual 3',5'-cyclic-AMP and -GMP phosphodiesterase 11A (PDE11A)	2q31.2	95, 96
Hyperostosis corticalis generalisata, benign form of worth, with torus palatinus	LRP5	Low density lipoprotein receptor-	11q13.2	97, 98

Disease	Gene	Product	Genomic Location	Reference
		related protein 5 (LRP5)		
Van Buchem disease, Type 2; HVB2	LRP5	Low density lipoprotein receptor-related protein 5 (LRP5)	11q13.3	99, 100
Osteopetrosis, autosomal dominant 1; OPTA1	LRP5	Low density lipoprotein receptor-related protein 5 (LRP5)	11q13.3	101, 102
Osteopetrosis, autosomal dominant 2; OPTA2	CLCN7	H(+)/Cl(-) exchange transporter 7 (CLCN7)	16p13.3	103, 104
ACTH-independent macronodular adrenal hyperplasia; AIMAH	GNAS	GNAS complex locus (GNAS) [Gs, alpha subunit, included]	20q13.32	105, 106
Hyper-IgE recurrent infection syndrome, autosomal dominant	STAT3	Signal transducer and activator of transcription 3 (STAT3)	17q21.2	107, 108
Coronary artery disease, autosomal dominant 2; ADCAD2 or CADO	LRP6	Low density lipoprotein receptor-related protein 6 (LRP6)	12p13.2	109, 110
Avascular necrosis of femoral head, primary; ANFH	COL2A1	Collagen, type II, alpha 1 (COL2A1)	12q13.11	111, 112
Spondyloepimetaphyseal dysplasia with joint laxity Type 2; SEMDJL2	KIF22	Kinesin-like protein KIF22 (KIF22)	16p11.2	113, 114
Spondyloepiphyseal dysplasia, Maroteaux type (pseudo-Morquio syndrome, Type 2)	TRPV4	Transient receptor potential cation channel, subfamily V, member 4 (TRPV4)	12q24.11	115, 116
Hypophosphatasia, adult	ALPL	Alkaline phosphatase, liver/bone/kidney or alkaline phosphatase, tissue-nonspecific isozyme (ALPL)	1p36.12	117, 118

Disease	Gene	Product	Genomic Location	Reference
Cleidocranial dysostosis; CLCD	RUNX2	Runt-related transcription factor 2 (RUNX2)	6p21.1	119, 120
Trichorhinophalangeal syndrome, type I; TRPS1	TRPS1	Zinc finger transcription factor Trps1(TRPS1)	8q23.3	121, 122

Table 3. Autosomal dominant diseases with bone mineral density loss.

Disease	Gene	Product	Genomic location	Reference
Vitamin D hydroxylation-deficient rickets, Type 1A; VDDR1A	CYP27B1	25-hydroxy-vitamin D-1 alpha hydroxylase, mitochondrial (CYP27B1)	12q13	123, 124
Hemochromatosis; HFE	HFE (C282Y y H63D)	Hereditary hemochromatosis protein (HFE)	6p22.2	125, 126
	BMP2 [HFE hemochromatosis, modifier of]	Bone morphogenetic protein 2 (BMP2)	20p12.3	
Beta-Thalassemia	beta-Thalassemia:HBB	Hemoglobin subunit beta (HBB)	11p15.4	47, 48
	Thalassemia, Hispanic gamma-delta-beta: LCRB	Locus control region, beta (LCRB)	11p15.5	
Osteoporosis-pseudoglioma syndrome; OPPG	LRP5	Low density lipoprotein receptor-related protein 5 (LRP5)	11q13.2	127, 128
Homocystinuria due to cystathionine beta-synthase deficiency	CBS/HIP4	Cystathionine beta-synthase (CBS)	21q22.3	45, 46
Homocysteinemia	MTHFR (C677T)	Methylenetetrahydrofolate reductase (MTHFR)	1p36.6	129, 130
	CBS	Cystathionine beta-synthase (CBS)	21q22.3	
	MS/MTR	Methionine synthase (MTR/METH)	1q23	

Disease	Gene	Product	Genomic location	Reference
Homocysteinemia	MTHFR (C677T)	Methylenetetrahydro folate reductase (MTHFR)	1p36.6	33, 131, 132
	CBS	Cystathionine beta-synthase (CBS)	21q22.3	
	MS/MTR	Methionine synthase (MTR/METH)	1q23	
Osteogenesis imperfecta, Type IX; OI9 [Osteogenesis imperfecta type II-B, III or IV PPIB related]	PPIB	Peptidyl-prolyl cis-trans isomerase B (PPIB)	15q22.31	35, 133
Propionic acidemia	PCCA	Propionyl-CoA carboxylase alpha chain, mitochondrial (PCCA)	13q32.3	134, 135
	PCCB	Propionyl-CoA carboxylase beta chain, mitochondrial (PCCB)	3q22.3	
Ehlers-Danlos syndrome, type VI; EDS6	PLOD1	Procollagen-lysine,2-oxoglutarate 5-dioxygenase 1 (PLOD1)	1p36.22	69, 136
Hypertrophic osteoarthropathy, primary, autosomal recessive, 1; PHOAR1	HPGD	15-hydroxy-prostaglandin dehydrogenase [NAD +] (HPGD)	4q34.1	137, 138
Pituitary adenoma, ACTH-secreting; CUDP	AIP	AH receptor-interacting protein (AIP)	11q13.2	139, 140
Gaucher disease, Type I; GDI	GBA	Glucosylceramidase (GLCM/GBA)	1q22	49, 50
Paget disease, juvenile; JPD	TNFRSF11B	Tumor necrosis factor receptor superfamily, member 11b (TNFRSF11B)	8q24.12	141, 142
Pycnodysostosis; PKND	CTSK	Cathepsin K	1q21.3	143, 144
Lipodystrophy, congenital generalized, type 4; CGL4	PTRF	Polymerase I and transcript release factor (PTRF)	17q21.2	145, 146

Disease	Gene	Product	Genomic location	Reference
Niemann-Pick disease, Type A	SMPD1	Sphingomyelin phosphodiesterase 1, acid lysosomal (SMPD1/ASM)	11p15.4	147, 148
Niemann-Pick disease, Type B	SMPD1	Sphingomyelin phosphodiesterase 1, acid lysosomal (SMPD1/ASM)	11p15.4	147, 149
Lathosterolosis	SC5DL	Lathosterol oxidase (SC5DL)	11q23.3	150, 151
Mucopolysaccharidosis Type IVA (Morquio syndrome A)	GALNS	N-acetyl-galactosamine-6-sulfatase (GALNS)	16q24.3	152-154
Mucopolysaccharidosis Type IVB (Morquio syndrome B)	GLB1	Beta-galactosidase1 (BGAL)	3p22.3	
Fibromatosis, juvenile hyaline; JHF	ANTXR2	Anthrax toxin receptor 2 (ANTXR2)	4q21	155, 156
Aromatase deficiency	CYP19A1	Cytochrome P450 19A1 (CYP19A1)	15q21.2	157, 158
Diastrophic dysplasia	SLC26A2	Sulfate transporter 2 (S26A2)	5q32	159, 160
Desbuquois dysplasia; DBQD	CANT1	Soluble calcium-activated nucleotidase 1 (CANT1)	17q25.3	161, 162
Torg-winchester syndrome	MMP2	72 kDa type IV collagenase (MMP2)	16q12.2	163, 164
Geroderma osteodysplasticum; GO	GORAB	RAB6-interacting golgin (GORAB)	1q24.2	165, 166
Lysinuric protein intolerance; LPI	SLC7A7	Y+L amino acid transporter 1 (YLAT1)	14q11.2	167, 168
Cerebroretinal microangiopathy with calcifications and cysts; CRMCC	CTC1	CST complex subunit CTC1	17p13.1	169, 170
Exudative vitreoretinopathy 4; EVR4	LRP5	Low density lipoprotein receptor-related protein 5 (LRP5)	11q13.2	171, 172
Nestor-Guillermo progeria syndrome; NGPS	BANF1	Barrier to autointegration factor 1 (BANF1)	11q13.1	173, 174

Disease	Gene	Product	Genomic location	Reference
Dyskeratosis congenita, autosomal recessive, 1; DKCB1	NOLA3 / NOP10	H/ACA ribonucleoprotein complex subunit 3 (NOP10/ NOLA3)	15q14	175, 176
Macrocephaly, alopecia, cutis laxa, and scoliosis	RIN2	Ras and Rab interactor 2 (RIN2)	20p11.23	177, 178
Hypertrophic osteoarthropathy, primary, autosomal recessive, 1; PHOAR1	HPGD	15-hydroxyprostaglandin dehydrogenase [NAD+] (PGDH)	4q34.1	137, 179
Multiple joint dislocations, short stature, craniofacial dysmorphism, and congenital heart defects	B3GAT3	Galactosylgalactosylxylosylprotein 3-beta-glucuronosyltransferase 3 (B3GAT3)	11q12.3	180, 181
Hyalinosis, infantile systemic; ISH	ANTXR2	Anthrax toxin receptor 2 (ANTXR2)	4q21.21	182, 183
Ovarian dysgenesis 1; ODG1	FSHR	Follicle stimulating hormone receptor (FSHR)	2p16.3	184, 185
Epiphyseal dysplasia, multiple, with early-onset diabetes mellitus	EIF2AK3	Eukaryotic translation initiation factor 2 alpha kinase 3 (EIF2AK3)	2p11.2	186, 187
Cerebrooculofacioskeletal syndrome 1; COFS1	ERCC6	DNA excision repair protein ERCC-6	10q11.23	188, 189
Wilson disease; WND	ATP7B	Copper-transporting ATPase 2 (ATP7B)	13q14.3	190, 191
Werner syndrome; WRN	WRN/RECQL2	Werner syndrome ATP-dependent helicase (WRN / RECQL2)	8p12	192, 193
Rothmund-thomson syndrome; RTS	RECQL4	ATP-dependent DNA helicase Q4 (RECQL4)	8q24.3	194, 195
Schwartz-Jampel syndrome, Type 1; SJS1	HSPG2	Basement membrane-specific heparan sulfate proteoglycan core protein (HSPG2)	1p36.12	196, 197

Disease	Gene	Product	Genomic location	Reference
Perrault syndrome; prlts	HSD17B4	Peroxisomal multifunctional enzyme type 2 (HSD17B4)	5q23.1	198, 199
Glycogen storage disease Ia; GSD1A	G6PC	Glucose-6-phosphatase, catalytic subunit (G6PC)	17q21.31	200, 201
Glycogen storage disease Ib; GSD1B	SLC37A4	Glucose-6-phosphate translocase (SLC37A4)	11q23.3	200, 201
Cranioectodermal dysplasia 1; CED1	IFT122	Intraflagellar transport protein 122 homolog (IFT122)	3q21.3	202, 203
Cerebrotendinous xanthomatosis; CTX	CYP27A1	Sterol 26-hydroxylase, mitochondrial (CYP27A1/CP27A)	2q35	204, 205
Arthropathy, progressive pseudorheumatoid, of childhood; PPAC	WISP3	WNT1-inducible-signaling pathway protein 3 (WISP3)	6q21	206, 207
Genitopatellar syndrome; GTPTS	KAT6B	Histone acetyltransferase KAT6B	10q22.2	208, 209
Congenital disorder of glycosylation, Type IIk; CDG2K	TMEM165	Transmembrane protein 165 (TMEM165/TM165)	4q12	210, 211
Cutis laxa, autosomal recessive, Type IA; ARCL1A	FBLN5	Fibulin-5 (FBLN5)	14q32.12	212, 213
Cutis laxa, autosomal recessive, Type IIB; ARCL2B	PYCR1	Pyrroline-5-carboxylate reductase 1, mitochondrial (PYCR1/P5CR1)	17q25.3	166, 214
Cutis laxa, autosomal recessive, Type IIIB; ARCL3B	PYCR1	Pyrroline-5-carboxylate reductase 1, mitochondrial (PYCR1/P5CR1)	17q25.3	212, 215
Niemann-Pick disease, Type B	SMPD1	Sphingomyelin phosphodiesterase (SMPD1)	11p15.4	149, 216
Trichothiodystrophy, photosensitive; TTDP	ERCC3	TFIIH basal transcription factor	2q14.3	217, 218

Disease	Gene	Product	Genomic location	Reference
		complex helicase XPB subunit (ERCC3)		
	GTF2H5	General transcription factor IIH, subunit 5 (GTF2H5)	6q25.3	
	ERCC2	TFIIH basal transcription factor complex helicase XPD subunit (ERCC2)	19q13.32	
Cerebral autosomal recessive arteriopathy with subcortical infarcts and leukoencephalopathy; CARASIL	HTRA1	Serine protease HTRA1	10q26.13	219, 220
Weill-Marchesani syndrome 1; WMS1	ADAMTS10	A disintegrin and metalloproteinase with thrombospondin motifs 10 (ADAMTS10/ATS10)	19p13.2	221, 222
Laron syndrome	GHR	Growth hormone receptor (GHR)	5p13-p12	223, 224
Mandibuloacral dysplasia with type A lipodystrophy; MADA	LMNA	Prelamin-A/C precursor (LMNA)	1q22	225, 226
Keutel syndrome	MGP	Matrix Gla protein (MGP)	12p12.3	227, 228
Hypophosphatasia, childhood	ALPL	Alkaline phosphatase, liver/bone/kidney or alkaline phosphatase, tissue-nonspecific isozyme (ALPL / PPBT)	1p36.12	229, 230
Fanconi-Sickel syndrome; FBS	SLC2A2	Solute carrier family 2, facilitated glucose transporter member 2 (SLC2A2 / GTR2)	3q26.2	231, 232
Lactose intolerance, adult type	MCM6	DNA replication licensing factor MCM6	2q21.3	233, 234
Trichohepatoenteric syndrome 1; THES1	TTC37	Tetratricopeptide repeat domain 37 (TTC37)	5q15	235, 236
Costello syndrome	HRAS	GTPase HRas (HRAS/ RASH) (HRAS / RASH)	11p15.5	237, 238

Disease	Gene	Product	Genomic location	Reference
Adrenal hyperplasia, congenital, due to 21-hydroxylase deficiency	CYP21A2	Steroid 21-hydroxylase (CYP21A2)	6p21.33	239, 240

Table 4. Autosomal recessive diseases with bone mineral density loss.

Disease	Gene	Product	Genomic location	Reference
Hypophosphatemic rickets, X-linked dominant; XLHR or HYP	PHEX	Phosphate-regulating neutral endopeptidase (PHEX/PEX)	Xp22.11	241, 242
Androgen insensitivity syndrome; AIS	AR	Androgen receptor (AR)	Xq12	243, 244
Fragile X mental retardation syndrome	FMR1	Fragile X mental retardation protein 1 (FMR1)	Xq27.3	245, 246
Fabry disease	GLA	Galactosidase, alpha (AGAL)	Xq22.1	51, 52
Occipital horn syndrome; OHS	ATP7A	Copper-transporting ATPase 1 (ATP7A)	Xq21.1	247, 248
Menkes disease	ATP7A	Copper-transporting ATPase 1 (ATP7A)	Xq21.1	249, 250
Dyskeratosis congenita, X-linked; DKCX	DKC1	H/ACA ribonucleoprotein complex subunit 4 (DKC1)	Xq28	251, 252
Hyperglycerolemia (glycerol kinase deficiency; GKD)	GK	Glycerol kinase (GK)	Xp21.2	253, 254
Premature ovarian failure 2B; POF2B	FLJ22792 / POF1B	Protein POF1B	Xq21.1-q21.2	255, 256
Terminal osseous dysplasia; TOD or ODPF	FLNA	Filamin-A (FLNA)	Xq28	257, 258

Table 5. X-linked recessive diseases with bone mineral density loss.

2.6. Genetic diseases of chromosomal origin and osteoporosis

Within the different categories of genetic diseases, we can include numeric or structural chromosomal abnormalities. Two of the most common chromosomal diseases are Turner's syndrome and Klinefelter's syndrome, both associated to X chromosome aneuploidy; in the first case, there is complete or partial absence of an X chromosome and less frequently, it can be caused by structural anomalies in the short arms of the X chromosome. In Klinefelter's syndrome, there is an additional X chromosome and occasionally, there may be more than one extra X chromosome. In both syndromes, the phenotypic spectrum includes gonadal dysgenesis, in Turner's syndrome there are fibrous bands instead of ovaries and in Klinefelter's, the testicles are hypoplastic, leading in both cases to hypogonadism and a partial or complete deficit in the sex hormones that would normally be produced by the ovaries and testicles. Due to their lack, the development of normal secondary sexual characteristics is stunted and the various metabolic processes dependent on the hormones are also compromised. One of these metabolic processes occurs in bone [259-262].

Undoubtedly, bone metabolism is complex and the processes of osteoblastogenesis, osteoclastogenesis and remodeling must occur in a balanced manner; it is important to mention that the entire family of steroid hormone receptors (estrogen, androgen, vitamin D and retinoids), are expressed in bone, both in osteoblasts and osteoclasts as well as in chondrocytes. Within this microenvironment, the action of these hormones on their receptors is key to appropriate skeletal development; as a matter of fact, individuals with genetic mutations encoding any of these receptors develop, among other manifestations, bad quality bone mass. These hormones and their receptors play a pivotal role in female and male bone growth and may also favor epiphyseal closure at the end of the growth period. It is known that one of effects of steroid hormones on bone metabolism is resorption inhibition since they promote osteoclast apoptosis and decrease the frequency of remodeling unit activation. Therefore, the integral treatment of both entities includes hormone replacement that to a certain extent, will improve bone mass and will prevent or delay the development of osteoporosis [263, 264].

3. Conclusion

Bone metabolism and the large amount of processes that it involves, such as osteoblastogenesis, osteoclastogenesis and bone remodeling, must be kept in constant balance. Each one of these aspects of the physiology of bone shows a particular gene expression patterns, which may even differ according to conditions and tissue needs. As previously mentioned the number of genes involved is very large and sometimes their expression might be modified by multiple environmental conditions. It is important to mention that the expression of these genes is ubiquitous and is not restricted to the bone tissue, which explains why the phenotypic characteristics of a large number of monogenic and some polygenic entities include alterations on bone mineral density and on the microarchitecture of this tissue; this includes several degrees of osteopenia,osteoporosis or increased bone mineral density. Even a good number of these genes have been identified through the study of human disease whose phenotype includes altered bone mineral density. Without a doubt, the investigation of several processes that regulate bone metabolism will continue generating new knowledge that will allow better understanding of bone physiology and physiopathology of multiple diseases and possibly new therapeutic options in diseases which compromise the quality and function of the bone.

http://dx.doi.org/10.5772/55546

Nomenclature

OPN-Osteopontin

ESR1-Estrogen Receptor Alpha

ESR2-Estrogen Receptor Beta

AR-Androgen Receptor

VDR-Vitamin D Receptor

PTHR1-Parathohormone Receptor

PTH-Parathormone

CASR-Calcium Sensing Receptor

CYP1A1-Cytochrome P450, Subfamily A, Polypeptide 1

PRL-Prolactin

LEP-Leptin

LEPR-Leptin Receptor

INS-Insulin

INSR-Insulin Receptor

ALOX12-Arachidonate 12-Lipoxygenase

ALOX15-Arachidonate 15-Lipoxygenase

BMP4-Bone Morphogenetic Protein 4

BMP7-Bone Morphogenetic Protein 7

IGF-1-Insulin-Like Growth Factor 1 (Somatomedin C)

SOST-Sclerostin

P53-Protein 53

RANK-Receptor Activator Of Nf-Kb2

RANK-L.-Receptor Activator Of Nf-Kb2 Ligand

IL1β-Interleucin 1 Beta

IL6-Interleucin 6

TNF-Tumor Necrosis Factor

TNFR2-Tumor Necrosis Factor Receptor

APOE-Apolipoprotein E

Author details

Margarita Valdés-Flores*, Leonora Casas-Avila and Valeria Ponce de León-Suárez

*Address all correspondence to: mvaldes@inr.gob.mx

Genetics Unit. National Rehabilitation Institute. Ministry of Health, Mexico

References

[1] Kok C, Sambrook PN. Secondary osteoporosis in patients with an osteoporotic fracture. Best Pract Res Clin Rheumatol 2009;23(6):769-79. Review.

[2] Krall EA, Dawson-Hugues B. Hereditable and life-style determinants of bone mineral density. J Bone Miner 1993;8(1):1-9.

[3] Obermayer-Pietsch B, Chararas C, Kotschan S, Walter D, Leb G. Genetic background of osteoporosis. Acta Med Austriaca 2000;27(1):18-22.

[4] Stewart TL, Ralston SH. Role of genetics in the pathogenesis of osteoporosis. J of Endocrinology 2000;166(2):235-245.

[5] Slemenda CW, Turner CH, Peacock M, et al. The genetics of proximal femur geometry, distribution of bone mass and bone mineral density. Osteoporos Int 1996;6(2): 178-182.

[6] Arden NK, Baker J, Hogg C, Baan K, Spector TD. The heritability of bone mineral density, ultrasound of the calcaneus and hip axis length: a study of postmenopausal twins. J Bone Miner Res 1996;11(4):530-534.

[7] Koller DL, Liu G, Econs MJ, et al. Genome screen for quantitative trait loci underlying normal variation in femoral structure. J Bone Miner Res 2001;16(6):985-991.

[8] Flicker L, Faulkner KG, Hopper JL, et al. Determinants of hip axis length in women aged 10–89 years: A twin study. Bone 1996;18(1):41-45.

[9] Deng HW, Mahaney MC, Williams JT, et al. Relevance of the genes for bone mass variation to susceptibility to osteoporotic fractures and its implications to gene search for complex human diseases. Genet Epidemiol 2002;22(1):12-25.

[10] Slemenda CW, Christian JC, Williams CJ, Norton JA, Johnston CCJr. Genetic determinants of bone mass in adult women: a reevaluation of the twin model and the potential importance of gene interaction on heritability estimates. J Bone Miner Res 1991;6(6):561-567.

[11] Flicker L, Hopper JL, Rodgers L, Kaymakci B, Green RM, Wark JD. Bone density determinants in elderly women: A twin study. J Bone Miner Res 1995;10(11):1607-1613.

[12] Harris M, Nguyen TV, Howard GM, Kelly PJ, Eisman JA. Genetic and environmental correlations between bone formation and bone mineral density: a twin study. Bone 1998;22(2):141-145.

[13] Xiong DH, Shen H, Zhao LJ, et al. Robust and comprehensive analysis of 20 osteoporosis candidate genes by very high-density single-nucleotide polymorphism screen among 405 white nuclear families identified significant association and gene-gene interaction. J Bone Miner Res 2006;21(11):1678-1695.

[14] Liu YZ, Liu YJ, Recker RR, Deng HW. Molecular studies of identification of genes for osteoporosis: the 2002 update. J Endocrinol 2003;177(2):147-96.

[15] Arvidson K, Abdallah BM, Applegate LA, et al. Bone regeneration and stem cells. J Cell Mol Med 2011;15(4):718-746. Review.

[16] Valdés-Flores M, Casas-Avila L, Falcón-Ramírez E, Ponce-de-León-Suárez V. Genetic aspects of osteoporosis. Rev Invest Clin 2012;64(3):294-307.

[17] Ralston SH, de Crombrugghe B. Genetic regulation of bone mass and susceptibility to osteoporosis. Genes Dev 2006;15:20(18):2492-2506. Review

[18] Rivadeneira F, Styrkársdottir U, Estrada K, et al. Genetic Factors for Osteoporosis (GEFOS) Consortium. Twenty bone-mineral-density loci identified by large-scale meta-analysis of genome-wide association studies. Nat Genet 2009;41(11):1199-1206.

[19] Richards JB, Kavvoura FK, Rivadeneira F, et al. Genetic Factors for Osteoporosis Consortium. Collaborative meta-analysis: associations of 150 candidate genes with osteoporosis and osteoporotic fracture. Ann Intern Med 2009;20;151(8):528-537.

[20] Sadat-Ali M, Al-Turki HA. Genetic influence of candidate osteoporosis genes in saudi arabian population: a pilot study. J Osteoporos 2012; doi: 10.1155/2012/569145.

[21] Langdahl BL, Uitterlinden AG, Ralston SH, et al. APOSS investigators; DOPS investigators; EPOS investigators; EPOLOS investigators; FAMOS investigators; LASA investigators; ERGO investigators; GENOMOS Study. Large-scale analysis of association between polymorphisms in the transforming growth factor beta 1 gene (TGFB1) and osteoporosis: the GENOMOS study. Bone 2008;42(5):969-981.

[22] Ralston SH. Genetics of osteoporosis. Proc Nutr Soc 2007;66(2):158-65. Review.

[23] Albagha OM, Ralston SH. Genetics and osteoporosis. Rheum Dis Clin North Am 2006;32(4):659-680. Review.

[24] Magaña JJ, Gómez R, Cisneros B, et al. Association of the CT gene (CA) polymorphism with BMD in osteoporotic Mexican women. Clin Genet 2006;70(5):402-408.

[25] Gómez R, Magaña JJ, Cisneros B, et al. Association of the estrogen receptor alpha gene polymorphisms with osteoporosis in the Mexican population. Clin Genet 2007;72(6):574-581.

[26] Magaña JJ, Gómez R, Cisneros B, Casas L, Valdés-Flores M. Association of interleukin-6 gene polymorphisms with bone mineral density in Mexican women. Arch Med Res 2008;39(6):618-624.

[27] Wang JT, Guo Y, Yang TL, et al. Polymorphisms in the estrogen receptor genes are associated with hip fractures in Chinese. Bone 2008;43(5):910-914.

[28] Massart F, Marini F, Bianchi G, et al. Age-specific effects of estrogen receptors' polymorphisms on the bone traits in healthy fertile women: the BONTURNO study. Reprod Biol Endocrinol 2009;7:32.

[29] Lee YH, Woo JH, Choi SJ, Ji JD, Song GG. Associations between osteoprotegerin polymorphisms and bone mineral density: a meta-analysis. Mol Biol Rep 2010;37(1): 227-234.

[30] Seremak-Mrozikiewicz A, Tatuśko J, Drews K, et al. Polymorphism of osteoprotegerin gene and osteoporosis in postmenopausal women. Ginekol Pol 2009;80(5):354-360.

[31] Jones ET, Hensinger RN. Spinal deformity in idiopathic juvenile osteoporosis. Spine (Phila Pa 1976). 1981;6(1):1-4.

[32] Lorenc RS. Idiopathic juvenile osteoporosis. Calcif Tissue Int 2002;70(5):395-7. Review.

[33] Van Dijk FS, Pals G, Van Rijn RR, Nikkels PG, Cobben JM. Classification of Osteogenesis Imperfecta revisited. Eur J Med Genet 2010;53(1):1-5.

[34] Zhang ZL, Zhang H, Ke YH, et al. The identification of novel mutations in COL1A1, COL1A2, and LEPRE1 genes in Chinese patients with osteogenesis imperfecta. J Bone Miner Metab 2012;30(1):69-77.

[35] Pyott SM, Schwarze U, Christiansen HE, et al. Mutations in PPIB (cyclophilin B) delay type I procollagen chain association and result in perinatal lethal to moderate osteogenesis imperfecta phenotypes. Hum Mol Genet 2011;20(8):1595-1609.

[36] Meyer HJ. Atypical osteogenesis imperfecta: Lobstein's disease. Arch Pediat 1955;72(6):182-186.

[37] Brude E. Ocular osteogenesis imperfecta. (Letter) Clin Genet 1986;29(2):187.

[38] Beighton P, Winship I, Behari D. The ocular form of osteogenesis imperfecta: a new autosomal recessive syndrome. Clin Genet 1985;28(1):69-75.

[39] Frontali M, Stomeo C, Dallapiccola B. Osteoporosis-pseudoglioma syndrome: report of three affected sibs and an overview. Am J Med Genet 1985;22(1):35-47.

[40] Gong Y, Slee RB, Fukai N, et al. LDL receptor-related protein 5 (LRP5) affects bone accrual and eye development. Cell 2001;107(4):513-523.

[41] Gong Y, Vikkula M, Boon L, et al. Osteoporosis-pseudoglioma syndrome, a disorder affecting skeletal strength and vision, is assigned to chromosome region 11q12-13. Am J Hum Genet 1996;59(1):146-151.

[42] Gardner-Medwin D. The natural history of Duchenne muscular dystrophy. In: Wise G, Blaw M, Procopis PG, (eds.) Topics in Child Neurology. New York: Spectrum; 1983. p 17–29.

[43] Pareyson D, Marchesi C. Diagnosis, natural history, and management of Charcot-Marie-Tooth disease. Lancet Neurol 2009;8:654–667.

[44] Dubowitz V. Ramblings in the history of spinal muscular atrophy. Neuromuscul Disord 2009;19(1):69-73.

[45] Lee SJ, Lee DH, Yoo HW, Koo SK, Park ES, Park JW, Lim HG, Jung SC. Identification and functional analysis of cystathionine beta-synthase gene mutations in patients with homocystinuria. J Hum Genet 2005;50(12):648-654.

[46] Tyagi N, Kandel M, Munjal C, et al. Homocysteine mediated decrease in bone blood flow and remodeling: role of folic acid. J Orthop Res 2011;29(10):1511-1516.

[47] Cao A, Galanello R. Beta-thalassemia. Genet Med 2010;12(2):61-76.

[48] Chatterjee R, Katz M, Bajoria R. Use of hormone replacement therapy for correction of high turnover bone disease in hypogonadal β-Thalassemia major patients presenting with osteoporosis: comparison with idiopathic premature ovarian failure. Hemoglobin 2011;35(5-6):653-658.

[49] Javier RM, Hachulla E, Rose C, et al. Vertebral fractures in Gaucher disease type I: data from the French "Observatoire" on Gaucher disease (FROG). Osteoporos Int 2011;22(4):1255-1261.

[50] Wenstrup RJ, Roca-Espiau M, Weinreb NJ, Bembi B. Skeletal aspects of Gaucher disease: a review. Br J Radiol 2002;75(Suppl 1):A2-12.

[51] Germain DP, Benistan K, Boutouyrie P, Mutschler C. Osteopenia and osteoporosis: previously unrecognized manifestations of Fabry disease. Clin Genet 2005;68(1): 93-95.

[52] Mersebach H, Johansson JO, Rasmussen AK, et al. Osteopenia: a common aspect of Fabry disease. Predictors of bone mineral density. Genet Med 2007;9(12):812-818.

[53] Haworth CS, Selby PL, Webb AK, Adams JE. Osteoporosis in adults with cystic fibrosis. J R Soc Med. 1998;91 Suppl 34:14-18.

[54] Javier RM, Jacquot J. Bone disease in cystic fibrosis: what's new? Joint Bone Spine. 2011;78(5):445-450.

[55] Paccou J, Zeboulon N, Combescure C, Gossec L, Cortet B. The prevalence of osteoporosis, osteopenia, and fractures among adults with cystic fibrosis: a systematic literature review with meta-analysis. Calcif Tissue Int. 2010;86(1):1-7.

[56] Aris R, Lester G, Ontjes D. Treatment of bone disease in cystic fibrosis. Curr Opin Pulm Med. 2004;10(6):524-30.

[57] Pollex RL, Hegele RA. Hutchinson-Gilford progeria syndrome. Clin Genet 2004;66(5):375-381.

[58] Iglesias BP, Guijarro AG, Civantos MS, Vega PB, Pavón PI, Monereo MS. Complicated osteoporosis in progeroid syndrome: treatment with teriparatide. J Clin Densitom 2012;15(1):116-119.

[59] Laine CM, Koltin D, Susic M, et al. Primary osteoporosis without features of OI in children and adolescents: clinical and genetic characteristics. Am J Med Genet A 2012;158A(6):1252-1261.

[60] Wekre LL, Eriksen EF, Falch JA. Bone mass, bone markers and prevalence of fractures in adults with osteogenesis imperfecta. Arch Osteoporos 2011;6(1-2):31-38.

[61] Sakai H, Visser R, Ikegawa S, et al. Comprehensive genetic analysis of relevant four genes in 49 patients with Marfan syndrome or Marfan-related phenotypes. Am J Med Genet A 2006;140(16):1719-1725.

[62] Villamizar C, Regalado ES, Fadulu VT, et al. Paucity of skeletal manifestations in Hispanic families with FBN1 mutations. Eur J Med Genet 2010;53(2):80-84

[63] Stheneur C, Collod-Béroud G, Faivre L, et al. Identification of 23 TGFBR2 and 6 TGFBR1 gene mutations and genotype-phenotype investigations in 457 patients with Marfan syndrome type I and II, Loeys-Dietz syndrome and related disorders. Hum Mutat 2008;29(11):E284-E95.

[64] Kirmani S, Tebben PJ, Lteif AN, et al. Germline TGF-beta receptor mutations and skeletal fragility: a report on two patients with Loeys-Dietz syndrome. Am J Med Genet A 2010;152A(4):1016-1019.

[65] Ben Amor IM, Edouard T, Glorieux FH, et al. Low bone mass and high material bone density in two patients with Loeys-Dietz syndrome caused by transforming growth factor beta receptor 2 mutations. J Bone Miner Res 2012;27(3):713-718.

[66] Kiliç E, Alanay Y, Utine E, Ozgen-Mocan B, Robinson PN, Boduroğlu K. Arterial tortuosity and aneurysm in a case of Loeys-Dietz syndrome type IB with a mutation p.R537P in the TGFBR2 gene. Turk J Pediatr 2012;54(2):198-202.

[67] van de Laar IM, Oldenburg RA, Pals G, et al. Mutations in SMAD3 cause a syndromic form of aortic aneurysms and dissections with early-onset osteoarthritis. Nat Genet 2011;43(2):121-126.

[68] van de Laar IM, van der Linde D, Oei EH, et al. Phenotypic spectrum of the SMAD3-related aneurysms-osteoarthritis syndrome. J Med Genet 2012;49(1):47-57.

[69] Stanitski DF, Nadjarian R, Stanitski CL, Bawle E, Tsipouras P. Orthopaedic manifestations of Ehlers-Danlos syndrome. Clin Orthop Relat Res 2000;376:213-221.

[70] Mayer K, Kennerknecht I, Steinmann B. Clinical utility gene card for: Ehlers-Danlos syndrome types I-VII and variants - update 2012. Eur J Hum Genet 2012; doi: 10.1038/ejhg.2012.162.

[71] Myllyharju J, Kivirikko KI. Collagens and collagen-related diseases. Ann Med 2001;33(1):7-21.

[72] Duan Y, De Luca V, Seeman E. Parathyroid hormone deficiency and excess: similar effects on trabecular bone but differing effects on cortical bone. J Clin Endocrinol Metab 1999;84(2):718-722.

[73] Bastepe M. The GNAS locus and pseudohypoparathyroidism. Adv Exp Med Biol 2008;626:27-40.

[74] Thiele S, de Sanctis L, Werner R, et al. Functional characterization of GNAS mutations found in patients with pseudohypoparathyroidism type Ic defines a new subgroup of pseudohypoparathyroidism affecting selectively Gsα-receptor interaction. Hum Mutat 2011;32(6):653-660.

[75] de Nanclares GP, Fernández-Rebollo E, Santin I, et al. Epigenetic defects of GNAS in patients with pseudohypoparathyroidism and mild features of Albright's hereditary osteodystrophy. J Clin Endocrinol Metab 2007;92(6):2370-2373.

[76] Cao LH, Wang LB, Wang SS, Ma HW, Ji CY, Luo Y. Identification of novel and recurrent mutations in the calcium binding type III repeats of cartilage oligomeric matrix protein in patients with pseudoachondroplasia. Genet Mol Res 2011;10(2):955-963.

[77] Jackson GC, Mittaz-Crettol L, Taylor JA, et al. Pseudoachondroplasia and multiple epiphyseal dysplasia: a 7-year comprehensive analysis of the known disease genes identify novel and recurrent mutations and provides an accurate assessment of their relative contribution. Hum Mutat 2012;33(1):144-157.

[78] Sinnema M, Maaskant MA, van Schrojenstein Lantman-de Valk HM, et al. Physical health problems in adults with Prader-Willi syndrome. Am J Med Genet A 2011;155A(9):2112-2124.

[79] Vestergaard P, Kristensen K, Bruun JM, et al. Reduced bone mineral density and increased bone turnover in Prader-Willi syndrome compared with controls matched for sex and body mass index--a cross-sectional study. J Pediatr 2004;144(5):614-619.

[80] Isidor B, Lindenbaum P, Pichon O, et al. Truncating mutations in the last exon of NOTCH2 cause a rare skeletal disorder with osteoporosis. Nat Genet 2011;43(4): 306-308.

[81] Simpson MA, Irving MD, Asilmaz E, et al. Mutations in NOTCH2 cause Hajdu-Cheney syndrome, a disorder of severe and progressive bone loss. Nat Genet 2011;43(4): 303-305.

[82] Prié D, Beck L, Friedlander G, Silve C. Sodium-phosphate cotransporters, nephrolithiasis and bone demineralization. Curr Opin Nephrol Hypertens 2004;13(6):675-681.

[83] Scheinman SJ, Tenenhouse HS. Nephrolithiasis, osteoporosis, and mutations in the type 2a sodium-phosphate cotransporter. N Engl J Med 2003;348(3):264-265.

[84] Karim Z, Gérard B, Bakouh N, et al. NHERF1 mutations and responsiveness of renal parathyroid hormone. N Engl J Med 2008;359(11):1128-1135.

[85] Arrabal-Polo MA, Arrabal-Martin M, de Haro-Munoz T, et al. Mineral density and bone remodelling markers in patients with calcium lithiasis. BJU Int 2011;108(11): 1903-1908.

[86] Arrabal-Polo MA, Arrabal-Martin M, Girón-Prieto MS, et al. Osteopenia/osteoporosis in patients with calcium nephrolithiasis. Urol Res 2012; doi:10.1007/s00240-012-0497-8.

[87] Norton N, Siegfried JD, Li D, Hershberger RE. Assessment of LMNA copy number variation in 58 probands with dilated cardiomyopathy. Clin Transl Sci 2011;4(5): 351-352.

[88] Sébillon P, Bouchier C, Bidot LD, et al. Expanding the phenotype of LMNA mutations in dilated cardiomyopathy and functional consequences of these mutations. J Med Genet 2003;40(8):560-567.

[89] Basel-Vanagaite L, Dokal I, Tamary H, et al. Expanding the clinical phenotype of autosomal dominant dyskeratosis congenita caused by TERT mutations. Haematologica 2008;93(6):943-934.

[90] Du HY, Pumbo E, Manley P, et al. Complex inheritance pattern of dyskeratosis congenita in two families with 2 different mutations in the telomerase reverse transcriptase gene. Blood 2008;111(3):1128-1130.

[91] Sasa GS, Ribes-Zamora A, Nelson ND, Bertuch AA. Three novel truncating TINF2 mutations causing severe dyskeratosis congenita in early childhood. Clin Genet 2012;81(5):470-478.

[92] Hofer AC, Tran RT, Aziz OZ, et al. Shared phenotypes among segmental progeroid syndromes suggest underlying pathways of aging. J Gerontol A Biol Sci Med Sci 2005;60(1):10-20.

[93] Groussin L, Jullian E, Perlemoine K, et al. Mutations of the PRKAR1A gene in Cushing's syndrome due to sporadic primary pigmented nodular adrenocortical disease. J Clin Endocrinol Metab 2002;87(9):4324-4329.

[94] Stratakis CA. New genes and/or molecular pathways associated with adrenal hyperplasias and related adrenocortical tumors. Mol Cell Endocrinol 2009;300(1-2):152-157.

[95] Horvath A, Boikos S, Giatzakis C, et al. A genome-wide scan identifies mutations in the gene encoding phosphodiesterase 11A4 (PDE11A) in individuals with adrenocortical hyperplasia. Nat Genet 2006;38(7):794-800.

[96] Carney JA, Gaillard RC, Bertherat J, Stratakis CA. Familial micronodular adrenocortical disease, Cushing syndrome, and mutations of the gene encoding phosphodiesterase 11A4 (PDE11A). Am J Surg Pathol 2010;34(4):547-555.

[97] Ihde LL, Forrester DM, Gottsegen CJ, et al. Sclerosing bone dysplasias: review and differentiation from other causes of osteosclerosis. Radiographics 2011;31(7): 1865-1882.

[98] van Egmond ME, Dikkers FG, Boot AM, van Lierop AH, Papapoulos SE, Brouwer OF. A rare cause of facial nerve palsy in children: Hyperostosis corticalis generalisata (Van Buchem disease). Three new pediatric cases and a literature review. Eur J Paediatr Neurol 2012; doi: 10.1016/j.ejpn.2012.03.002.

[99] Scopelliti D, Orsini R, Ventucci E, Carratelli D. Van Buchem disease. Maxillofacial changes, diagnostic classification and general principles of treatment. Minerva Stomatol 1999;48(5):227-234.

[100] van Wesenbeeck L, Cleiren E, Gram J, et al. Six novel missense mutations in the LDL receptor-related protein 5 (LRP5) gene in different conditions with an increased bone density. Am J Hum Genet 2003;72(3):763-771.

[101] Grodum E, Gram J, Brixen K, Bollerslev J. Autosomal dominant osteopetrosis: bone mineral measurements of the entire skeleton of adults in two different subtypes. Bone 1995;16(4):431-434.

[102] Bollerslev J, Nielsen HK, Larsen HF, Mosekilde L. Biochemical evidence of disturbed bone metabolism and calcium homeostasis in two types of autosomal dominant osteopetrosis. Acta Med Scand 1988;224(5):479-483.

[103] Bénichou O, Cleiren E, Gram J, Bollerslev J, de Vernejoul MC, Van Hul W. Mapping of autosomal dominant osteopetrosis type II (Albers-Schönberg disease) to chromosome 16p13.3. Am J Hum Genet 2001;69(3):647-654.

[104] Kantaputra PN, Thawanaphong S, Issarangporn W, et al. Long-term survival in infantile malignant autosomal recessive osteopetrosis secondary to homozygous p.Arg526Gln mutation in CLCN7. Am J Med Genet A 2012;158A(4):909-916.

[105] Lahera Vargas M, da Costa CV. Prevalence, etiology and clinical findings of Cushing's syndrome. Endocrinol Nutr 2009;56(1):32-39.

[106] Beauregard C, Dickstein G, Lacroix A. Classic and recent etiologies of Cushing's syndrome: diagnosis and therapy. Treat Endocrinol 2002;1(2):79-94.

[107] Heimall J, Freeman A, Holland SM. Pathogenesis of hyper IgE syndrome. Clin Rev Allergy Immunol 2010;38(1):32-38.

[108] Moneret-Vautrin DA, Kanny G, Thinus G. Hyperglobulinemia E syndrome with recurrent infections (Job's syndrome). Rev Med Interne 1999;20(2):133-140.

[109] Mani A, Radhakrishnan J, Wang H, et al. LRP6 mutation in a family with early coronary disease and metabolic risk factors. Science 2007;315(5816):1278-1282.

[110] van Meurs JB, Trikalinos TA, Ralston SH, et al. Large-scale analysis of association between LRP5 and LRP6 variants and osteoporosis. JAMA 2008;299(11):1277-1290.

[111] Ugwonali OF, Sarkissian H, Nercessian OA. Bilateral osteonecrosis of the femoral head associated with pregnancy: four new cases and a review of the literature. Orthopedics 2008;31(2):183.

[112] Zhao F, Li Z, Zhang N, et al. Differences between transient osteoporosis of the hip and bone marrow edema associated with osteonecrosis of the femoral head. Zhongguo Xiu Fu Chong Jian Wai Ke Za Zhi 2008;22(10):1157-1160.

[113] Boyden ED, Campos-Xavier AB, Kalamajski S, et al. Recurrent dominant mutations affecting two adjacent residues in the motor domain of the monomeric kinesin KIF22 result in skeletal dysplasia and joint laxity. Am J Hum Genet 2011;89(6):767-772. Erratum in: Am J Hum Genet 2012;90(1):170.

[114] Min BJ, Kim N, Chung T, et al. Whole-exome sequencing identifies mutations of KIF22 in spondyloepimetaphyseal dysplasia with joint laxity, leptodactylic type. Am J Hum Genet 2011;89(6):760-766.

[115] Dai J, Kim OH, Cho TJ, et al. Novel and recurrent TRPV4 mutations and their association with distinct phenotypes within the TRPV4 dysplasia family. J Med Genet 2010;47(10):704-709.

[116] Nishimura G, Dai J, Lausch E, et al. Spondylo-epiphyseal dysplasia, Maroteaux type (pseudo-Morquio syndrome type 2), and parastremmatic dysplasia are caused by TRPV4 mutations. Am J Med Genet A 2010;152A(6):1443-1449.

[117] Watanabe H, Hashimoto-Uoshima M, Goseki-Sone M, Orimo H, Ishikawa I. A novel point mutation (C571T) in the tissue-non-specific alkaline phosphatase gene in a case of adult-type hypophosphatasia. Oral Dis 2001;7(6):331-5.

[118] Sutton RA, Mumm S, Coburn SP, Ericson KL, Whyte MP. "Atypical femoral fractures" during bisphosphonate exposure in adult hypophosphatasia. J Bone Miner Res 2012;27(5):987-994.

[119] Wang GX, Sun RP, Song FL. A novel RUNX2 mutation (T420I) in Chinese patients with cleidocranial dysplasia. Genet Mol Res 2010;9(1):41-47.

[120] El-Gharbawy AH, Peeden JN Jr, Lachman RS, Graham JM Jr, Moore SR, Rimoin DL. Severe cleidocranial dysplasia and hypophosphatasia in a child with microdeletion of the C-terminal region of RUNX2. Am J Med Genet A 2010;152A(1):169-174.

[121] Shao C, Tian J, Shi DH, et al. A novel mutation in TPRS1 gene caused tricho-rhino-phalangeal syndrome in a Chinese patient with severe osteoporosis. Chin Med J (Engl) 2011;124(10):1583-1585.

[122] Gai Z, Gui T, Muragaki Y. The function of TRPS1 in the development and differentiation of bone, kidney, and hair follicles. Histol Histopathol 2011;26(7):915-921.

[123] Kitanaka S, Takeyama K, Murayama A, Kato S. The molecular bases of vitamin D-dependent rickets type I. Endocr J 2001;48(4):427-432.

[124] Portale AA, Miller WL. Human 25-hidroxyvitamin D-1alpha-hydroxilase: cloning, mutation and gene expression. Pediatr Nefrol 2000;14(7):620-625.

[125] Valenti L, Varenna M, Fracanzani AL, Rossi V, Fargion S, Sinigaglia L. Association between iron overload and osteoporosis in patients with hereditary hemochromatosis Osteoporos Int 2009;20(4):549–555.

[126] Nakchbandi IA, van der Merwe SW. Current understanding of osteoporosis associated with liver disease. Nat Rev Gastroenterol Hepatol 2009;6:660-670.

[127] Narumi S, Numakura C, Shiihara T, et al. Various types of LRP5 mutations in four patients with osteoporosis-pseudoglioma syndrome: identification of a 7.2-kb microdeletion using oligonucleotide tiling microarray. Am J Med Genet A 2010;152A(1): 133-140.

[128] Laine CM, Chung BD, Susic M, et al. Novel mutations affecting LRP5 splicing in patients with osteoporosis-pseudoglioma syndrome (OPPG). Eur J Hum Genet 2011;19(8):875-81.

[129] El Maghraoui A, Ghozlani I, Mounach A, et al. Homocysteine, folate, and vitamin b(12) levels and vertebral fracture risk in postmenopausal women. J Clin Densitom 2012;15(3):328-333.

[130] Bucciarelli P, Martini G, Martinelli I, et al. The relationship between plasma homocysteine levels and bone mineral density in post-menopausal women. Eur J Intern Med 2010;21(4):301-305.

[131] Takagi M, Ishii T, Barnes AM, et al. A novel mutation in LEPRE1 that eliminates only the KDEL ER- retrieval sequence causes non-lethal osteogenesis imperfecta. PLoS One 2012;7(5):e36809. doi: 10.1371/journal.pone.0036809.

[132] Willaert A, Malfait F, Symoens S, et al. Recessive osteogenesis imperfecta caused by LEPRE1 mutations: clinical documentation and identification of the splice form responsible for prolyl 3-hydroxylation. J Med Genet 2009;46(4):233-241.

[133] van Dijk FS, Nesbitt IM, Zwikstra EH, et al. PPIB mutations cause severe osteogenesis imperfecta. Am J Hum Genet 2009;85(4):521-527.

[134] Kraus JP, Spector E, Venezia S, et al. Mutation analysis in 54 propionic acidemia patients. J Inherit Metab Dis 2012;35(1):51-63.

[135] Pérez B, Angaroni C, Sánchez-Alcudia R, et al. The molecular landscape of propionic acidemia and methylmalonic aciduria in Latin America. J Inherit Metab Dis 2010;33(Suppl 2):S307-S314.

[136] Yen JL, Lin SP, Chen MR, Niu DM. Clinical features of Ehlers-Danlos syndrome. J Formos Med Assoc 2006;105(6):475-480.

[137] Uppal S, Diggle CP, Carr IM, et al. Mutations in 15-hydroxyprostaglandin dehydrogenase cause primary hypertrophic osteoarthropathy. Nat Genet. 2008;40(6):789-793. Erratum in: Nat Genet 2008;40(7):927.

[138] Shimizu C, Kubo M, Kijima Het al. A rare case of acromegaly associated with pachydermoperiostosis. J Endocrinol Invest 1999;22(5):386-389.

[139] Georgitsi M, Raitila A, Karhu A, et al. Molecular diagnosis of pituitary adenoma predisposition caused by aryl hydrocarbon receptor-interacting protein gene mutations. Proc Natl Acad Sci USA 2007;104(10):4101-4105.

[140] Minetto M, Reimondo G, Osella G, Ventura M, Angeli A, Terzolo M. Bone loss is more severe in primary adrenal than in pituitary-dependent Cushing's syndrome.Osteoporos Int 2004;15(11):855-861.

[141] Chong B, Hegde M, Fawkner M, et al. International Hyperphosphatasia Collaborative Group. Idiopathic hyperphosphatasia and TNFRSF11B mutations: relationships between phenotype and genotype. J Bone Miner Res 2003;18(12):2095-2104.

[142] Whyte MP, Singhellakis PN, Petersen MB, Davies M, Totty WG, Mumm S. Juvenile Paget's disease: the second reported, oldest patient is homozygous for the TNFRSF11B "Balkan" mutation (966_969delTGACinsCTT), which elevates circulating immunoreactive osteoprotegerin levels. J Bone Miner Res 2007;22(6):938-946.

[143] Yates CJ, Bartlett MJ, Ebeling PR. An atypical subtrochanteric femoral fracture from pycnodysostosis: a lesson from nature. J Bone Miner Res 2011;26(6):1377-1379.

[144] Toral-López J, González-Huerta LM, Sosa B, Orozco S, González HP, Cuevas-Covarrubias SA. Familial pycnodysostosis: identification of a novel mutation in the CTSK gene (cathepsin K). J Investig Med 2011;59(2):277-280.

[145] Hayashi YK, Matsuda C, Ogawa M, et al. Human PTRF mutations cause secondary deficiency of caveolins resulting in muscular dystrophy with generalized lipodystrophy. J Clin Invest 2009;119(9):2623-2633.

[146] Shastry S, Delgado MR, Dirik E, Turkmen M, Agarwal AK, Garg A. Congenital generalized lipodystrophy, type 4 (CGL4) associated with myopathy due to novel PTRF mutations. Am J Med Genet A 2010;152A(9):2245-2253.

[147] Desnick JP, Kim J, He X, Wasserstein MP, Simonaro CM, Schuchman EH. Identification and characterization of eight novel SMPD1 mutations causing types A and B Niemann-Pick disease. Mol Med 2010;16(7-8):316-321.

[148] Bachor E, Knop E, Karmody CS, Northrop C, Carranza A, Schuknecht HF. Temporal bone histopathology of Niemann-Pick disease type A. Am J Otolaryngol 1997;18(5): 349-362.

[149] Volders P, Van Hove J, Lories RJ, et al. Niemann-Pick disease type B: an unusual clinical presentation with multiple vertebral fractures. Am J Med Genet 2002;109(1): 42-51.

[150] Brunetti-Pierri N, Corso G, Rossi M, et al. Lathosterolosis, a novel multiple-malformation/mental retardation syndrome due to deficiency of 3beta-hydroxysteroid-delta5-desaturase. Am J Hum Genet 2002;71(4):952-958. Erratum in: Am J Hum Genet 2003;73(2):445.

[151] Rossi M, D'Armiento M, Parisi I, et al. Am J Med Genet A 2007;143A(20):2371-2381.

[152] Pajares S, Alcalde C, Couce ML, et al. Molecular analysis of mucopolysaccharidosis IVA (Morquio A) in Spain. Mol Genet Metab 2012;106(2):196-201.

[153] Tomatsu S, Montaño AM, Oikawa H, et al. Mucopolysaccharidosis type IVA (Morquio A disease): clinical review and current treatment. Curr Pharm Biotechnol 2011;12(6):931-945.

[154] Menkès CJ, Rondot P. Idiopathic osteonecrosis of femur in adult Morquio type B disease. J Rheumatol 2007;34(11):2314-2316.

[155] Krishnamurthy J, Dalal BS, Sunila, Gubanna MV. Juvenile hyaline fibromatosis. Indian J Dermatol. 2011;56(6):731-3.

[156] El-Kamah GY, Fong K, El-Ruby M, et al. Spectrum of mutations in the ANTXR2 (CMG2) gene in infantile systemic hyalinosis and juvenile hyaline fibromatosis. Br J Dermatol. 2010;163(1):213-215.

[157] Oz OK, Zerwekh JE, Fisher C, et al. Bone has a sexually dimorphic response to aromatase deficiency. J Bone Miner Res 2000;15(3):507-514.

[158] Vandenput L, Ohlsson C. Estrogens as regulators of bone health in men. Nat Rev Endocrinol 2009;5:437-443.

[159] Dwyer E, Hyland J, Modaff P, Pauli RM. Genotype-phenotype correlation in DTDST dysplasias: Atelosteogenesis type II and diastrophic dysplasia variant in one family. Am J Med Genet A 2010;152A(12):3043-3050.

[160] Forlino A, Piazza R, Tiveron C, et al. A diastrophic dysplasia sulfate transporter (SLC26A2) mutant mouse: morphological and biochemical characterization of the resulting chondrodysplasia phenotype. Hum Mol Genet 2005;14(6):859-871.

[161] Faivre L, Cormier-Daire V, Young I, et al. Long-term outcome in Desbuquois dysplasia: a follow-up in four adult patients. Am J Med Genet A 2004;124A(1):54-59.

[162] Faden M, Al-Zahrani F, Arafah D, Alkuraya FS. Mutation of CANT1 causes Desbuquois dysplasia. Am J Med Genet A 2010;152A(5):1157-1160.

[163] Mosig RA, Dowling O, DiFeo A, et al. Loss of MMP-2 disrupts skeletal and craniofacial development and results in decreased bone mineralization, joint erosion and defects in osteoblast and osteoclast growth. Hum Mol Genet 2007;16(9):1113-1123.

[164] Zankl A, Bonafé L, Calcaterra V, Di Rocco M, Superti-Furga A. Winchester syndrome caused by a homozygous mutation affecting the active site of matrix metalloproteinase 2. Clin Genet 2005;67(3):261-266.

[165] Newman WG, Clayton-Smith J, Metcalfe K, et al. Geroderma osteodysplastica maps to a 4 Mb locus on chromosome 1q24. Am J Med Genet A 2008;146A(23):3034-3037.

[166] Yildirim Y, Tolun A, Tüysüz B. The phenotype caused by PYCR1 mutations corresponds to geroderma osteodysplasticum rather than autosomal recessive cutis laxa type 2. Am J Med Genet A 2011;155A(1):134-140.

[167] Sebastio G, Sperandeo MP, Andria G. Lysinuric protein intolerance: reviewing concepts on a multisystem disease. Am J Med Genet C Semin Med Genet 2011;157(1): 54-62.

[168] Gömez L, García-Cazorla A, Gutiérrez A, et al. Treatment of severe osteoporosis with alendronate in a patient with lysinuric protein intolerance. J Inherit Metab Dis 2006;29(5):687.

[169] Briggs TA, Abdel-Salam GM, Balicki M, et al. Cerebroretinal microangiopathy with calcifications and cysts (CRMCC). Am J Med Genet A 2008;146A(2):182-190.

[170] Toiviainen-Salo S, Linnankivi T, Saarinen A, Mäyränpää MK, Karikoski R, Mäkitie O. Cerebroretinal microangiopathy with calcifications and cysts: characterization of the skeletal phenotype. Am J Med Genet A 2011;155A(6):1322-1328.

[171] Jiao X, Ventruto V, Trese MT, Shastry BS, Hejtmancik JF. Autosomal recessive familial exudative vitreoretinopathy is associated with mutations in LRP5. Am J Hum Genet 2004;75(5):878-884.

[172] Qin M, Hayashi H, Oshima K, Tahira T, Hayashi K, Kondo H. Complexity of the genotype-phenotype correlation in familial exudative vitreoretinopathy with mutations in the LRP5 and/or FZD4 genes. Hum Mutat 2005;26(2):104-112.

[173] Cabanillas R, Cadiñanos J, Villameytide JA, et al. Néstor-Guillermo progeria syndrome: a novel premature aging condition with early onset and chronic development caused by BANF1 mutations. Am J Med Genet A 2011;155A(11):2617-2625.

[174] Osorio FG, Ugalde AP, Mariño G, Puente XS, Freije JM, López-Otín C. Cell autonomous and systemic factors in progeria development. Biochem Soc Trans 2011;39(6): 1710-1714.

[175] Walne AJ, Vulliamy T, Marrone A, et al. Genetic heterogeneity in autosomal recessive dyskeratosis congenita with one subtype due to mutations in the telomerase-associated protein NOP10. Hum Mol Genet 2007;16(13):1619-1629.

[176] Vulliamy TJ, Dokal I. Dyskeratosis congenita: the diverse clinical presentation of mutations in the telomerase complex. Biochimie 2008;90(1):122-130.

[177] Basel-Vanagaite L, Sarig O, Hershkovitz D, et al. RIN2 deficiency results in macrocephaly, alopecia, cutis laxa, and scoliosis: MACS syndrome. Am J Hum Genet 2009;85(2):254-263.

[178] Syx D, Malfait F, Van Laer L, et al. The RIN2 syndrome: a new autosomal recessive connective tissue disorder caused by deficiency of Ras and Rab interactor 2 (RIN2). Hum Genet 2010;128(1):79-88.

[179] Sinibaldi L, Harifi G, Bottillo I, et al. A novel homozygous splice site mutation in the HPGD gene caused mild primary Hypertrophic osteoarthropathy. Clin Exp Rheumatol 2010;28(2):153-157.

[180] Sajnani AK, Yiu CK, King NM. Larsen syndrome: a review of the literature and case report. Spec Care Dentist 2010;30(6):255-260.

[181] Knoblauch H, Urban M, Tinschert S. Autosomal recessive versus autosomal dominant inheritance in Larsen syndrome: report of two affected sisters. Genet Couns 1999;10(3):315-320.

[182] Lindvall LE, Kormeili T, Chen E, et al. Infantile systemic hyalinosis: Case report and review of the literature. J Am Acad Dermatol 2008;58(2):303-307.

[183] Dowling O, Difeo A, Ramirez MC, et al. Mutations in capillary morphogenesis gene-2 result in the allelic disorders juvenile hyaline fibromatosis and infantile systemic hyalinosis. Am J Hum Genet 2003;73(4):957-966.

[184] Lussiana C, Guani B, Mari C, Restagno G, Massobrio M, Revelli A. Mutations and polymorphisms of the FSH receptor (FSHR) gene: clinical implications in female fecundity and molecular biology of FSHR protein and gene. Obstet Gynecol Surv 2008;63(12):785-795.

[185] Doherty E, Pakarinen P, Tiitinen A, Kiilavuori A, Huhtaniemi I, Forrest S, Aittomäki K. A Novel mutation in the FSH receptor inhibiting signal transduction and causing primary ovarian failure. J Clin Endocrinol Metab 2002;87(3):1151-1155.

[186] Delépine M, Nicolino M, Barrett T, Golamaully M, Lathrop GM, Julier C. EIF2AK3, encoding translation initiation factor 2-alpha kinase 3, is mutated in patients with Wolcott-Rallison syndrome. Nat Genet 2000;25(4):406-409.

[187] Liu J, Hoppman N, O'Connell JR, Wang H, Streeten EA, McLenithan JC, Mitchell BD, Shuldiner AR. A functional haplotype in EIF2AK3, an ER stress sensor, is associated with lower bone mineral density. J Bone Miner Res 2012;27(2):331-341.

[188] Jaakkola E, Mustonen A, Olsen P, et al. ERCC6 founder mutation identified in Finnish patients with COFS syndrome. Clin Genet. 2010;78(6):541-547.

[189] Natale V. A comprehensive description of the severity groups in Cockayne syndrome. Am J Med Genet A 2011;155A(5):1081-1095.

[190] Selimoglu MA, Ertekin V, Doneray H, Yildirim M. Bone mineral density of children with Wilson disease: efficacy of penicillamine and zinc therapy. J Clin Gastroenterol 2008;42(2):194-198.

[191] Hegedus D, Ferencz V, Lakatos PL, et al. Decreased bone density, elevated serum osteoprotegerin, and beta-cross-laps in Wilson disease. J Bone Miner Res 2002;17(11): 1961-1967.

[192] Ogata N, Shiraki M, Hosoi T, Koshizuka Y, Nakamura K, Kawaguchi H. A polymorphic variant at the Werner helicase (WRN) gene is associated with bone density, but not spondylosis, in postmenopausal women. J Bone Miner Metab 2001;19(5):296-301.

[193] Uhrhammer NA, Lafarge L, Dos Santos L, et al. Werner syndrome and mutations of the WRN and LMNA genes in France. Hum Mutat 2006;27(7):718-719.

[194] Mohaghegh P, Hickson ID. Premature aging in RecQ helicase-deficient human syndromes. Int J Biochem Cell Biol 2002;34(11):1496-1501.

[195] Mehollin-Ray AR, Kozinetz CA, Schlesinger AE, Guillerman RP, Wang LL. Radiographic abnormalities in Rothmund-Thomson syndrome and genotype-phenotype correlation with RECQL4 mutation status. AJR Am J Roentgenol 2008;191(2):W62-W66.

[196] Stum M, Davoine CS, Vicart S, et al. Spectrum of HSPG2 (Perlecan) mutations in patients with Schwartz-Jampel syndrome. Hum Mutat 2006;27(11):1082-1091.

[197] Mallineni SK, Yiu CK, King NM. Schwartz-Jampel syndrome: a review of the literature and case report. Spec Care Dentist 2012;32(3):105-111.

[198] Pierce SB, Walsh T, Chisholm KM, et al. Mutations in the DBP-deficiency protein HSD17B4 cause ovarian dysgenesis, hearing loss, and ataxia of Perrault Syndrome. Am J Hum Genet 2010;87(2):282-288.

[199] Jenkinson EM, Clayton-Smith J, et al. Perrault syndrome: further evidence for genetic heterogeneity. J Neurol 2012;259(5):974-976.

[200] Cabrera-Abreu J, Crabtree NJ, Elias E, Fraser W, Cramb R, Alger S. Bone mineral density and markers of bone turnover in patients with glycogen storage disease types I, III and IX. J Inherit Metab Dis 2004;27(1):1-9.

[201] Lee PJ, Patel JS, Fewtrell M, Leonard JV, Bishop NJ. Bone mineralisation in type 1 glycogen storage disease. Eur J Pediatr 1995;154(6):483-487.

[202] Zaffanello M, Diomedi-Camassei F, Melzi ML, Torre G, Callea F, Emma F. Sensenbrenner syndrome: a new member of the hepatorenal fibrocystic family. Am J Med Genet A 2006;140(21):2336-2340.

[203] Walczak-Sztulpa J, Eggenschwiler J, Osborn D, et al. Cranioectodermal Dysplasia, Sensenbrenner syndrome, is a ciliopathy caused by mutations in the IFT122 gene. Am J Hum Genet 2010;86(6):949-956.

[204] Gallus GN, Dotti MT, Mignarri A, et al. Four novel CYP27A1 mutations in seven Italian patients with CTX. Eur J Neurol 2010;17(10):1259-1262.

[205] Keren Z, Falik-Zaccai TC. Cerebrotendinous xanthomatosis (CTX): a treatable lipid storage disease. Pediatr Endocrinol Rev 2009;7(1):6-11.

[206] Dalal A, Bhavani G SL, Togarrati et al. Analysis of the WISP3 gene in Indian families with progressive pseudorheumatoid dysplasia. Am J Med Genet A 2012; doi:10.1002/ajmg.a.35620.

[207] Delague V, Chouery E, Corbani S, et al. Molecular study of WISP3 in nine families originating from the Middle-East and presenting with progressive pseudorheumatoid dysplasia: identification of two novel mutations, and description of a founder effect. Am J Med Genet A. 2005;138A(2):118-126.

[208] Penttinen M, Koillinen H, Niinikoski H, Mäkitie O, Hietala M. Genitopatellar syndrome in an adolescent female with severe osteoporosis and endocrine abnormalities. Am J Med Genet A 2009;149A(3):451-455.

[209] Campeau PM, Kim JC, Lu JT, et al. Mutations in KAT6B, encoding a histone acetyltransferase, cause Genitopatellar syndrome. Am J Hum Genet. 2012;90(2):282-289.

[210] Foulquier F, Amyere M, Jaeken J, et al. TMEM165 deficiency causes a congenital disorder of glycosylation. Am J Hum Genet 2012;91(1):15-26.

[211] Woods AG, Woods CW, Snow TM. Congenital disorders of glycosylation. Adv Neonatal Care 2012;12(2):90-95.

[212] Noordam C, Funke S, Knoers NV, et al. Decreased bone density and treatment in patients with autosomal recessive cutis laxa. Acta Paediatr 2009;98(3):490-494.

[213] Callewaert B, Su CT, Van Damme T, et al. Comprehensive clinical and molecular analysis of 12 families with type 1 recessive cutis laxa. Hum Mutat 2012; doi: 10.1002/humu.22165.

[214] Reversade B, Escande-Beillard N, Dimopoulou A, et al. Mutations in PYCR1 cause cutis laxa with progeroid features. Nat Genet 2009;41(9):1016-1021.

[215] Lin DS, Yeung CY, Liu HL, et al. A novel mutation in PYCR1 causes an autosomal recessive cutis laxa with premature aging features in a family. Am J Med Genet A. 2011;155A(6):1285-1289.

[216] Rodríguez-Pascau, L., Gort, L., Schuchman, et al. Identification and characterization of SMPD1 mutations causing Niemann-Pick types A and B in Spanish patients. Hum. Mutat 2009;30:1117–1122.

[217] Lambert WC, Gagna CE, Lambert MW. Trichothiodystrophy: Photosensitive, TTD-P, TTD, Tay syndrome. Adv Exp Med Biol 2010;685:106-110.

[218] Hashimoto S, Egly JM. Trichothiodystrophy view from the molecular basis of DNA repair/transcription factor TFIIH. Hum Mol Genet 2009;18(R2):R224-R230.

[219] Fukutake T. Cerebral autosomal recessive arteriopathy with subcortical infarcts and leukoencephalopathy (CARASIL): from discovery to gene identification. J Stroke Cerebrovasc Dis 2011 Mar-Apr;20(2):85-93.

[220] Hara K, Shiga A, Fukutake T, et al. Association of HTRA1 mutations and familial ischemic cerebral small-vessel disease. N Engl J Med 2009;360(17):1729-1739.

[221] Giordano N, Senesi M, Battisti E, Mattii G, Gennari C. Weill-Marchesani syndrome: report of an unusual case. Calcif Tissue Int 1997;60(4):358-360.

[222] Dagoneau N, Benoist-Lasselin C, Huber C, et al. ADAMTS10 mutations in autosomal recessive Weill-Marchesani syndrome. Am J Hum Genet 2004;75(5):801-806.

[223] Eshed V, Benbassat CA, Laron Z. Effect of alendronate on bone mineral density in adult patients with Laron syndrome (primary growth hormone insensitivity).Growth Horm IGF Res 2006;16(2):119-124.

[224] Benbassat CA, Eshed V, Kamjin M, Laron Z. Are adult patients with Laron syndrome osteopenic? A comparison between dual-energy X-ray absorptiometry and volumetric bone densities. J Clin Endocrinol Metab 2003;88(10):4586-4589.

[225] Agarwal AK, Kazachkova I, Ten S, Garg A. Severe mandibuloacral dysplasia-associated lipodystrophy and progeria in a young girl with a novel homozygous Arg527Cys LMNA mutation. J Clin Endocrinol Metab 2008;93(12):4617-4623.

[226] Kosho T, Takahashi J, Momose T, et al. Mandibuloacral dysplasia and a novel LMNA mutation in a woman with severe progressive skeletal changes. Am J Med Genet A 2007;143A(21):2598-2603.

[227] Cranenburg EC, VAN Spaendonck-Zwarts KY, Bonafe L, et al. Circulating matrix γ-carboxyglutamate protein (MGP) species are refractory to vitamin K treatment in a new case of Keutel syndrome. J Thromb Haemost 2011;9(6):1225-1235.

[228] Cranenburg EC, Schurgers LJ, Vermeer C. Vitamin K: the coagulation vitamin that became omnipotent. Thromb Haemost 2007;98(1):120-125.

[229] Goseki-Sone M, Sogabe N, Fukushi-Irie M, et al. Functional analysis of the single nucleotide polymorphism (787T>C) in the tissue-nonspecific alkaline phosphatase gene associated with BMD. J Bone Miner Res 2005;20(5):773-782.

[230] Girschick HJ, Schneider P, Kruse K, Huppertz HI. Bone metabolism and bone mineral density in childhood hypophosphatasia. Bone 1999;25(3):361-367.

[231] Grünert SC, Schwab KO, Pohl M, Sass JO, Santer R. Fanconi-Bickel syndrome: GLUT2 mutations associated with a mild phenotype. Mol Genet Metab 2012;105(3): 433-437.

[232] Pena L, Charrow J. Fanconi-Bickel syndrome: Report of life history and successful pregnancy in an affected patient. Am J Med Genet A 2011; 155(2):415-417.

[233] Obermayer-Pietsch BM, Gugatschka M, Reitter S, et al. Adult-type hypolactasia and calcium availability: decreased calcium intake or impaired calcium absorption? Osteoporos Int 2007;18(4):445-451.

[234] Honkanen R, Pulkkinen P, Järvinen R, et al. Does lactose intolerance predispose to low bone density? A population-based study of perimenopausal Finnish women. Bone 1996;19(1):23-28.

[235] Hartley JL, Zachos NC, Dawood B, et al. Mutations in TTC37 cause trichohepatoenteric syndrome (phenotypic diarrhea of infancy). Gastroenterology 2010;138(7): 2388-2398, 2398.e1-2.

[236] Fabre A, Martinez-Vinson C, Roquelaure B, et al. Novel mutations in TTC37 associated with tricho-hepato-enteric syndrome. Hum Mutat 2011;32(3):277-281.

[237] Digilio MC, Sarkozy A, Capolino R, et al. Costello syndrome: clinical diagnosis in the first year of life. Eur J Pediatr 2008;167(6):621-628.

[238] White SM, Graham JM Jr, Kerr B, et al. The adult phenotype in Costello syndrome. Am J Med Genet A 2005;136(2):128-135. Erratum in: Am J Med Genet A 2005;139(1): 55.

[239] Bachelot A, Chakhtoura Z, Samara-Boustani D, Dulon J, Touraine P, Polak M. Bone health should be an important concern in the care of patients affected by 21 hydroxylase deficiency. Int J Pediatr Endocrinol 2010;2010: 326275.

[240] Arlt W, Willis DS, Wild SH, et al. United Kingdom Congenital Adrenal Hyperplasia Adult Study Executive (CaHASE). Health status of adults with congenital adrenal hyperplasia: a cohort study of 203 patients. J Clin Endocrinol Metab 2010;95(11): 5110-5121.

[241] Francis F, Hennig S, Korn B, et al. A gene (PEX) with homologies to endopeptidases is mutated in patients with X–linked hypophosphatemic rickets. Nature Genet 1995;11(2):130-136.

[242] Sato K, Tajima T, Nakae J, et al. Three novel PHEX gene mutations in Japanese patients with X-linked hypophosphatemic rickets. Pediatr Res 2000;48(4):536-40.

[243] Boehmer AL, Brinkmann O, Brüggenwirth H, et al. Genotype versus phenotype in families with androgen insensitivity syndrome. J Clin Endocrinol Metab 2001;86(9): 4151-4160. Erratum in: J Clin Endocrinol Metab 2002;87(7):3109.

[244] Melo KF, Mendonca BB, Billerbeck AE, et al. Clinical, hormonal, behavioral, and genetic characteristics of androgen insensitivity syndrome in a brazilian cohort: five novel mutations in the androgen receptor gene. J Clin Endocrinol Metab 2003;88:3241-3250.

[245] D'Hulst C, Kooy RF. Fragile X syndrome: from molecular genetics to therapy. J Med Genet 2009;46(9):577-584.

[246] Hjalgrim H, Fisher Hansen B, Brondum-Nielsen K, Nolting D, Kjaer I. Aspects of skeletal development in fragile X syndrome fetuses. Am J Med Genet 2000;95(2): 123-129.

[247] Bazzocchi A, Femia R, Feraco P, Battista G, Canini R, Guglielmi G. Occipital horn syndrome in a woman: skeletal radiological findings. Skeletal Radiol 2011;40(11): 1491-1494.

[248] Dagenais SL, Adam AN, Innis JW, Glover TW. A novel frameshift mutation in exon 23 of ATP7A (MNK) results in occipital horn syndrome and not in Menkes disease. Am J Hum Genet 2001;69(2):420-427.

[249] Gérard-Blanluet M, Birk-Møller L, Caubel I, Gélot A, Billette de Villemeur T, Horn N. Early development of occipital horns in a classical Menkes patient. Am J Med Genet A 2004;130A(2):211-213. Review. Erratum in: Am J Med Genet A 2005;134(3):346.

[250] Kanumakala S, Boneh A, Zacharin M. Pamidronate treatment improves bone mineral density in children with Menkes disease. J Inherit Metab Dis 2002;25(5):391-398.

[251] Mason PJ, Bessler M. The genetics of dyskeratosis congenita. Cancer Genet 2011;204(12):635-645.

[252] Heiss NS, Knight SW, Vulliamy TJ, et al. X-linked dyskeratosis congenita is caused by mutations in a highly conserved gene with putative nucleolar functions. Nat Genet 1998;19(1):32-38.

[253] Scherleue A, Greenberg F, McCabe ERB. Dysmorphic features in patients with glycerol-kinase deficiency. J Pediatr 1995;126:764-767.

[254] Walker AP, Muscatelli F, Stafford AN, et al. Mutations and phenotype in isolated glycerol kinase deficiency. Am J Hum Genet 1996;58(6):1205-1211.

[255] Goswami D, Conway GS. Premature ovarian failure. Horm Res 2007;68(4):196-202.

[256] Persani L, Rossetti R, Cacciatore C. Genes involved in human premature ovarian failure. J Mol Endocrinol 2010;45(5):257-79. Review. Erratum in: J Mol Endocrinol 2010;45(6):405.

[257] Brunetti-Pierri N, Lachman R, Lee K, et al. Terminal osseous dysplasia with pigmentary defects (TODPD): Follow-up of the first reported family, characterization of the radiological phenotype, and refinement of the linkage region. Am J Med Genet A 2010;152A(7):1825-1831.

[258] Sun Y, Almomani R, Aten E, et al. Terminal osseous dysplasia is caused by a single recurrent mutation in the FLNA gene. Am J Hum Genet 2010;87(1):146-153.

[259] Hsu LY. Phenotype/karyotype correlations of Y chromosome aneuploidy with emphasis on structural aberrations in postnatally diagnosed cases. Am J Med Genet 1994; 53:108-40.

[260] Tuck-Muller CM, Chen H, Martinez JE, et al. Isodicentric Y chromosome: cytogenetic, molecular and clinical studies and review of the literature. Hum Genet 1995;96:119-29.

[261] Ksglaede L, Petersen JH, Main KM, Skakkebaek NE, Juul A. High normal Testosterone levels in infants with non-mosaic Klinefelter's syndrome. Eur J Endocrinol 2007;157:345-350.

[262] Corona G, Petrone L, Paggi F, et al. Sexual dysfunction in subjects with Klinefelter's syndrome. Int J Androl 2009a;32:1-8.

[263] Khosla S, Oursler MJ, Monroe DG. Estrogen and the skeleton. Trends Endocrinol Metab 2012;23(11):576-581.

[264] Delhon I, Gutzwiller S, Morvan F, et al. Absence of estrogen receptor-related-alpha increases osteoblastic differentiation and cancellous bone mineral density. Endocrinology 2009;150(10):4463-4472.

Chapter 3

Serum Leptin and Bone Turnover Markers in Postmenopausal Osteoporosis

Mehreen Lateef, Mukhtiar Baig and Abid Azhar

Additional information is available at the end of the chapter

http://dx.doi.org/10.5772/54527

1. Introduction

Osteoporosis is a very important health problem worldwide. It is defined as a disease characterized by low bone mass and micro-architectural deterioration of bone tissue, leading to enhanced bone fragility and consequent increase in fracture risk [1]. Osteoporosis is a silent disease and the health and financial impact of the disease result from fracture, particularly hip fracture, for which subjects with osteoporosis are at an increased risk [2]. In the UK, one in two women and one in five men suffer a fracture after the age of 50, with an annual cost to the health services of around £2 billion [3,4].

In 1990, the number of osteoporotic fractures estimated in Europe was 2.7 million, with an estimated direct cost in 2004 of €36 billion (£24.5 billion), of which €24.3 billion (£16.6 billion) were accounted for by hip fracture. Costs are expected to rise to €76.8 billion (£52.4 billion) by the year 2050 [5]. Similar projections are made for many other regions of the world because of the increasing numbers of the elderly. In the USA, the annual cost of incident fractures due to osteoporosis or low bone mass is predicted to rise from $16.9 billion in 2006 to around $25.3 billion by the year 2025 [4]. The direct costs of medical care of hip fractures were over $65 million in 2004 [6].

There are many hormones involved in bone and mineral metabolism, such as oestrogens, testosterone and parathormone (PTH). The adipocyte also plays an important role in regulating bone metabolism by releasing estrogens, and the adipokines, like leptin, resistin, adiponectin, and many others. After the discovery of leptin receptors in bone many studies have been done to explore its involvement in bone metabolism. Some studies have shown that leptin is expressed and secreted from primary cultures of human osteoblasts during the mineralization period, and that it may stimulate osteogenesis in human bone marrow in vitro [7,8].

Furthermore, leptin may reduce ovariectomy-induced osteoporosis in rats and may also be involved in foetal and growing bone metabolism [9, 10].

Leptin, a fat-derived cytokine-like hormone, was discovered in 1994 by Friedman and colleagues [11]. A 16-kDa hormone, encoded by the OB gene, is predominantly expressed in adipose tissue [12] and circulates as a free and as a protein-bound entity. According to structural studies leptin belongs to the growth hormone four-helical cytokine subfamily. The leptin receptor was identified in the db locus of mouse chromosome 4. As a member of the IL-6 receptor family, the leptin receptor contains an extracellular-binding domain, a single transmembrane domain and a cytoplasmatic signaling domain [13]. Intracellular signaling is mediated through a non-covalently associated tyrosine kinase of the JAK kinase family [14]. Alternate gene splicing results in five known isoforms of the leptin receptor. The longest form of the receptor (ObR) is the only isoform capable of complete signal transduction. Conversely, the shorter isoforms of the leptin receptor have been suggested to participate in leptin clearance and/or to facilitate transport of leptin across the blood-brain barrier [14]. Circulating levels of leptin correlate with BMI and the content of fat mass. After crossing the blood–brain barrier, leptin reaches the hypothalamus, where it acts as a crucial regulator of feeding. Leptin is mainly regarded as a "starvation-hormone" signaling from the adipose tissue (AT) to the brain, indicating the size of the AT-stores [15].

Food intake and energy expenditure are controlled by leptin through an interaction with various neuropeptides in the hypothalamus. Neuropeptide Y (NPY) and agouti-related peptide (AGRP) expressions are inhibited, whereas pro-opiomelanocortin (POMC) expression is stimulated by leptin with increased food intake [16, 17]. Moreover, leptin interacts with neuromedin U (NMU); a novel and recently identified hypothalamic neuropeptide involved also in the regulation of appetite and locomotor activity [18]. Besides energy metabolism, leptin demonstrates pleiotropic effects in such areas as hematopoesis, blood pressure, T lymphocyte function, reproduction and bone mass regulation [14, 19]. Several endocrine and paracrine factors play a role in the fat-bone relationship. A number of local cytokines secreted by the adipose tissue, including leptin, have also been related to BMD variations [20]. Leptin because of its diverse role in bone is being considered one of the main functional connections between fat and bone.

Leptin, known to regulate appetite & energy expenditure may also contribute to mediate the effects of fat mass on bone. Interestingly, obesity seems to protect from osteoporosis. This observation led to researchers at bone formation in mouse models of obesity. Much effort has been dedicated to the relationship between leptin and bone. This interest stems from the well-founded knowledge that body weight is a major determinant of bone density [21]. It is known that obesity is generally accompanied by increased bone strength. Obese persons have stronger bones and lose bone tissue at a slower pace [22]. Leptin has been proposed to regulate increased body weight as well as increased bone density. Mice that have congenital absence of leptin (ob/ob) have been shown to be obese and have very high bone density. Leptin makes them lose both fat and bone [23]. The bone mass phenotype of ob/ob mice can be rescued by intracerebroventricular (ICV) infusion of leptin, suggesting that leptin exerts an indirect influence on bone mass. There is a report which has shown that when leptin injected into the brain of animals it will inhibit bone formation at doses lower than those that cause loss of body weight [24]. A lot of studies have been done to explore the relationship of serum leptin with bone mass density and biochemical bone markers in osteoporosis. In this chapter, the mechanism of action of leptin on bone is reviewed and role of serum leptin in postmenopausal females is discussed with respect to its relation with bone mass density and biochemical bone markers.

2. Leptin and its mechanism of action on bone

Leptin acts on bone by two different mechanisms. The first is the indirect mechanism revealed by Ducy et al (2000) in mutant mice and rats that either cannot produce or cannot respond to leptin [25]. Leptin secreted from fat cells is carried by the ObRa receptors of vascular endothelial cells across the blood-brain-barrier where it activates ObRb receptors in the hypothalamus. These signals then stimulate expression of HOBIF (hypothalamic osteoblast inhibitory factor) which when released, lowers the matrix-making ability of osteoblasts [25-29] and because of this reason obese Ob (Lep)–/– mice, which should have low bone mass due to lack of leptin, and thus estrogen, actually have an abnormally high bone mass.

The second direct mechanism of leptin action is by promoting differentiation of bone marrow stromal cells into osteoblasts [8] and by inhibiting osteoclast generation [30]. Bone marrow stromal cells (BMSC) can differentiate into either adipocytes or osteoblast cell lineage. Bone marrow adipocytes may serve as a direct source of leptin, which can inhibits adipogenesis differentiation of BMSC and stimulates differentiation of osteoblasts [31] while Kim et al. (2003) have shown that very high leptin levels led to BMSC apoptosis [32]. Reseland et al. (2001) have found that human osteoblasts start making and secreting leptin when they are either in the late, matrix-mineralizing stage or when changing to osteocytes [7]. Leptin has also stimulates the proliferation of cultured human osteoblasts [33], and it has been shown to cause human bone marrow stromal cells to express alkaline phosphatase, collagen-I, and osteocalcin and to mineralize matrix [8]. These tissue culture experiments support the dual effect of leptin within the bone microenvironment depending on the local leptin concentration.

In the last decade Ducy et al. (2000a,b) [25,27] have not found any long isoforms of the leptin receptors (Ob-R) on osteoblasts, so they assumed that leptin acted centrally as a very potent inhibitor of bone formation. Although the long isoform of Ob-R is abundantly expressed in the hypothalamus, and in a large number of peripheral tissues [14]. BMSC, osteoblasts, osteoclasts and chondrocytes also express leptin receptors [8]. In osteoblasts, leptin acts through the osteoprotegerin (OPG)/RANKL (Receptor Activator for Nuclear factor κB Ligand) signaling pathway. Treatment with leptin changes the OPG/RANKL expression profile favoring OPG [30]. Consequently, osteoclastogenesis is very likely suppressed by leptin through the OPG/RANKL pathway. In agreement with the previous findings, Burguera et al [10] have also confirmed the previous findings that administration of leptin reduced ovariectomy induced bone loss in rats by increasing osteoprotegerin mRNA in osteoblasts. Cornish et al in 2001 have found that leptin given peripherally increased bone strength in mice and also increased proliferation of osteoblasts in vitro [34]. The results of these studies showed that direct peripheral action of leptin on bone is to enhance the strength of the bone in contrast to its central effect.

In order to evaluate its central effect, leptin was injected into the brain in the form of an intra-cerebelo-ventricular infusion [25, 27, 35]. Bone loss occurred in both wild-type mice and leptin deficient mice confirming that bone mass is partly regulated via the central, hypothalamic relay [25]. However, bone formation was inhibited at lower doses of leptin than those necessary to cause the loss of body weight. Ob/ob mice have low sympathetic activity, which led to the assumption that the central effect of leptin on bone is mediated by the sympathetic nervous system (SNS) [36]. The effect of leptin on the sympathetic nervous system is an important aspect in the regulation of energy homeostasis as well as several other physiological functions [37].

3. Serum leptin and Bone Mass Density (BMD)

It is widely recognized that BMD measurement can predict fracture risk in the same way as cholesterol predicts cardiovascular disease [38]. In fact, the strength of BMD measurement to predict fracture is approx 3 fold higher than strength of serum cholesterol to predict cardiovascular disease [39]. Bone mass measurement has been found to be a single best predictor of fracture risk and is required to the early diagnosis of osteoporosis [37,38,39].

It is observed in a study by Lateef et al 2010 that BMD is found to be significantly lower in postmenopausal females with and without osteoporosis as compared to premenopausal females [40] and there is a negative correlation between age and BMD found in post menopausal ostreoporotic females indicating bone loss with age and menopause [41]. A rapid bone loss is commonly seen in elderly individuals and tends to worsen with advancing age. The aging population is inevitably proven to be more osteoporotic unless it is intervened first with diagnostic tools and after preventive therapy [42].

Another study of Lateef et al 2011 showed that plasma leptin levels were positively correlated with bone mineral density (BMD) values in osteoporotic females [43]. Some reports have suggested a correlation between serum leptin concentration and BMD while other showed no such association [44-48]. It has been shown that plasma leptin levels are positively correlated with BMD at all skeleton sites measured in postmenopausal osteoporosis [49]. It is interesting to note that the obese are usually protected against osteoporosis and have increased bone mineral density [50]. This has been attributed to the mechanical effects of their excessive weight on bone tissue. It has been shown that obese postmenopausal women have a tendency to have increased bone mineral density compared with lean women [51-53]. The study of Di Carlo et al. (2007) documented a significant correlation between serum leptin and BMD in early postmenopausal women but the correlation was lost during progression of the postmenopausal period [54]. Thomas et al. (2001) have observed that serum leptin correlated with BMD

http://dx.doi.org/10.5772/54527

in women but not in men [31]. Sato et al. (2001) have found a positive correlation between serum leptin and calcaneus BMD in men, but the relationship became inverse when adjusted for body weight [18]. Pasco et al. (2001) have demonstrated a significant positive association between BMD and serum leptin in non-obese women [55]. Results of Blain et al (2002) reported that leptin is an independent predictor of whole body and femoral neck BMD in postmenopausal women [56]. Nagy et al. (2001) found a negative correlation between serum leptin levels and radial and femoral BMD in postmenopausal women [57]. Hadji et al. (2001) reported that bone mass is not correlated with the serum leptin level in pre or postmenopausal women [58]. Rauch et al. (1998) also reported no correlation between bone mass and serum leptin levels by examining total and trabecular bone density at the distal radius in adult women [59]. In leptin literature, several studies have examined the relationship between serum leptin and BMD in various cohorts, but the results remain contradictory. This fact reflects the intricacy of the relationship of leptin and bone.

A study by Hamrick and Ferrari (2008) has documented that the effect of leptin is reduced with increased age and higher BMI in both humans and laboratory animals in spite of high serum leptin levels [60]. It has been postulated that the under-responsiveness to leptin, or leptin resistance, is mediated either by impaired transport of leptin through the blood-brain barrier, lower expression of leptin receptors and/or by the inhibition of the intracellular leptin signaling [61]. In plasma, leptin is bound to soluble leptin receptor (SLR), the product of an alternate splicing of leptin receptor mRNA or proteolytic cleavage [14]. Whereas serum leptin levels correlate positively with BMI, SLR is correlated negatively [14,62]. The inverse relationship between SLR and BMI reflects a feedback regulation between the body weight and leptin or leptin receptor expressions. It is observed in a study by Welt et al. (2004) when low serum leptin levels in women with hypothalamic amenorrhea (induced either by exercise or by low body weight) were treated with recombinant human leptin for three months, it led to an increase of osteocalcin, bone alkaline phosphates and IGF-1, whereas urinary N-telopeptide did not change [63].They have demonstrated that leptin administration in individuals with leptin deficiency appeared to improve the growth hormone axis and markers of bone formation [63].

4. Osteoporosis and bone turnover markers (BTMs)

Bone markers are product derived from the bone remodeling process. During this process, compounds are released either from bone or from the cells involved in the bone remodeling process (osteoblasts and osteoclasts.) Markers of bone turnover are biochemical products measured usually in blood or urine that reflect the metabolic activity of bone but which themselves have no function in controlling skeletal metabolism [64]. Biochemical markers of bone turnover are broadly divided into two categories: markers of bone resorption, which reflect osteoclast activity and are for the most part degradation products of type I collagen; markers of bone formation, which reflect osteoblast activity and are byproducts of collagen synthesis, matrix proteins or osteoblastic enzymes (Table 1) [65].

Bone formation	Detected in
Byproducts of collagen synthesis	
Procollagen type I C-terminal propeptides (P1CP)	Serum
Procollagen type I N-terminal propeptides (PINP)	Serum/Plasma
Matrix protein	
Osteocalcins (OC)	Serum/Plasma
Osteoblast enzyme	
Bone alkaline phosphatases (BALP)	Serum
Bone resorption	Detected in
Collagen degradation products	
Hydroxyprolin	Urine
Pyridinolin(PYD)	Urine
Deoxypyridinoline (DPD)	Urine
Cross-linked telopeptides of type I collagen	
N-terminal cross-linked telopeptide (NTX)	Urine and serum/plasma
C-terminal cross-linked telopeptide (CTX)	Urine and serum/plasma
Osteoclast enzymes	
Tartrate-resistant acid phosphatases (TRACP)	Serum

Table 1. List of important biochemical markers of bone turnover

5. Markers of bone formation

Bone formation markers are direct or indirect products of active osteoblasts expressed during different phases of osteoblast development and reflecting different aspects of osteoblast function and bone formation. All markers are measured in serum or plasma [66].

5.1. Alkaline phosphatase

Alkaline phosphatase (ALP) is a ubiquitous enzyme that plays an important role in osteoid formation and mineralization. The total ALP serum pool consists of several dimeric isoforms which originate from various tissues such as liver, bone, intestine, spleen, kidney and placenta. In adults with normal liver function, approximately 50% of the total ALP activity in serum arises from liver and 50% arise from bone [67].

5.2. Bone specific alkaline phosphatase

Bone specific alkaline phosphatase (BALP) is one of several isoenzymes of the alkaline phosphatase (ALP) family. The entire family is encoded by four gene loci, three tissue specific genes (bone,kidney,liver and other tissues). Although the nonspecific ALPs are the products of a single gene, the ioenzymes present in tissues such as bone, kidney or liver vary greatly because of variations in their carbohydrate side chains. These post translational modifications are exploited to distinguish the various ALP-isoforms from each other, employing methods including gel electrophoresis, heat denaturation, chemical inhibition or binding through specific monoclonal antibodies [68]. For therapeutic monitoring of patients, B-ALP measurements are good indicators of the metabolic activity of bone. Rising ALP concentrations may indicate estrogen deficiency [69,70].

5.3. Osteocalcin

Osteocalcin (OC) is a small, hydroxyapetite-binding protein synthesized by osteoblasts and to a lesser extent by hypertrophic chondrocytes. It contains three gamma- carboxyglutamic acid (Gla) residues which are responsible for calcium binding properties of protein. The precise function of osteocalcin has yet to be determined but recent studies suggest that OC is involved in bone remodeling via a negative mechanism. Serum osteocalcin is considered as a specific marker of osteoblast function, as its levels correlate with bone formation rates. However, the peptide is rapidly degraded in serum and both intact peptides and OC fragments of various sizes coexist in the circulation [70]. Osteocalcin is normally considered as bone formation marker. However, because it is released during bone formation from bone forming cells and during bone resorption from bone matrix, it reflects the overall turnover of bone. Assays have been developed to detect the intact protein and or the main breakdown product called N-mid fragment. OC serum levels follow a circadian rhythm with high values in early morning, but usually not influenced by food intake. Serum osteocalcin levels reportedly vary significantly during the menstrual cycle with the highest level observerd during luteal phase [71].

5.4. Amino & carboxyterminal procollagen propeptides of type I collagen

The amino and carboxy terminal procollagen propeptides of type I collagen (PINP, PICP) are cleaved by specific extracellular endopeptidases from newly translated collagen type I pepetide. As these extension peptides are generated in a stoichiometric relationship with collagen biosynthesis, they are considered quantitative measures of newly formed type I collagen. However, because type I collagen is also a component of several soft tissues (fibrocartilage, tendon, skin, gingival, intestine, heart valve, and large vessels) there is potential contribution to circulating procollagens from soft tissue synthesis of type I collagen. Both PICP and PINP demonstrate a cardian rhythm with peak values in the early morning, and are usually not influenced by food intake. Serum levels of amino and carboxy terminal procollagen propeptides of type I collagen (PINP, PICP) are measured by type and site specific immunoassays [66]. Moderate correlations between serum PICP levels and the rate of bone formation have been reported [72].

5.5. Markers of bone resorption

Most biochemical markers of bone resorption are degradation products of bone collagen, but noncollagenous proteins such as bone sialoprotein or tartarate resistant acid phosphatase have also been investigated [73].

5.6. Hydroxy proline

Hydroxyproline is an amino acid common to and characteristic of all forms of collagen, and urinary hydroxyproline excretion is the oldest test of bone resorption. However, this test lacks specificity for bone resorption because excreted hydroxyproline also comes from other tissues, particularly from skin collagen (which can turn over rapidly in certain disorders), from newly synthesized collagen that is not incorporated into tissue, and from dietary collagen and gelatin. Because it is less specific than newer tests, it is no longer widely used [74].

5.7. Pyridinoline (Pyr) and Deoxypyridinoline (DPD)

The pyridinum crosslinks pyridinoline (PYD) and deoxypyridinolin (DPD) are the main crosslinks in skeletal tissues but act as stabilizers of mature croslinks in type I, II & III collagens of all major connective tissues (bone, dentin, ligaments, tendons, vascular walls, muscle and intestine) except skin. While PYD predominates in most tissues, DPD is most abundant in bone and therefore is considered the more specific marker [75].

5.8. Crosslinked Telopeptides

The term "crosslinked telopeptides" refers to the measurement of collagen degradation products associated with the crosslink regions in type I collagen. Fragments derived from the C terminus are also released into circulation as a result of the osteoclast-mediated degradation of type I collagen and can be measured by various assays [76, 77]. The immuno reactive epitopes are located on peptide fragments derived from the N terminal (NTX-1) and C terminal (CTX-1 and ICTP) telopeptides of the collagen type I molecule. The NTX-1 and CTX-1 epitopes can be measured in both serum and in urine [78, 79].

6. Tatartarate Resistant Acid Phosphatase (TRACP)

Tartarate resistant acid phosphate is synthesized and secreted by osteoclasts during active bone resorption. The process of resorption occurs after the attachment of osteoclasts to the bone surface and follows the secretion of acid and enzymes into a space created between the osteoclast and the bone. The acidic environment is produced by the action of carbonic anhydrase and an H-ATPase proton pump. TRACP, one of the enzymes secreted into this space, has been located in the adjacent osteoclast membrane (known as the ruffled border) [80]. Its activity in serum reflects bone resorption rates and more recently it has been possible to measure the isoenzyme by very specific immunoassays

The use of biochemical markers of bone remodeling in the monitoring of patients on treatment for osteoporosis is generally well-recognized [81,82]. However, optimum treatment targets specific to various therapies and the benefits of monitoring in terms of improvement in fracture outcomes or in adherence to oral therapies are not established [83].

The changes in BMD and BTMs following the initiation of osteoporosis treatment independently correlate with fracture risk reduction [84]. The advantage of BTM over BDM is that the change in BTMs following treatment explains a greater proportion of treatment as compared to BMD does, in terms of fracture risk reduction [85,86]. Also, the change in BMD is small and slow whereas the changes in BTMs are large and occur early after initiation of therapy. Repeat BMD is not advocated within 12 months after initiation of therapy as the changes do not generally attain significance within that time, and in fact 18-24 months may be appropriate for repeat BMD measurements [87]. BTMs on the other hand show significant change by 3-6 months. For example, bone resorption markers can be measured 3 months after initiation of oral bisphosphonates, and bone formation markers 6 months after start of therapy [88, 89). Changes in BTMs may be useful in monitoring osteoporosis treatment to confirm compliance with oral therapies and efficacy of treatment [90].

There are many studies which have demonstrated BTMs and their contribution to fracture risk, but the results of these studies have been inconsistent [91-95]. Many studies which have shown positive results with BTMs included bone resorption markers, with increased resorption marker predicting an increased fracture risk. While for BTMs to predict fracture risk independently of BMD, it is needed to clarify their relationships to other established risk factors.

The changes in BTMs following therapy are well documented. There is a decrease in BTMs following initiation of anti-resorptive therapy, reflecting inhibition of osteoclastic activity [96-100]. For example, with bisphosphonate treatment, there is a decrease in bone resorption markers within days following intravenous therapy, and within weeks following oral therapy.

Vasikaran et al [83] supports the role of BTMs in the management of patients with osteoporosis and also emphasized on the adoption of international reference standards for enhancing laboratory consistency and to facilitate their inclusion in routine clinical practice.

The problem in BTMs use is their wide biological and analytical variability, Glover et al [101] emphasized that reference ranges should be defined and standardized with emphasis on sample size and age range of the population. Sandhu & Hampson (2011) describe that the best established clinical use for BTMs is in monitoring treatment efficacy and compliance [102]. In a study by Kim et al observed that BMT can be used to determine BMD response to antiresorptive therapy in Korean postmenopausal osteoporotic females [103].

The Scientific Advisory Council of Osteoporosis Canada including multidisciplinary working group stated about the bone turnover markers in the management of postmenopausal osteoporosis that as far as potential uses of bone turn over markers (BTMs) are concerned, they can be used to predict bone loss and fracture in untreated postmenopausal women. They can also be used to monitor osteoporosis therapy, and up to some extent enhance the adherence to therapy but BTMs should not be used for diagnosis of osteoporosis as s separate and independent factor. Similarly it must not be used to select the most appropriate type of osteoporotic therapy for the treatment. [104].

7. Relationship of leptin with bone markers in post menopausal osteoporotic females

Data in the literature are inconsistent and conflicting about the relationship of leptin with bone markers in post menopausal osteoporotic females. The study of Goulding & Taylor (1998) was the first to examine relationships among plasma levels of leptin, and dynamic biochemical markers of bone cell activity in postmenopausal women [46]. This study demonstrated no association between circulating plasma levels of leptin and biochemical markers of either osteoclastic or osteoblastic activity. They concluded that leptin itself does not play any significant direct role in controlling bone cell activity in postmenopausal women.

Scariano et al reported positive association between serum leptin and bone specific alkaline phosphatase in postmenopausal women and elderly men after adjustment for BMD, age and BMI [105]. The association of circulating leptin levels with bAP, a specific marker of osteoblast activity suggests that leptin levels influence osteoblast activity in vivo in elderly women and men. In a cross sectional study by Filip R & Raszewski G (2009) a positive association between leptin and osteocalcin in older patients with hip fracture [106]. Rauch et al. and Lateef et al also found no relationship between plasma leptin level and bone turnover markers in adult women and postmenopausal osteoporotic females respectively [40,59]. Filip & Raszewski et al, found no correlations of serum leptin with lumber spine BMD, femoral neck BMD, biochemical markers of bone turnover with leptin, in overweight and obese postmenopausal women, even after stratification of the study group by BMI ratio value (25–29 9, 30–39 9 and ≥ 40), or by waist: hip ratio (WHR), ratio value (< 0 85 and ≥ 0 85) [106]. In a small study, Iwamoto et al. (2000) found correlations between serum leptin and bone remodelling markers only in premenopausal women [107]. Peng et al (2008) reported no association between serum leptin and bone turnover biochemical markers in men [108].

In postmenopausal osteoporotic patients with increased bone turnover, serum leptin concentration is not correlated with BMD or with the biomarkers of bone formation or bone resorption [109]. According to few studies performed in China no correlation found between serum leptin and bone turnover biochemical markers in post-menopausal Chinese women [110-112]. Similarly, no correlation observed between leptin and bone turnover markers in Chinese adolescent dancers and control group in one more study (101) Blain, et al (2002) reported that serum leptin level was positively correlated with weight, fat mass, BMI, E2, creatinine clearance, and BAP level and inversely correlated with urine CTx [56]. They supported the suggestion that circulating leptin exerts its protective effect on bone through limiting the excessive bone resorption coupled with bone formation that is associated with bone loss after menopause.

Prouteau et al (2006) suggested a regulatory role of leptin on type I collagen metabolism [113]. The negative association between bone resorption (CTx levels) and serum leptin levels observed at baseline (stable body weight) was further confirmed by the biochemical changes

http://dx.doi.org/10.5772/54527

occurring in responses to weight loss and weight regain. The drop in leptin levels was strongly related to the increase in bone resorption marker occurring in response to weight loss. Similarly, after weight regain the rise in leptin levels was associated with a concomitant decrease in bone resorption. The reasons for these discrepancies need to be clarified.

8. Conclusion

The relationship of leptin and bone turnover markers in post menopausal osteoporosis has not yet been clarified. Although several studies have been done but still there is need to explore their exact connection. Many studies have recommended that in the treatment of the post-menopausal women, biochemical markers of bone turnover may be useful as adjuncts to BMD and other diagnostic tests. They can be mainly used to monitor response to treatment and also used as relatively economical tools for studying bone metabolism. The exact roles of BTM need to be established in clinical practice. It is suggested that repeated measurements of bone markers during anti-resorptive therapy may help to improve the management of osteoporotic patients.

Both a peripheral and a central action of leptin on bone metabolism have been suggested. Peripherally, leptin is thought to exert positive effects on bone formation, whereas it is thought to reduce bone formation via a central control mechanism when binding to its specific receptors located on the hypothalamic nuclei [26]. It has been suggested that circulating leptin may act positively to maintain bone mass but these effects of serum leptin are not mediated due to these biochemical markers. Despite a preliminary understanding of leptin–bone mass interactions, the exact roles of leptin on bone metabolism have not yet been elucidated.

The role of BTMs in monitoring osteoporosis treatment to confirm compliance with oral therapies, and efficacy of treatment has been established. Further studies with reference to serum leptin and BTMs in post menopausal osteoporotic females are needed to clarify their association and significance of that association in treatment targets for various therapies and optimal monitoring regimes.

Author details

Mehreen Lateef[1*], Mukhtiar Baig[2] and Abid Azhar[3]

*Address all correspondence to: meher_khan555@hotmail.com; drmukhtiarbaig@yahoo.com; abid.azhar@kibge.edu.pk

1 Pharmaceutical Research Centre, Pakistan Council of Scientific and Industrial Research Complex Laboratories Complex, PCSIR, Karachi, Pakistan

2 Department of Biochemistry, Bahria University Medical and Dental College (BUMDC), Karachi, Pakistan

3 Karachi Institute of Biotechnology and Genetic Engineering (KIBGE), Karachi, Pakistan

References

[1] Consensus Development Conference Diagnosis, prophylaxis and treatment of osteoporosis. American Journal of Medical Sciences 1993; 94:646–65.

[2] Davey DA. Osteoporosis, osteopenia and fracture risk: Widening the therapeutic horizons. South African Medical Journal 2012; 102: 285-288.

[3] Dennison E, Cole Z, Cooper C, et al. Diagnosis and epidemiology of osteoporosis. CurrentOpinion ofRheumatology 2005; 17:456-461.

[4] Burge RT. The cost of osteoporotic fractures in the UK: Projections for 2000-2020. Journal of Medical Economics 2001;4: 51.

[5] Kanis JA, Johnell O. Requirements for DXA for the management of osteoporosis in Europe. Osteoporosis International 2005; 16:229–238.

[6] Lim S, Koo BK, Lee EJ, Park JH, Kim MH, Shin KH, et al. Incidence of hip fractures in Korea. Journal of Bone & Mineral Metabolism 2008; 26: 400-405.

[7] Reseland J, Syversen U, Bakke I. et al. Leptin is expressed in and secreted from primary cultures of human osteoblasts and promotes bone mineralization. Journal of Bone & Mineral Research 2001;16:1426–1433.

[8] Thomas T, Gori F, Khosla S, Jensen MD, Burguera B, Riggs BL. Leptin acts on human marrow stromal cells to enhance diff erentiation to osteoblasts and to inhibit differentiation to adipocytes. Endocrinology 1999; 140:1630–1638.

[9] Steppan CM, Crawford DT, Chidsey-Fink KL, et al.Leptin is a potent stimulator of bone growth in ob/ob mice. Regulatory Peptides 2000; 92, 73–78.

[10] Burguera B, Hofbauer LC, Thomas, T. et al. Leptin reduces ovariectomy-induced bone loss in rats. Endocrinology 2001; 142, 3546–3553.

[11] Zhang Y, Proenca R, Maffei M, et al. Positional cloning of the mouse obese gene and its human homologue. Nature 1994; 372: 425-432.

[12] Coen G. Leptin and bone metabolism. Journal of Nephrology 2004;17: 187-189.

[13] Tartaglia LA, Dembski M, Weng X,et al. Identification and expression cloning of a leptin receptor, OB-R. Cell 1995; 83: 1263-1271.

[14] Zhang F, Chen Y., Heiman M, et al. Leptin: structure, function and biology. Vitamins & Hormones 2005; 71: 345-365.

[15] Krysiak R, Handzlik-Orlik G, Okopien B. The role of adipokines in connective tissue diseases. European Journal of Nutrition 2012;51:513–528.

[16] Wardlaw SL. Obesity as a neuroendocrine disease: lessons to be learned from proopiomelanocortin and melanocortin receptor mutations in mice and men.Journal ofClinicalEndocrinology andMetabolism 2001; 86: 1442.

[17] Patel MS, Elefteriou F. The new field of neuroskeletal biology. CalcifedTissue International 2007; 80: 337-347.

[18] Sato S, Hanada R, Kimura A, et al. Central control of bone remodelling by neuromedin U. NaturalMedicine 2007; 13: 1234-1240.

[19] Sirotkin AV, Mlynček M, Makarevich AV, et al. Leptin affects proliferation-, apoptosis- and protein kinase A-related peptides in human ovarian granulosa cells. PhysiologicalResearch 2008; 57:437-442.

[20] Reid I. Relationships among body mass, its components, and bone. Bone 2002; 13: 547-555.

[21] Mazess RB, Barden, HS, Ettinger M, Johnston C, Dawson-Hughes B, Baran D, Powell, M. &Notelovitz, M. Spine and femur density using dual-photon absorptiometry in US white women. Journal of Bone and Mineral Research 1987; 2: 211-219.

[22] Tremollieres F, Pouilles JM,Ribot C.Vertebral postmenopausal bone loss is reduced in overweight women: a longitudinal study in 155 early postmenopausal women. Journal of ClinicalEndocrinology & Metabolism 1993; 77: 683-686.

[23] Elias CF, Purohit D. Leptin signaling and circuits in puberty and fertility. Cellular and Molecular Life Sciences 2012.DOI 10.1007/s00018-012-1095-1(Accessed 12 August 2012).

[24] Mundy GR. Secondary osteoporosis: the potential relevance of leptin and low body weight. Annals of Internal Medicine 2000; 21: 828-830.

[25] Ducy P, Amling M, Takeda S. Leptin inhibits bone formation through a hypothalamic relay. Cell 2000; 100:197–207.

[26] Amling M, Takeda S, Karsenty GA. Neuro(endo)crine regulation of bone remodeling. Bioessays 2000; 22: 970–975.

[27] Ducy P, Schinke T, Karsenty G. The osteoblast: a sophisticated fibroblast under central surveillance. Science 2000; 289:1501–1504.

[28] Karsenty G. Leptin controls bone formation through a hypothalamic relay. Recent ProgHorm Res 56:401–415, 2001.

[29] Takeda S &Karsenty G. Central control of bone formation. Journal ofBone& MineralMetabolism 2001;19:195–198.

[30] Holloway WR, Collier FM, Aitken CJ, Myers DE, Hodge JM, Malakellis M, et al.. Leptin inhibits osteoclast generation. Journal of Bone and Mineral Research 2002; 17:200–209.

[31] Thomas T, Burguera B, Melton LJ. Role of serum leptin, insulin, and estrogen levels as potential mediators of the relationship between fat mass and bone mineral density in men versus women.Bone 2001; 29:114–120.

[32] Kim GS, Hong JS, Kim SW, et al. Leptin induces apoptosis via ERK/cPLA2/cytochrome c pathway in human bone marrow stromal cells. Journal of Biological Chemistry 2003; 13: 21920-21929.

[33] Evans BAJ, Elford C, Gregory JW. Leptin control of bone metabolism; direct or indirect action? Bone 2001; 28:149.

[34] Cornish J, Callon KE, Bava U. The direct actions of leptin on bone cells increase bone strength in vivo: an explanation of low frequency fracture rates in obesity. Bone 2001;28:S88.

[35] Karsenty G. Convergence between bone and energy homeostasis: leptin regulation of bone mass. Cell Metabolism 2006; 4: 341-348.

[36] Takeda S, Elefteriou F, Levasseur R, et al. Leptin regulates bone formation via the sympathetic nervous system. Cell 2002; 111: 305-317.

[37] Harlan SM. Rahmouni K. Neuroanatomical determinants of the sympathetic nerve responsesevoked by leptin. Clinical Autonomic Research Doc 10.1007/s10286-012-0168-4 (Accessed June 2012).

[38] Sergio RagiEIS, LewiecklME. Peripheral bone densitometry: clinical applications. ArquivosBrasileiros de Endocrinologia&Metabologia2006; 50 :596-602.

[39] Marshall D, Johnell O, Wedel H. Meta-analysis of how well measured of bone mineral density predict occurrence of osteoporotic fractures. British Medical Journal 1996; 312: 1254-1259.

[40] Lateef M, Baig M, Azhar A. Estimation of osteocalcin and telopeptide-C in postmenopausal osteoporotic females. Osteoporosis International 2010;21:751-755.

[41] Hans D, Fuerst T, Lang T, Majumdar S, Lu Y, Genant HK & Gluer C.How we can measure bone quality? Bailliers Clinical Rheumatology 1997; 11: 495-515.

[42] Gluer CC. Quantitative ultrasound techniques for the assessment of osteoporosis: expert agreement and current status. Journal of Bone & Mineral Research 1997; 12: 1280-1288.

[43] Lateef M, Baig, M, Azhar A. Relationship of leptin with BMD in postmeopausal osteoporosis. In Kanis JA &Lindlay A. (eds) Osteoporosis International: Abstracts of 1st IOF-ESCEO Preclinical Symposium and ECCEO-IOF Congress, 22-23 March 2011, Valencia, Spain.

[44] Ensurd, KE, Palermo, L, Black DM.Cauley, J, Jergas, M, Orwoll, ES, Nevitt, MC, Fox KM. & Cummings SR. Hip and calcaneous bone loss increase with advancing age:

longitudinal results from the study of osteoporotic fractures. Journal of Bone and Mineral Research 1995; 10: 1778-1787.

[45] Miller PD,Zapalowski, C, Kulak CA. &Bilezikian JP.Bone Densitometry: the best way to detect osteoporosis and to monitor therapy. Journal of Clinical Endocrinologyand Metabolism 1999;84: 1867-1871.

[46] GouldingA,Taylor RW. Plasma Leptin values in relation to bone mass and density and to dynamic biochemical markers of bone resorption and formation in postmenopausal women. Calcified Tissue International 1998; 63: 456 -458.

[47] Rouch F, Blum WF, Klein K. Allolio, B. &Schonau, E. Does leptin have an effect on bone in adult women? Calcified Tissue International 1998; 63: 453-455.

[48] Iwamoto I, Douchi T, Kosha S, Murakami, M. Fujino T. & Nagata Y. Relationship between serum leptin level and regional bone mineral density, bone metabolic markers in healthy women. ActaObstetriciaetGynecologicaScandinavica 2000; 79: 1060-1064.

[49] Yamauchi M, Sugimoto T, Yamaguchi T. Plasma leptin concentrations are associated with bone mineral density and the presence of vertebral fractures in postmenopausal women. ClinicalEndocrinology 2001; 55:341–347.

[50] Albala C, Yanez M, Deveto E, Sostin C, Zeballos, L. & Santos JL. (1996). Obesity as protective factor for postmenopausal factor postmenopausal osteoporosis. International Journal of Obesity and Related Metabolic Disorders 1996; 20:1027-1032.

[51] Riggs BL, Melton J. Involutional osteoporosis. New EnglandJournal ofMedicine 1986; 314: 676-685.

[52] Ribot C, Tremollierrs F, Pouilles JM, Bonneu M, Germain F,Louvet JP. Obesity and postmenopausal bone loss: the influence of obesity on vertebral density and bone turnover in postmenopausal women. Bone 1987; 8: 327-331.

[53] Dequeker J,Boonen S. Extraskeletal Risk and Protective Factors for fractures In Geuseus P.(ed)Osteoporosis in clinical practice In *Springer*: London; 1998. p55-58.

[54] Di Carlo C, Tommaselli GA, Gargano V, Sammartino A, Bifulco G, Tauchmanova L et al. Effects of estrogen-progestin therapy on serum levels of RANKL, osteoprotegerin, osteocalcin, leptin, and ghrelin in postmenopausal women. Menopause 2007; 14:7–9.

[55] Pasco JA, Henry MJ, Kotowicz J A, et al. Serum leptin levels are associated with bone mass in no obese women. Journal of Clinical Endocrinology andMetabolism; 86: 1884-1887.

[56] Blain H, Vuillemin A, Guillemin F,et al. Serum leptin level is a predictor of bone mineral density in postmenopausal women. Journal of Clinical Endocrinology and Metabolism 2002; 87, 1030–1035

[57] Nagy Z, Speer G, Takács I, Bajnok Č, Lakatos P. Serum leptin levels and bone mineral density in postmenopausal women In Journal ofBone andMineral Research: Pro-

gram and abstracts from the Twenty-Third Annual Meeting of the American Society for Bone and Mineral Research; October 12–16, 2001; Phoenix, Arizona.

[58] Hadji P, Bock K, Gottschalk M, Kalder M, Emons G, Shulz KD. The influence of serum leptin concentrations on bone mass assessed by quantitative ultrasonometry (QUS) in pre- and postmenopausal women In Journal ofBone andMineral Research: Program and abstracts from the Twenty-Third Annual Meeting of the American Society for Bone and Mineral Research, October 12–16, 2001; Phoenix, Arizona.

[59] Rauch F, Blum WF, Klein K, Allolio B, Schönau E. Does Leptin Have an Effect on Bone in Adult Women? Calcified Tissue International 1998;63:453–455.

[60] Hamrick MW, Ferrari SI. Leptin and the sympathetic connection of fat to bone. Osteoporosis International 2008; 19:905-912.

[61] Munzberg H, Bjornholm M, Bates SH, et al. Leptin receptor action and metabolisms of leptin resistance. Cellullar& MolecularLife Sciences 2005; 62: 642-652.

[62] Anderlová K, Křemen J, Doležalová R, et al., The influence of very-low-calorie-diet on serum leptin, soluble leptin receptor, adiponectin and resistin levels in obese women. Physiological Research 2006; 55: 277-283.

[63] Welt CK, Chan JI, Bullen J, et al. Recombinant human leptin in women with hypothalamic amenorrhea. New England Journal of Medicine 2004; 351: 987-997.

[64] VasikaranS, Eastell R, Bruyère O, et al. Markers of bone turnover for the prediction of fracture risk and monitoring of osteoporosis treatment: a need for international reference standards. Osteoporosis International 2011; 22: 391–420.

[65] Eastell R, Hannon RA. Biomarkers of bone health and osteoporosis risk. Proceedings of the Nutrition Society 2008; 67:157-162.

[66] Delmas PD. Markers of bone turnover for monitoring treatment of osteoporosis with antiresorptive drugs. Osteoporosis International 2000;11::S66- 76.

[67] Green S, Antiss CL, Fishman WH. Automated differential isoenzyme analysis II. The fractionation of serum alkaline phosphatase into liver, intestinal and other components. Enzymologia 1997; 41: 9 -26.

[68] Seibel MJ. Biochemical markers of bone metabolism in the assessment of osteoporosis: useful or not? EndocrinologicalInvestigation 2003; 26: 464-471.

[69] Gundberg CM,Nishimoto SK. InSeibel MJ, Robbins SP, Bilezzikian, JP, (eds) Vitamin K dependent proteins of bone and cartilage. Dynamics of bone and cartilage metabolism In Academic Press, San Diego; 1999;p43-58.

[70] Vesper HW. Analytical and preanalytical issues in measurement of biochemical bone markers. Laboratory Medicine 2005; 36: 424-429.

[71] Gundberg CM, Markowitz ME, Mizruchi M, Rosen JF. Osteocalcin in human serum: a circadian rhythm. *Journal ofClinical andEndocrinologicalMetabolism*1985;60:736-739.

[72] Parafitt AM, Simon LS, Villanueva AR, &Krane SM. Procollagen type I carboytermi-nal extension propeptide in serum as a marker of collagen biosynthesis in bone.Jour-nal ofBone & Mineral Research 1987; 5: 427 -436.

[73] Risteli J, Risteli L. Products of bone collagen metabolism. In: Seibel MJ, Robbins SP, Bilzekian JP, eds. *Dynamics of Bone and Cartilage Metabolism: Principles and Clinical Ap-plications*. London: Academic Press; 1999:275-287.

[74] Singer FR, Eyre DR. Using biochemical markers of bone turnover in clinical practice. Cleveland Clinic Journal of Medicine 2008; 75: 739-750.

[75] Calvo MS, Eyre DR, Gundberg CM. Molecular basis and clinical applicationof biolog-ical markers of bone turnover. Endocrinol Review 1996;17:333–368.13.

[76] Garnero P, Gineyts E, Riou JP, Delmas PD. Assessment of boneresorption with a new marker of collagen degradation in patients with metabolic bone disease. Journal of Clinical andEndocrinologyMetabolism 1994;79:780–785.

[77] Christgau S, Rosenquist C, Alexandersen P, et al. Clinical evaluationof the Serum CrossLaps One Step ELISA, a new assay measuring theserum concentration of bone-derived degradation products oftype I collagen C-telopeptides. ClinicalChemistry 1998; 44:2290–2300.

[78] Hanson DA, Weis MA, Bollen AM, Maslan SL, Singer FR, Eyre DR. A specific immu-noassay for monitoring human bone resorption:quantitation of type I collagen cross-linked N-telopeptides in urine.Journal ofBone MineralResearch 1992; 7:1251–1258.

[79] Clemens JD, Herrick MV, Singer FR, Eyre DR. Evidence that serumNTx (collagen-type I N-telopeptides) can act as an immunochemicalmarker of bone resorption. ClinicalChemistry 1997; 43:2058–2063.

[80] Price CP. Tartarate Resistant Acid Phosphatase as a marker of bone resorption. Clini-cal Chemistry1995; 41: 641-643.

[81] Brown JP, Albert C, Nassar BA, Adachi JD, Cole D, Davison KS, Dooley KC, Don-Wauchope A, Douville P et al., Bone turnover markers in the management of post-menopausal osteoporosis. Clinical Biochemistry 2009; 42:929–942.

[82] Bergmann P, Body JJ, Boonen S, Boutsen Y, Devogelaer JP, Goemaere S, et al. Evi-dence-based guidelines for the use of biochemical markers of bone turnover in the selection and monitoring of bisphosphonate treatment in osteoporosis: a consensus document of the Belgian Bone Club. International Journal of Clinical Practise 2009; 63:19-26.

[83] VasikaranS, Eastell R, Bruyère O et al. Markers of bone turnover for the prediction of fracture risk and monitoring of osteoporosis treatment: a need for international reference standards. Osteoporosis International 2011; 22:391–420.

[84] Riggs BL, Melton LJ, O'Fallon WM. Drug therapy for vertebral fractures in osteoporosis: evidence that decreases in bone turnover and increases in bone mass both determine antifracture efficacy. Bone 1996; 18:197S-201S.

[85] Delmas PD,Seeman E. Changes in bone mineral density explain little of the reduction in vertebral or nonvertebral fracture risk with anti-resorptive therapy. Bone 2004; 34:599-604.

[86] Delmas PD. Markers of bone turnover for monitoring treatment of osteoporosis with antiresorptive drugs. Osteoporosis International 2000; 11:S66- 76.

[87] Clinical guideline for the prevention and treatment of osteoporosis in postmenopausal women and older men (RACGP) 2012 http://www.racgp.org.au/guidelines/musculoskeletaldiseases/osteoporosis (accessed on Feb 2010)

[88] Chung SH, Kim TH, Lee HH. Relationship between Vitamin D level and bone mineral density in postmenopausal women from Bucheon area. Jounal ofKorean Society of Osteoporosis 2009; 7:198-202.

[89] Meunier PJ, Roux C, Seeman E, Ortolani S, Badurski JE, Spector TD, et al. The effects of strontium ranelate on the risk of vertebral fracture in women with postmenopausal osteoporosis. New England Journal ofMedicine 2004; 50:459-468.

[90] Lee J, Vasikaran S. Current Recommendations for Laboratory Testing and Use of Bone Turnover Markers in Management of Osteoporosis. Annals ofLaboratory Medicine 2012; 32:105-112.

[91] Tromp AM, Ooms ME, Popp-Snijders C, Roos JC, Lips P. Predictors of fractures in elderly women. OsteoporosisInternational 2000; 11:134-140.

[92] Chapurlat RD, Garnero P, Bréart G, Meunier PJ, Delmas PD. Serum type I collagen breakdown product (serum CTX) predicts hip fracture risk in elderly women: the EPIDOS study. Bone 2000; 27:283-286.

[93] Garnero P, Sornay-Rendu E, Claustrat B, Delmas PD. Biochemical markers of bone turnover,endogenous hormones and the risk of fractures in postmenopausal women: the OFELY Study. Journal of Bone& Mineral Research 2000; 15: 1526-1536.

[94] Garnero P, Cloos P, Sornay-Rendu E, Qvist P, Delmas PD. Type I collagen racemization and isomerization and the risk of fracture in postmenopausal women: the OFELY prospective study. Journal of Bone& Mineral Research 2002; 17:826-33.

[95] Meier C, Nguyen TV, Center JR, Seibel MJ, Eisman JA. Bone resorption and osteoporotic fractures in elderly men: the dubbo osteoporosis epidemiology study.Journal of Bone& Mineral Research 2005; 20:579-587.

[96] Garnero P, Shih WJ, Gineyts E, Karpf DB, Delmas PD. Comparison of new biochemical markers of bone turnover in late postmenopausal osteoporotic women in response to alendronate treatment. Journal of ClinicalEndocrinology & Metabolism 1994; 79:1693-1700.

[97] Bell NH, Bilezikian JP, Bone HG, Kaur A, Maragoto A, Santora AC. Alendronate increases bone mass and reduce bone markers in postmenopausal African-American women.Journal of ClinicalEndocrinology & Metabolism 2002; 87:2792- 2797.

[98] Greenspan SL, Parker RA, Ferguson L, Rosen HN, Maitland-Ramsey L, Karpf DB. Early changes in biochemical markers of bone turnover predict the long-term response to alendronate therapy in representative elderly women: a randomized clinical trial. Journal of ClinicalEndocrinology & Metabolism 1998; 13: 1431-1438.

[99] Garnero P, Gineyts E, Arbault P, Christiansen C, Delmas PD. Different effects of bisphosphonate and estrogen therapy on free and peptide-bound bone cross-links excretion. Journal of ClinicalEndocrinology & Metabolism1995; 10:641-649.

[100] Rosen HN, Moses AC, Garber J, Ross DS, Lee SL, Greenspan SL. Utility of biochemical markers of bone turnover in the follow-up of patients treated with bisphosphonates. CalcifedTissue International 1998; 63:363-368.

[101] Glover SJ, Garnero P, Naylor K, et al. Establishing a reference range for bone turnover markers in young, healthy women. Bone 2008; 42:623 -630.

[102] Sandhu KS, Hampson G. The pathogenesis, diagnosis, investigation and management of osteoporosis. Journal of ClinicalPathology 2011; 64:1042-1050.

[103] Kim SW, Park DJ, Park KS et al. Early changes in biochemical markers of bone turnover predict bone mineral dnsity response to antiresorptive therapy in Korean postmenopausal women with osteoporosis. Endocrine Journal 2005;52:667-674.

[104] Brown JP, Albert C, Nassar BA, Adachi JD, Cole D, Davison KS, et al. Bone turnover markers in the management of postmenopausal osteoporosis. Clinical Biochemistry 2009; 42:929-442.

[105] Scariano JK, Garry PJ, Montova GD et al. Serum leptin levels, bone mineral density and osteoblast alkaline phosphatase activity in elderly men and women. Mechanism of Ageing and Development 2003; 24:281-286.

[106] Filip R &Raszewski G. Bone mineral density and bone turnover in relation to serum leptin, -α ketoglutarate and sex steroids in overweight and obese postmenopausal women. Clinical Endocrinology 2009; 70, 214–220.

[107] Iwamoto I, Douchi T, Kosha S, et al. Relationships between serum leptin level and regional bone mineral density, bone metabolic markers in healthy women. ActaObstetriciaetGynecologicaScandinavica2000; 79: 1060-1064.

[108] Peng XD, Xie H, Zhao Q, et al.Relationships between serum adiponectin, leptin, resistin, visfatin levels and bone mineral density, and bone biochemical markers in Chinese men. ClinicaChimicaActa 2008; 387: 31-35.

[109] Shaarawy M, Abassi AE, Hassan H, et al.Relationship between serumleptinconcentrations and bonemineraldensity as well as biochemicalmarkers of boneturnover in women with postmenopausalosteoporosis. Fertility & Sterility 2003; 79: 919-924.

[110] Zhang H, Xie H, Zhao Q et al. Relationships between serum adiponectin, apelin, leptin, resistin, visfatin levels and bone mineral density, and bone biochemical markers in post-menopausal Chinese women. Journal of Endocrinological Investigation 2010; 33:707-711.

[111] Wu N, Wang QP, Li H, et al. Relationships between serum adiponectin, leptin concentrations and bone mineral density, and bone biochemical markers in Chinese women. ClinicaChemicaActa 2010; 411:771-775.

[112] Yang LC, Lan Y, Hu J et al. Correlation of serumleptinlevel with bonemineraldensity and boneturnovermarkers in Chineseadolescentdancers. Biomedicaland EnviromentalScience; 2009; 22:369-373.

[113] Prouteau S, L Benhamou L, Courteix D. Relationships between serum leptin and bone markers during stable weight, weight reduction and weight regain in male and female judoists. European Journal of Endocrinology 2006; 154: 389–395.

Chapter 4

Modification of Sex Hormones with RGD-Peptide: A Strategy of Improving HRT and Other Secondary Osteoporosis Therapy

Ming Zhao, Yuji Wang, Jianhui Wu and Shiqi Peng

Additional information is available at the end of the chapter

http://dx.doi.org/10.5772/54361

1. Introduction

In the time of transition from premenopausal state to postmenopausal state the capacity of ovary producing sex hormones including estrogens, progesterone and testosterone cuts down [1]. Due to the menopause the level of serum oestrogen dramatically decreases, which increases the production of bone-resorbing cytokines and osteoblasts and then increases the number and activity of osteoclast, thereby increasing the bone loss [2]. Hormonal replacement therapy (HRT) is able to prevent bone loss for sex hormones-deficient menopausal women and consequently is of clinical importance for the treatment of osteoporosis. [1-3] In Europe and USA the osteoporosis prevention of 25-50% of the post-menopausal women rely on HRT [2,5, 6]. In past years, however, the large international studies, such as the randomized Woman Health Initiative, the observational Million Women Study and the Women's International Study of long Duration, discussed both of the adverse and beneficial effects of post-menpausal HRT [7]. In respect of the adverse effects, the discussion was focused on HRT induced risk of breast cancer [8-11], venous thromboembolism [12], stroke and myocardial infarction [13], as well as coronary heart diseases [14]. To limit these adverse effects a series of regimens of HRT, such as continuous combination of oestrogen and progestogen or continuous oestrogen and interruptted progestogen [15], and with dehydroepiandrosterone as a new strategic tool [16], were developed. In general these regimens confer no positive result, and thus new strategies are still needed.

Osteoporosis relates to both the decrease of the formation of osteoblast-modulated bone and the increase of the resorption osteoclast-modulated bone. Estrogen directly up-modulates the activity and the proliferation of osteoblasts, and/or regulats the gene expression in osteoblasts and osteoclasts [17-20]. Bone resorption is regulated by the adhesion of osteoclasts to the surface of the bone, which is mediated by the receptor $\alpha_v\beta_3$ integrin and its recognition to RGD (Arg-Gly-Asp) containing protein of osteoclasts [21]. These suggest that the activity and proliferation of osteoblasts and the adhesiveness of osteoclasts can be simultaneously up-regulated with estrogen and down-regulated with RGD peptide, respectively. On the other hand, it was explored that the covalent modifications of hydrocortisone and estrone with kyotorphin (a dipeptide, Tyr-Arg) may increase the analgesic activities of hydrocortisone and estrone [22], as well as the covalent modifications of hydrocortisone and prednisolone with urotoxins (Gly-Asp-Gly, His-Gly-Gly, His-Gly-Lys and His-Gly-Lys-$NHNH_2$) may increase the immunosuppressive activities of hydrocortisone and prednisolone [23]. Similarly, the anti-osteoporosis activities of estrone and estradiol were enhanced by growth hormone releasing peptides (GHRPs: Tyr-Gly-Gly-Phe-Met-NH_2, Tyr-Gly-Gly-Phe-Met, Tyr-Gly-Gly-Phe-Leu-NH_2, Tyr-Gly-Gly-Phe-Leu, Tyr-Gly-Gly-Phe-Gly-NH_2 and Tyr-Gly-Gly-Phe-Gly) [24-26]. In this context a strategy to enhance anti-osteoporosis potency and reduce adverse effects of HRT was practiced by covalent modifications of sex hormone with RGD-peptides.

2. Covalent modifications of estrogen with RGD-peptides and ip treated ovariectomy mice

Estrogens including estrone, estradiol, estriol, conjugated estrogen and tibolone have been widely used in HRT. Upon the promotion of the enzyme both estrone and estradiol can be converted to ertriol. Conjugated estrogen is an oral estrogen isolated from the urine of gravid horse and contains estrone monosodium sulfate (50.0% - 63.0%), equilin monosodium sulfate (22.5% - 32.5%), a few of 17α-estradiol monosodium sulfate and equilenin monosodium sulfate. Tibolone is an analog of norethynodrel. Of these estrogens, estrone and estradiol are the common parents and estradiol is the major agents of HRT. Thus estradiol and estrone were covalently modified by RGD-peptides (**1-9**, Figure 1) and evaluated with ip treated ovariectomy mice [27].

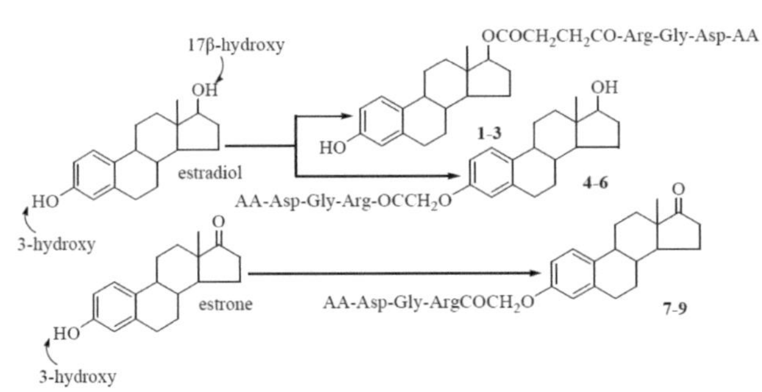

Figure 1. Structures of conjugates of estradiol-RGD-tetrapeptides. In **1**, **4,7** AA = Ser, in **2**, **5, 8** AA = Val, in **3**, **6, 9** AA = Phe.

2.1. Covalent modification of estradiol with RGD-tetrapeptides decreasing bone turnover

Using succinyl group as the linker the covalent modifications of the 17β-hydroxy of estradiol with RGD-tetrapeptides provided conjugates **1-3**, and using carbonylmethyl group as the linker the covalent modifications of the 3-hydroxy of estradiol or estrone with RGD-tetrapeptides provided conjugates **4-9** (Figure 1). The changes of the levels of the serum calcium and serum alkaline phosphatase (ALP) of the mice receiving ip injection of **1-6** for 4 weeks are shown in Figure 2. After the treatments of conjugates **1-6** the levels of serum calcium and serum ALP of the treated mice are significantly lower than that of ovariotomy and estradiol treated mice. This means that the ip injection efficacy of conjugates **1-6** in decreasing the serum calcium and serum ALP is significantly higher than that of estradiol. Due to serum ALP been the biomarker of bone turnover low serum ALP means conjugates **1-6** benefits the inhibition of bone turnover.

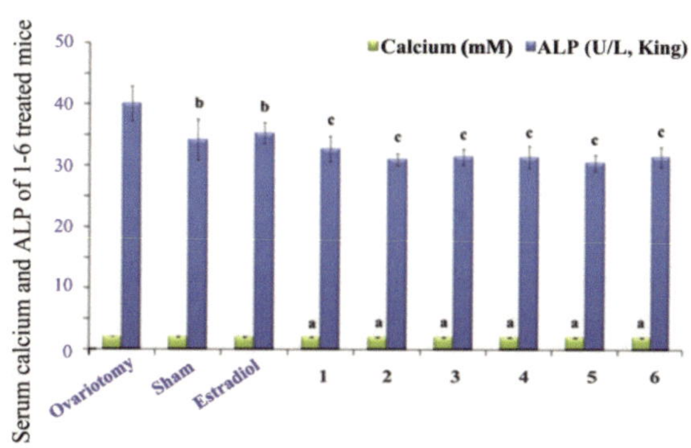

Figure 2. Serum calcium and serum ALP of **1-6** treated mice. Dose = 110.3 μmol/kg, n=12, a) Compared to ovariotomy P<0.05; b) Compared to ovariotomy P<0.01; c) Compared to ovariotomy and estradiol P<0.01. The statistical analysis of the data was carried out by use of an ANOVA test and p<0.05 was considered significant.

2.2. Covalent modification of estradiol with RGD-tetrapeptides inhibiting bone loss

The effects of ip injection of **1-6** for 4 weeks on the bone loss of the mice are shown in Figure 3. The level of bone loss is represented with the weight of dry femur and the weight of femur ash. The data indicate that the weight of dry femur and the weight of femur ash of **1-6** treated mice are significantly higher than those of ovariotomy and estradiol treated mice. This means that ip injection efficacy of **1-6** in inhibiting the bone loss is significantly higher than that of estradiol, and the covalent modification of estradiol with RGD-tetrapeptides benefits the inhibition of bone loss.

2.3. Covalent modification of estrone with RGD-tetrapeptides inhibiting bone turnover

Using carbonylmethyl group as the linker the covalent modifications of the 3-hydroxy of estrone with RGD-tetrapeptides provided conjugates **7-9** (Figure 4). The effects of ip injection

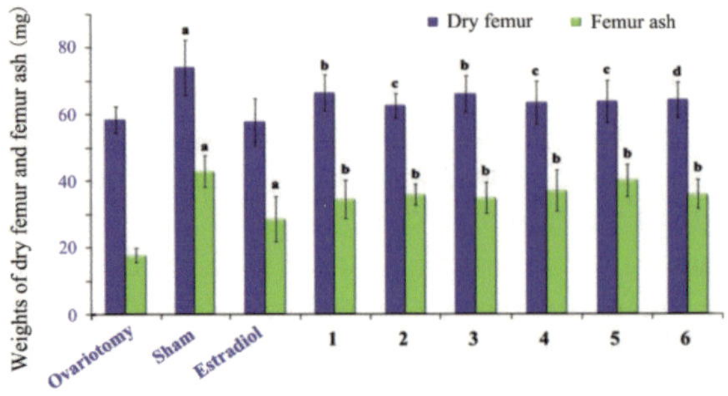

Figure 3. Weight of dry femur and femur ash of **1-6** treated mice. Dose =110.3 μmol/kg, n=12; a) Compared to ovariotomy P<0.01; b) Compared to ovariotomy and estradiol P<0.01; c) Compared to ovariotomy and estradiol P<0.05; d) Compared to ovariotomy P<0.01, to estradiol P<0.05. The statistical analysis of the data was carried out by use of an ANOVA test and p<0.05 was considered significant.

of **7-9** for 4 weeks on serum calcium and serum ALP of the mice are shown in Figure 4. The serum calcium and serum ALP of **7-9** treated mice are significantly lower than that of ovariotomy and estrone treated mice. This means that the ip injection efficacy of conjugates **7-9** in decreasing the serum calcium and serum ALP is significantly higher than that of estrone. Due to serum ALP reflecting the level of bone turnover and low serum ALP corresponding with low bone turnover, **7-9** benefits the inhibition of bone turnover.

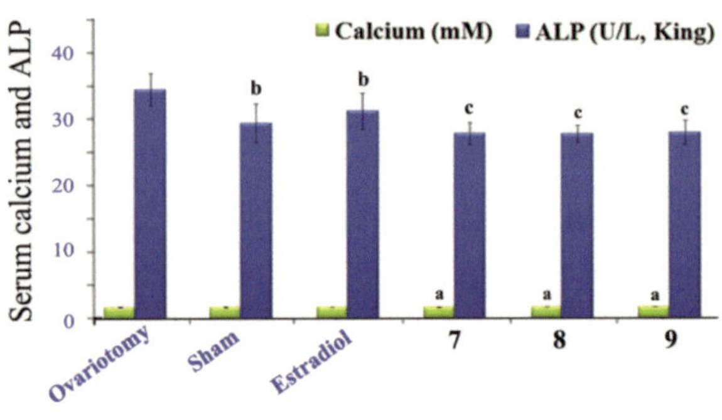

Figure 4. Serum calcium and ALP of **7-9** treated mice. Dose = 110.3 μmol/kg, n=12, a) Compared to ovariotomy P<0.05; b) Compared to ovariotomy P<0.01; c) Compared to ovariotomy and estrone P<0.01. The statistical analysis of the data was carried out by use of an ANOVA test and p<0.05 was considered significant.

2.4. Covalent modification of estrone with RGD-tetrapeptides preventing bone loss

The effect of ip injection of **7-9** for 4 weeks on the bone loss of the mice is shown in Figure 5. The weight of dry femur and the weight of femur ash of **7-9** treated mice are significantly higher than that of ovariotomy and estrone treated mice. Due to the weight of dry femur and the weight of femur ash reflecting the level of bone loss of osteoporosis mice this comparison means that ip injection efficacy of **7-9** in inhibiting bone loss is significantly higher than that of estrone and the covalent modification enhances the inhibition of estrone in bone loss.

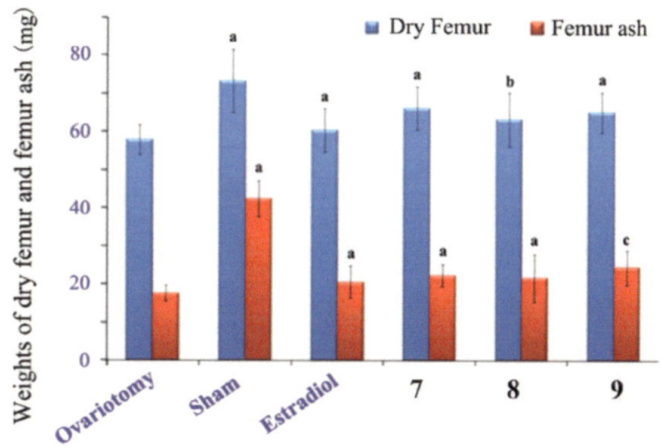

Figure 5. Weight of dry femur and femur ash of conjugates **7-9** treated mice. Dose =110.3 μmol/kg, n=12; a) Compared to ovariotomy P<0.01; b) Compared to ovariotomy P<0.05; c) Compared to ovariotomy P<0.01, to estrone P<0.05. The statistical analysis of the data was carried out by use of an ANOVA test and p<0.05 was considered significant.

2.5. Covalent modification of estrogen with RGD-tetrapeptides inducing no endometrial cell hyperplasia

The effects of ip injection of **1-9** for 4 weeks on endometrial cell hyperplasia of the mice were also observed. The weight of the uteri of ovariotomy, estradiol and estrone treated mice is significantly higher than that of **1-9** treated mice. Due to the weight of the uteri reflecting the level of endometrial cell hyperplasia of treated mice this comparison means that ip injection efficacy of **1-9** in inducing endometrial cell hyperplasia is significantly lower than that of estradiol and estrone and the covalent modification induces no observable endometrial cell hyperplasia.

2.6. Summary of covalent modification of estrogen with RGD-tetrapeptides

With RGD-tetrapeptides modifying one hydroxyl group of estradiol and estrone resulted in 9 conjugates. On ovariotomy mouse model and at 110.3 μmol/kg of ip dose their anti-osteoporosis activities were significantly higher than that of estradiol and estrone themselves. In contrast to estradiol and estrone themselves, the anti-osteoporosis therapy of these conjugates induced no endometrial cell hyperplasia. It is commonly accepted that osteoporosis relates to both the decrease in bone formation modulated by osteoblasts and the increase in bone resorption modulated by osteoclasts. In HRT, estradiol and estrone are used to treat the decrease in skeletal muscle and bone by the direct modulation of osteoblastic activity and proliferation or by the regulation of gene expression in osteoblasts and osteoclasts. Bone resorption is regulated by the binding of osteoclasts to the bone surface and, therefore, depends upon osteoclast adhesiveness. This bone adhesion process is mediated by RGD-tetrapeptides binding integrin receptor on cell surface. This action of RGD-tetrapeptides should be responsible for both the increased anti-osteoporosis activity and the decreased endometrial cell hyperplasia of the conjugates. Due to ovariotomy mouse model simulates the bone loss condition of postmenopausal women these RGD-tetrapeptides modified estradiol and estrone should be promising candidates for HRT use.

3. Covalent modification of estrogen with RGD-octapeptides and orally treated ovariectomy mice

It was explored that the modification of RGD-tetrapeptides with oligopeptides usually increased their bioactivities [28, 29], suggesting the modification of RGD-tetrapeptides with RGD-tetrapeptides may result in increase of the activity of down-regulating proliferation of osteoblasts and the adhesiveness of osteoclasts. In this context estradiol and estrone were modified with RGD-octapeptides (**10-21**, Figure 6) to evaluate the oral activity on ovariectomy mice [30, 31].

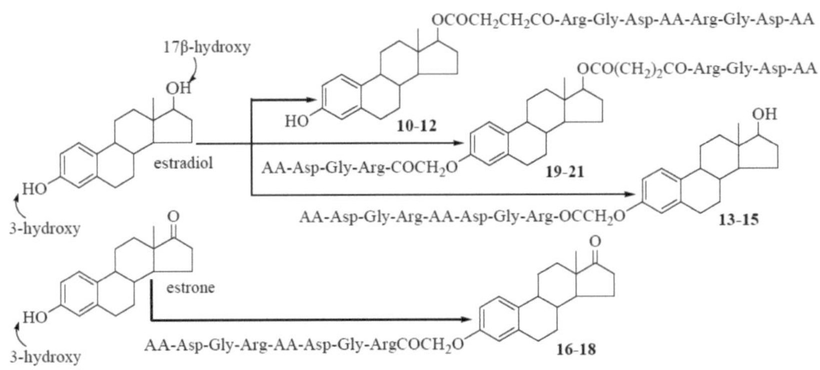

Figure 6. Structures of conjugates of RGD-octapeptides and estradiol. In **10, 13, 16, 19** AA = Ser, in **11, 14, 17, 20** AA = Val, in **12, 15, 18, 21** AA = Phe.

3.1. Covalent modification of estradiol with RGD-octapeptides inhibiting bone turnover

Using succinyl group as the linker the 17β-hydroxy of estradiol was modified with RGD-octapeptides and provided **10-12**, using carbonylmethyl group as the linker the 3-hydroxy of estradiol was modified with RGD-octapeptides and provided **13-15** (Figure 6). The effect of oral administration of **10-15** for 4 weeks on serum calcium and serum ALP of the mice are shown in Figure 7. The data indicate that the serum calcium and serum ALP of **10-15** treated mice are significantly lower than that of ovariotomy and estradiol treated mice. This means that the frequency of bone turnover of **10-15** orally treated mice is significantly lower than that of estradiol treated mice, the efficacy of oral **10-15** in inhibiting bone turnover is significantly higher than that of estradiol.

http://dx.doi.org/10.5772/54361

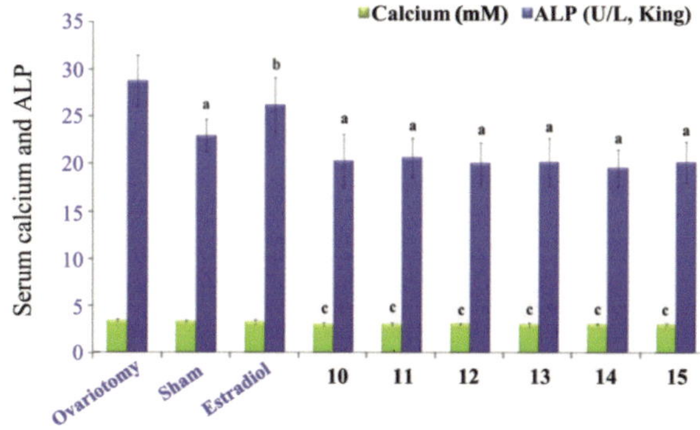

Figure 7. Serum calcium and ALP of **10-15** treated mice. Dose = 110.3 nmol/kg, n=12, a) Compared to ovariotomy and estradiol P<0.01; b) Compared to ovariotomy P<0.01; c) Compared to ovariotomy P<0.01, to estradiol P<0.05. The statistical analysis of the data was carried out by use of an ANOVA test and p<0.05 was considered significant.

3.2. Covalent modification of estradiol with RGD-octapeptides preventing bone loss

The effect of orally administration of **10-15** for 4 weeks on the bone loss of the treated mice is shown in Figure 8, of which the activity is represented with dry femur weight and femur ash weight. The data indicate that both the weights of dry femur and femur ash of **10-15** treated mice are significantly higher than that of ovariotomy and estradiol treated mice. This means that when orally dosed **10-15** effectively inhibit the mice to lose femur and their efficacy is significantly higher than that of estradiol, and the covalent modification of estradiol benefits the inhibition of bone loss.

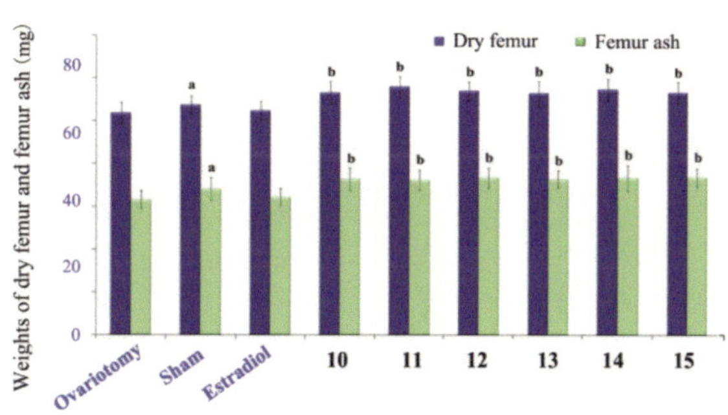

Figure 8. Weight of dry femur and femur ash of conjugates **10-15** treated mice. Dose =110.3 nmol/kg, n=12; a) Compared to ovariotomy P<0.05; b) Compared to ovariotomy and estradiol P<0.01. The statistical analysis of the data was carried out by use of an ANOVA test and p<0.05 was considered significant.

3.3. Covalent modification of estrone with RGD-octapeptides inhibiting bone turnover

Using carbonylmethyl group as the linker the 3-hydroxy of estrone was modified with RGD-octapeptides and provided **16-18** (Figure 6). The effects of oral administration of **16-18** for 4 weeks on serum calcium and serum ALP of the mice are shown in Figure 9. The data indicate that the serum calcium and serum ALP of **16-18** treated mice are significantly lower than that of ovariotomy and estrone treated mice. This means that the frequency of bone turnover of **16-18** orally treated mice is significantly lower than that of estrone treated mice, the efficacy of oral **16-18** in inhibiting bone turnover is significantly higher than that of estrone.

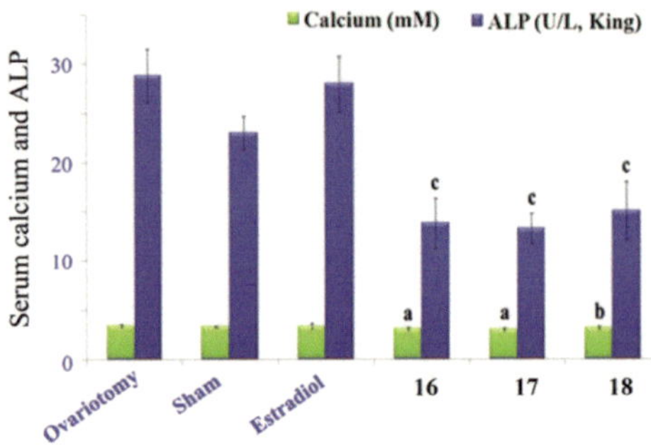

Figure 9. Serum calcium and serum ALP of **16-18** treated mice. Dose = 110.3 nmol/kg, n=12, a) Compared to ovariotomy P<0.01, to estrone P<0.05; b) Compared to ovariotomy P<0.05; c) Compared to ovariotomy and estrone P<0.01. The statistical analysis of the data was carried out by use of an ANOVA test and p<0.05 was considered significant.

3.4. Covalent modification of estrone with RGD-octapeptides preventing bone loss

The effect of orally administration of **16-18** for 4 weeks on the bone loss of the treated mice is shown in Figure 10, their activities are represented with dry femur weight and femur ash weight. The data indicate that both the weights of dry femur and femur ash of **16-18** treated mice are significantly higher than that of ovariotomy and estradiol treated mice. This means that upon oral administration **16-18** effectively inhibit the mice losing femur, their efficacies are significantly higher than that of estrone, and the covalent modification of estrone prevents the bone loss.

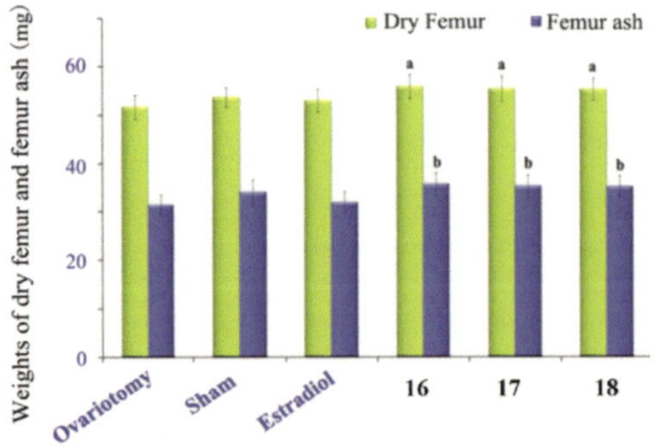

Figure 10. Weight of dry femur and femur ash of conjugates **16-18** treated mice. Dose =110.3 nmol/kg, n=12; a) Compared to ovariotomy and estrone P<0.01; b) Compared to ovariotomy P<0.01, to estrone P<0.05. The statistical analysis of the data was carried out by use of an ANOVA test and p<0.05 was considered significant.

http://dx.doi.org/10.5772/54361

3.5. Covalent modification of estradiol with two RGD-octapeptides inhibiting bone turnover

Using succinyl group as the linker of the 17β-hydroxy and using carbonylmethyl group as the linker of the 3-hydroxy estradiol was simultaneously modified with RGD-tetrapeptides and provided **19-21** (Figure 6). The effects of oral administration of **19-21** for 4 weeks on serum calcium and serum ALP of the mice are shown in Figure 11. The data indicate that the serum calcium and serum ALP of **19-21** treated mice are significantly lower than that of ovariotomy and estradiol treated mice. This means that the frequency of bone turnover of **19-21** orally treated mice is significantly lower than that of estradiol treated mice, the efficacy of oral **19-21** in inhibiting bone turnover is significantly higher than that of estradiol.

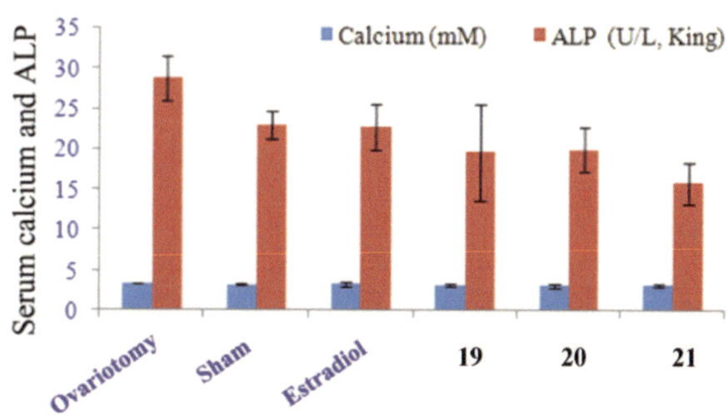

Figure 11. Serum calcium and serum ALP of **19-21** treated mice. Dose = 110.3 nmol/kg, n=12. The statistical analysis of the data was carried out by use of an ANOVA test and p<0.05 was considered significant. For serum calcium a) Compared to ovariotomy P<0.05; For serum ALP b) compared to ovariotomy and estradiol P<0.01.

3.6. Covalent modification of estradiol with two RGD-octapeptides preventing bone loss

The effect of orally administration of **19-21** for 4 weeks on the bone loss of the treated mice is shown in Figure 12, their activities are represented with dry femur weight and femur ash weight. The data indicate that both the weights of dry femur and femur ash of **19-21** treated mice are significantly higher than that of ovariotomy and estradiol treated mice. This means that upon oral administration **19-21** effectively inhibit the mice losing femur, their efficacies are significantly higher than that of estradiol, and the covalent modification of estrone prevents the bone loss.

3.7. Covalent modification of estradiol with RGD-octapeptides inducing no endometrial cell hyperplasia

The effect of orally administration of **10-21** for 4 weeks on the endometrial cell hyperplasia of the mice was observed, of which the inhibition is represented with uteri weight. The data indicate that the weight of the uteri of **10-21** treated mice is significantly lower than that of ovariotomy and estradiol treated mice. This means that, in contrast to estradiol and estrone, oral administration of **10-21** induces no observable endometrial cell hyperplasia, and the covalent modification of estradiol and estrone with RGD-octapeptides limits the dose-related adverse effects of estradiol.

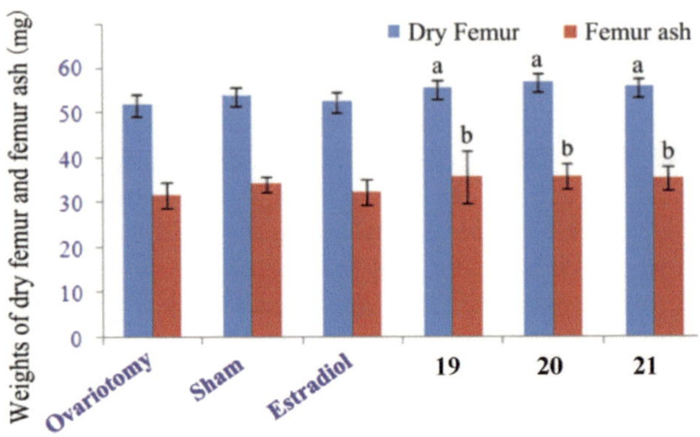

Figure 12. Weight of dry femur and femur ash of conjugates **19-21** treated mice. Dose =110.3 nmol/kg, n=12, weights of dry femurs and femur ashes are represented as X±SD mg; a) Compared to ovariotomy, estradiol $P<0.01$; b) Compared to ovariotomy $P<0.01$, to estradiol $P<0.05$.

3.8. Covalent modification of estradiol with RGD-octapeptides having no thrombosis risk

The effect of orally administration of **10-21** for 4 weeks on thrombosis risk of the mice was observed, of which the risk is represented with tail bleeding time. The data indicate that the tail bleeding time of **10-21** treated mice is significantly longer than that of ovariotomy, estradiol and estrone treated mice. This means that, in contrast to estradiol and estrone, oral administration of **10-21** induces no observable thrombosis risk, and the covalent modification of estradiol and estrone with RGD-octapeptides limits the dose-related adverse effects of estradiol.

3.9. Summary of covalent modification of estrogen with RGD-octapeptides

With RGD-octapeptides modifying one hydroxyl group of estradiol and estrone or with RGD-tetrapeptides simultaneously modifying two hydroxyl groups of estradiol resulted in 12 conjugates. On ovariotomy mouse model and at 110.3 nmol/kg of oral dose their anti-osteoporosis activities were significantly higher than that of estradiol and estrone themselves. In contrast to estradiol and estrone themselves, the anti-osteoporosis therapy of these conjugates induced no endometrial cell hyperplasia and thrombosis risk. Comparing to RGD-tetrapeptide modified estradiol and estrone the effective dose of RGD-octapeptide modified estradiol and estrone is 1000 folds lower. This means that the anti-osteoporosis efficacy of RGD-octapeptide modified estradiol and estrone is 1000 folds higher than that of RGD-tetrapeptide modified estradiol and estrone. Reasonably, this dramatically enhanced efficacy could attitude to the introduction of RGD-octapeptides. Furthermore, due to ovariotomy mouse model simulates the bone loss condition of postmenopausal women and high activity these RGD-octapeptides modified estradiol and estrone should be preferentially promising candidates for HRT use.

http://dx.doi.org/10.5772/54361

4. Direct covalent modification of androgen with RGD-tetrapeptides

In the improvements of the efficacy of HRT, the anti-osteoporosis efficacy of androgen is found to be higher than that of estrogen, inducing no endometrial cell hyperplasia and having no thrombosis risk. Particularly in the research of androgen, 17β-amino-11α-hydroxyandrost-1,4-diene-3-one is disclosed as a new androgen. Comparing to estrone and estrogen 17β-amino-11α-hydroxyandrost-1,4-diene-3-one has higher anti-osteoporosis activity and raises no endometrial cell hyperplasia and thrombosis risk. Thus 17β-amino-11α-hydroxyandrost-1,4-diene-3-one is selected as the androgen and directly and covalently modified with RGD-tetrapeptides (**22-24**, Figure 13) [32].

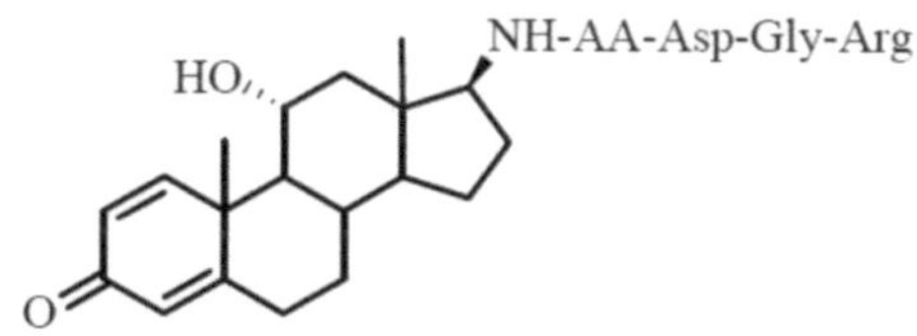

22-24

Figure 13. Structures of conjugates of androgen and RGD-tetrapeptides. In **22** AA = Ser, in **23** AA = Val, in **24** AA = Phe.

4.1. Direct covalent modification of androgen with RGD-tetrapeptides inhibiting bone turnover

The direct covalent modification of the 17β-amino of 17β-amino-11α-hydroxyandrost-1,4-diene-3-one (androgen) with RGD-tetrapeptides provided **22-24** (Figure 13). The effect of oral administration of **22-24** plus intramuscular prednisone for 4 weeks on serum calcium and serum ALP of the mice is shown in Figure 14. The data indicate that the serum calcium and serum ALP of oral administration of **22-24** plus intramuscular prednisone treated mice are significantly lower than that of prednisone alone and oral administration of estradiol plus intramuscular prednisone treated mice. This means that the frequency of bone turnover of **22-24** orally treated mice is significantly lower than that of androgen treated mice, the efficacy of oral **22-24** in inhibiting bone turnover is significantly higher than that of estradiol.

4.2. Direct covalent modification of androgen with RGD-tetrapeptides preventing bone loss

The effect of oral administration of **22-24** plus intramuscular prednisone for 4 weeks on the bone loss of the treated mice is shown in Figure 15, their activities are represented with dry femur weight and femur ash weight. The data indicate that both the weights of dry femur and femur ash of oral adminis-tration of **22-24** plus intramuscular prednisone treated mice are significantly higher than that of intramuscular prednisone alone and oral administration of estradiol plus intramuscular prednisone treated mice. This means that upon oral administra-

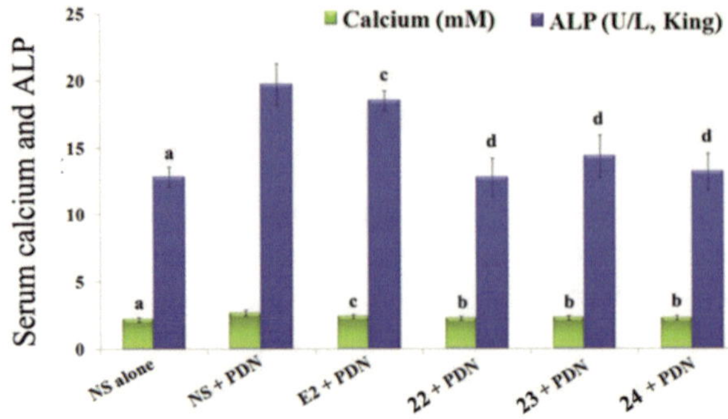

Figure 14. Serum calcium and ALP of **22-24** treated mice. ip Dose of prednisone (PDN): 6.3 mg/kg, twice a week; oral dose of **22-24**: 110 nmol/kg, once a day; oral dose of estradiol (E2): 110 nmol/kg, once a day; n = 12. a) Compared to NS + PND and E2 + PND p< 0.01; b) Compared to NS + PND p< 0.01, to E2 + PND p< 0.05; c) Compared to NS + PND p< 0.05; d) Compared to NS + PND and E2 + PND p< 0.01. The statistical analysis of the data was carried out by use of an ANOVA test and p<0.05 was considered significant.

tion **22-24** effectively inhibit the mice losing femur, their efficacies are significantly higher than that of estradiol, and the direct covalent modification of androgen prevents the bone loss.

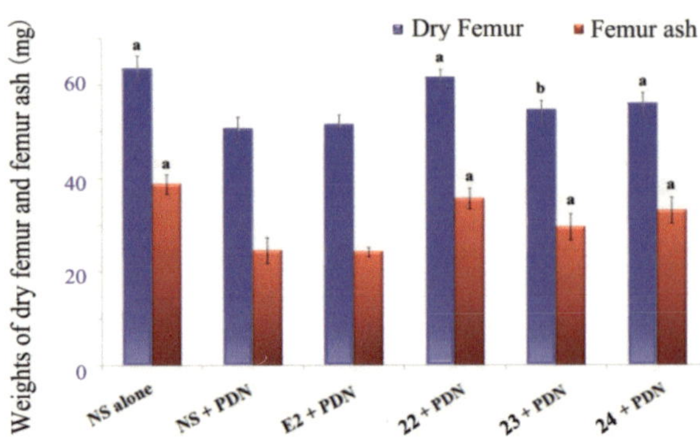

Figure 15. Weight of dry femur and femur ash of conjugates **22-24** treated mice. ip Dose of prednisone (PDN): 6.3 mg/kg, twice a week; oral dose of **22-24**: 110 nmol/kg, once a day; oral dose of estradiol (E2): 110 nmol/kg, once a day; n = 12. a) Compared to NS + PND and E2 + PND p< 0.01; b) Compared to NS + PND and E2 + PND p< 0.05. The statistical analysis of the data was carried out by use of an ANOVA test and p<0.05 was considered significant.

4.3. Direct covalent modification of androgen with RGD-tetrapeptides increasing total vBMD

CT measured 3D bone geometry and the size-independent vBMD, as well as pQCT quantitatively measured 3D bone geometry and size-independent vBMD were used to represent the anti-osteoporosis efficacy of **22-24** and are shown in Figure 16. The data indicates that the total vBMD of the femurs of NS plus intramuscular prednisone treated mice is significantly lower than that of the femurs of NS alone treated mice. This means that intramuscular administration of prednisone effectively induces the mice to decrease the total vBMD. The total vBMDs of the

http://dx.doi.org/10.5772/54361

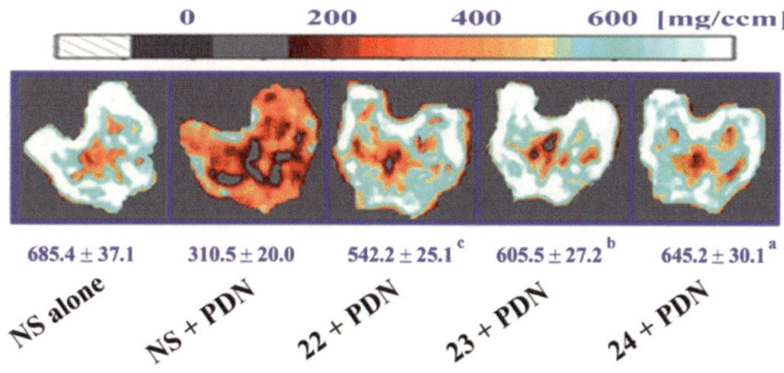

Figure 16. Total vBMD and images of pQCT scanning at a distance from the proximal femur growth palate corresponding to < 6 % of the total length of the femur of **22-24** treated mice. ip Dose of prednisone (PDN): 6.3 mg/kg, twice a week; oral dose of **22-24**: 110 nmol/kg, once a day; n = 12. a) Compared to NS alone , NS + PND, 23 + PDN and 22 + PDN $p< 0.01$; b) Compared to NS alone , NS + PND and 22 + PDN c) Compared to NS alone and NS + PND $p< 0.01$. The statistical analysis of the data was carried out by use of an ANOVA test and $p<0.05$ was considered significant.

femurs of oral administration of **22-24** plus intramuscular prednisone treated mice are significantly higher than that of the femurs of NS plus intramuscular prednisone treated mice. This means that upon oral administration **22-24** effectively prevent intramuscular administration of prednisone treated mice decreasing total vBMD.

4.4. Direct covalent modification of androgen with RGD-tetrapeptides increasing trabecular vBMD

Figure 17 indicates that the trabecular vBMD of the femurs of NS plus intramuscular administration of prednisone treated mice is significantly lower than that of the femurs of NS alone treated mice. This means that prednisone effectively induces the mice to decrease trabecular vBMD. The trabecular vBMDs of the femurs of oral administration of **22-24** plus intramuscular administration of prednisone treated mice are significantly higher than those of the femurs of NS plus intramuscular administration of prednisone treated mice. This means that upon oral administration **22-24** effectively prevent intra-muscular administration of prednisone treated mice decreasing trabecular vBMD.

4.5. Direct covalent modification of androgen with RGD-tetrapeptides inducing no endomtrial cell hyperplasia

The effect of oral administration of **22-24** plus intramuscular administration of prednisone for 4 weeks on the endometrial cell hyperplasia of the mice was observed, and their inhibition activities are represented with uteri weight. The data indicate that the weight of the uteri of oral administration of **22-24** plus intramuscular administration of prednisone treated mice is significantly lower than that of intramuscular administration of prednisone alone and oral administration of estradiol plus intramuscular administration of prednisone treated mice. This means that, in contrast to oral administration of estradiol, oral administration of **19-21** induces no observable endometrial cell hyperplasia, and the direct covalent modification of androgen with RGD-tetrapeptides induces no dose-related adverse effects of estradiol.

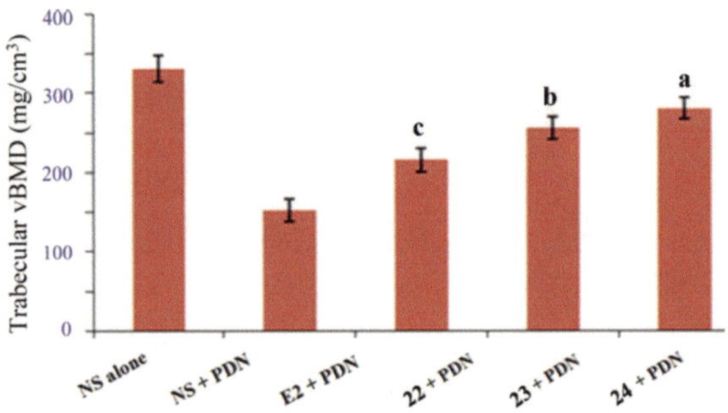

Figure 17. Trabecular vBMD of the femurs of the treated mice at a distance from the proximal femur growth palate corresponding with < 6 % of the total length of the femurs of **22-24** treated mice. a) Trabecular vBMD is represented with mean ± SD mg/cm^3, n = 12, PDN = prednisone, dose = 110 nmol/kg. b) Compared to NS + PDN, **22 +** PDN and **23 +** PDN p< 0.01; c) Compared to NS + PDN and **22 +** PDN p< 0.01; d) Compared to NS + PDN p< 0.01.

4.6. Direct covalent modification of androgen with RGD-tetrapeptides having no thrombosis risk

The effect of oral administration of **22-24** plus intramuscular administration of prednisone for 4 weeks on thrombosis risk of the mice was observed, and the risk is represented with tail bleeding time. The data indicate that the tail bleeding time of oral administration of **22-24** plus intramuscular administration of prednisone treated mice is significantly longer than that of ntramuscular administration of prednisone alone and oral administration of estradiol plus intramuscular administration of prednisone treated mice. This means that, in contrast to oral administration of estradiol, oral administration of **22-24** induces no observable thrombosis risk, and the direct covalent modification of androgen with RGD-tetrapeptides induces no dose-related adverse effects of estradiol.

4.7. Summary of direct covalent modification of androgen with RGD-tetrapeptides

RGD-octapeptides directly modifying the 17*β*-amino group of 17*β*-amino-11*α*-hydroxyandrost-1,4-diene-3-one was performed by amidation and resulted in 3 conjugates. On prednisone treated mouse model and at 110 nmol/kg of oral dose their anti-osteoporosis activities were significantly higher than that of estradiol. In contrast to estradiol, the anti-osteoporosis therapy of these conjugates induced no endometrial cell hyperplasia and thrombosis risk. Comparing to RGD-tetrapeptide modified estradiol the effective dose of RGD-octapeptide modified 17*β*-amino-11*α*-hydroxyandrost-1,4-diene-3-one is 1000 folds lower. This means that the anti-osteoporosis efficacy of RGD-octapeptide modified 17*β*-amino-11*α*-hydroxyandrost-1,4-diene-3-one is 1000 folds higher than that of RGD-tetrapeptide modified estradiol. Reasonably, this dramatically enhanced efficacy could attitude to the introduction of 17*β*-amino-11*α*-hydroxyandrost-1,4-diene-3-one. In addition to premenopausal women and in older men, secondary osteoporosis is common in the patients treated with glucocorticoids and in prostate cancer patients receiving androgen deprivation therapy (ADT) in particular. Glucocorticoids are ubiquitously prescribed in the fields of rheumatol-

http://dx.doi.org/10.5772/54361

ogy, respirology, neurology, hematology, dermatology, gastroenterology, and transplant medicine. Chronic exposure to pharmacological doses of glucocorticoids causes multiple deleterious effects on osteopenia, osteoporosis and bone fracture. Prostate cancer is one of the most common diseases in the older men. After the surgery or radiation therapy the male patients with localized or metastatic prostate cancer are generally given ADT. Though male patients on ADT usually have good prognosis, osteoporosis is a very common consequence of this therapy and up to 20% of the patients will fracture within 5 years. To prevent osteoporotic fracture in the female patients treated with glucocorticoids and the male patients receiving ADT novel effective agents are needed. The ability of these RGD-octapeptides modified 17β-amino-11α-hydroxyandrost-1,4-diene-3-one to prevent prednisone treated mouse developing osteoporosis suggests that these conjugates should be promising candidates of secondary osteoporosis therapies.

5. Indirect covalent modification of androgen with RGD-tetrapeptides

For androgen a parallel covalent modification with the direct covalent modification is an indirect strategy. In brief, between the 17β-amino group of 17β-amino-11α-hydroxyandrost-1,4-diene-3-one and RGD-tetrapeptides as a linker, succinyl group, is inserted to provide RGD-tetrapeptides indirectly modified androgen (Figure 18) [33].

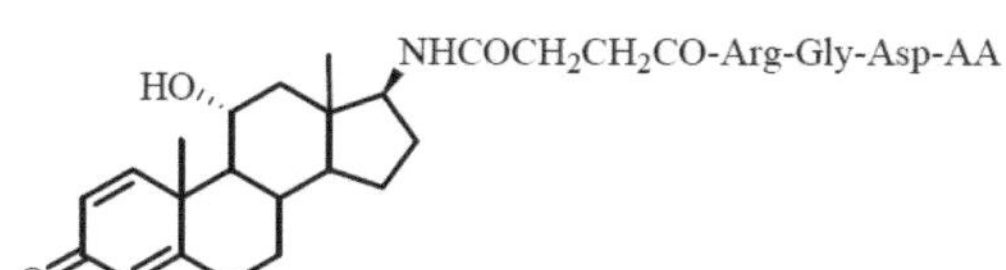

25-27

Figure 18. Structures of conjugates of androgen, succinyl group and RGD-tetrapeptides. In **25** AA = Ser, in **26** AA = Val, in **27** AA = Phe.

5.1. Indirect covalent modification of androgen with RGD-tetrapeptides inhibiting bone turnover

The effect of oral administration of **25-27** plus intramuscular administration of prednisone for 4 weeks on serum calcium and serum ALP of the mice is shown in Figure 19. The data indicate that the serum calcium and serum ALP of oral administration of **25-27** plus intramuscular administration of prednisone treated mice are significantly lower than those of intramuscular administration of prednisone alone and oral administration of estradiol plus intramuscular administration of prednisone treated mice. This means that the frequency of bone turnover of oral administration of **25-27** treated mice is significantly lower than that of oral administration of estradiol treated mice, the efficacy of oral administration of **25-27** in inhibiting bone turnover is significantly higher than that of oral administration of estradiol.

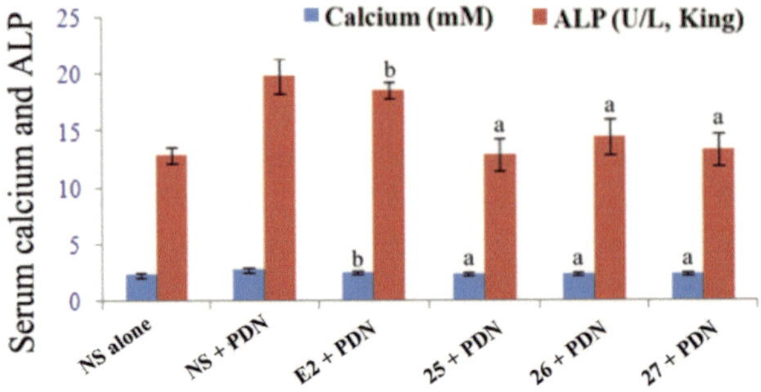

Figure 19. Serum calcium and ALP of **25-27** treated mice. ip Dose of prednisone (PDN): 6.3 mg/kg, twice a week; oral dose of **25-27**: 110 nmol/kg, once a day; oral dose of estradiol (E2): 110 nmol/kg, once a day; n = 12. **For serum Ca^{+2}:** a) Compared to NS + PND p< 0.01, to E2 + PND p< 0.05; b) Compared to NS + PND p< 0.05. **For serum ALP:** a) Compared to NS + PND and E2 + PND p< 0.01; b) Compared to NS + PND p< 0.05.

5.2. Indirect covalent modification of androgen with RGD-tetrapeptides preventing bone loss

The effect of oral administration of **25-27** plus intramuscular administration of prednisone for 4 weeks on the bone loss of the treated mice is shown in Figure 20, their activities are represented with dry femur weight and femur ash weight. The data indicate that both the weights of dry femur and femur ash of oral administration of **25-27** plus intramuscular administration of prednisone treated mice are significantly higher than those of intramuscular administration of prednisone alone and oral administration of estradiol plus intramuscular administration of prednisone treated mice. This means that upon oral administration **25-27** effectively inhibit the mice to losing femur, their efficacies are significantly higher than that of oral administration of estradiol, and the direct covalent modification of androgen prevents the bone loss.

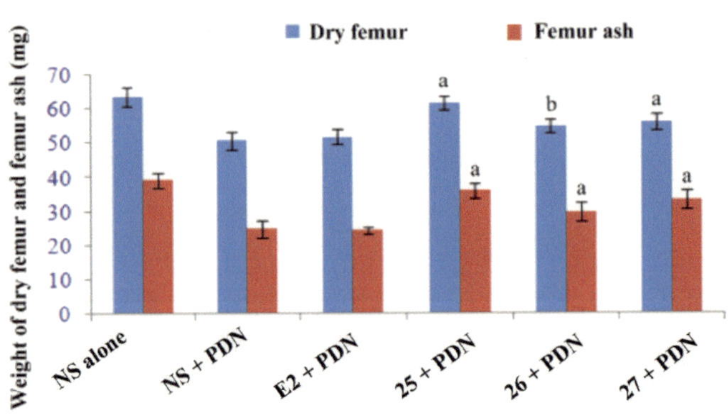

Figure 20. Weight of dry femur and femur ash of conjugates **25-27** treated mice. ip Dose of prednisone (PDN): 6.3 mg/kg, twice a week; oral dose of **25-27**: 110 nmol/kg, once a day; oral dose of estradiol (E2): 110 nmol/kg, once a day; n = 12. **For dry femur:** a) Compared to NS + PND and E2 + PND p< 0.05; b) Compared to NS + PND and E2 + PND p< 0.05. **For femur ash:** a) Compared to NS + PND and E2 + PND p< 0.01.

http://dx.doi.org/10.5772/54361

5.3. Indirect covalent modification of androgen with RGD-tetrapeptides increasing total vBMD

CT measured 3D bone geometry and the size-independent vBMD, as well as pQCT quantitatively measured 3D bone geometry and size-independent vBMD were used to represent the anti-osteoporosis efficacy of **25-27** and are shown in Figure 21. The data indicates that the total vBMD of the femurs of NS plus intramuscular administration of prednisone treated mice is significantly lower than that of the femurs of NS alone treated mice. This means that intramuscular administration of prednisone effectively induces the mice to decrease the total vBMD. The total vBMDs of the femurs of oral administration of **25-27** plus intramuscular administration of prednisone treated mice are significantly higher than that of the femurs of NS plus intramuscular administration of prednisone treated mice. This means that upon oral administration **25-27** effectively inhibit intramuscular administration of prednisone treated mice decreasing total vBMD.

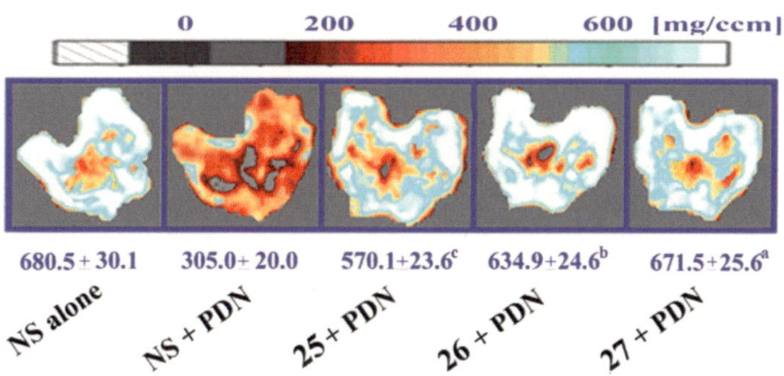

Figure 21. Total vBMD and images of pQCT scanning at a distance from the proximal femur growth palate corresponding to < 6 % of the total length of the femur of **25-27** treated mice.

5.4. Indirect covalent modification of androgen with RGD-tetrapeptides increasing trabecular vBMD

Figure 22 indicates that the trabecular vBMD of the femurs of NS plus intramuscular administration of prednisone treated mice is significantly lower than that of the femurs of NS alone treated mice. This means that prednisone effectively induces the mice to decrease trabecular vBMD. The trabecular vBMDs of the femurs of oral administration of **25-27** plus intramuscular administration of prednisone treated mice are significantly higher than that of the femurs of NS plus intramuscular administration of prednisone treated mice. This means that upon oral administration **25-27** effectively inhibit intramuscular administration of prednisone treated mice decreasing trabecular vBMD.

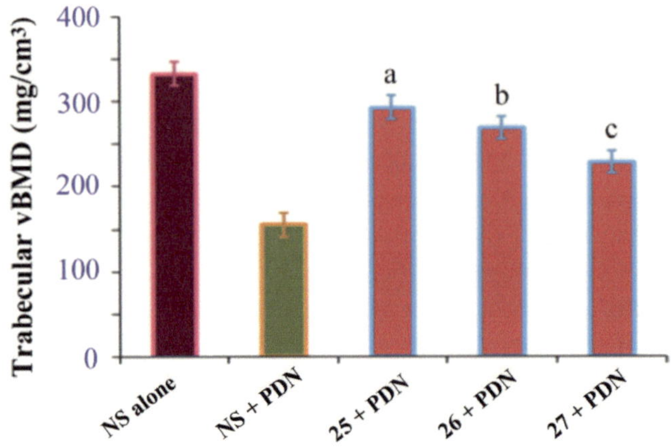

Figure 22. Trabecular vBMD in the femurs of treated mice at a distance from the proximal femur. Growth plate corresponds with < 6% of the total length of the femur of the treated mice. Trabecular vBMD is represented with mean ± SD mg/cm^3, n = 12, PDN = prednisone, dose of **25-27** = 110 nmol/kg. a) Compared to NS + PDN, **25 +** PDN and **26 +** PDN p< 0.01; b) Compared to NS + PDN and **27 +** PDN p< 0.01; c) Compared to NS + PDN p< 0.01.

5.5. Indirect covalent modification of androgen with RGD-tetrapeptides inducing no endomtrial cell hyperplasia

The effect of oral administration of **25-27** plus intramuscular administration of prednisone for 4 weeks on the endometrial cell hyperplasia of the mice was observed, and their inhibition activities are represented with uteri weight. The data indicate that the weight of the uteri of oral administration of **25-27** plus intramuscular administration of prednisone treated mice is significantly lower than that of intramuscular administration of prednisone alone and oral administration of estradiol plus intramuscular administration of prednisone treated mice. This means that, in contrast to oral administration of estradiol, upon oral administration **25-27** induces no observable endometrial cell hyperplasia, and the direct covalent modification of androgen with RGD-octapeptides induces no dose-related adverse effects of estradiol.

5.6. Indirect covalent modification of androgen with RGD-tetrapeptides having no thrombosis risk

The effect of oral administration of **25-27** plus intramuscular administration of prednisone for 4 weeks on thrombosis risk of the mice was observed, and the risk is represented with tail bleeding time. The data indicate that the tail bleeding time of oral administration of **25-27** plus intramuscular administration of prednisone treated mice is significantly longer than that of ntramuscular administration of prednisone alone and oral administration of estradiol plus intramuscular administration of prednisone treated mice. This means that, in contrast to oral administration of estradiol, upon oral administration **25-27** induces no observable thrombosis risk, and the indirect covalent modification of androgen with RGD-octapeptides induces no dose-related adverse effects of estradiol.

http://dx.doi.org/10.5772/54361

5.7. Summary of indirect covalent modification of androgen with RGD-tetrapeptides

RGD-tetrapeptides indirectly modifying the 17β-amino group of 17β-amino-11α-hydroxyandrost-1,4-diene-3-one was performed by inserting a succinyl functional group and resulted in 3 conjugates. On prednisone treated mouse model and at 110 nmol/kg of oral dose their anti-osteoporosis activities were significantly higher than that of estradiol. In contrast to estradiol, the anti-osteoporosis therapy of these conjugates induced no endometrial cell hyperplasia and thrombosis risk. In respect to inhibiting the prednisone treated mice to lose total vBMD, trabecular vBMD, femur ash weight, femur Ca^{2+} and bone mineral content 110 nmol/kg of RGD-tetrapeptides indirectly modified 17β-amino-11α-hydroxyandrost-1,4-diene-3-one was more effective than 110 nmol/kg of RGD-tetrapeptides directly modified 17β-amino-11α-hydroxyandrost-1,4-diene-3-one, and this increased efficacy could be attributed to the insertion of a succinyl group. Similarly, the ability of these RGD-octapeptides indirectly modified 17β-amino-11α-hydroxyandrost-1,4-diene-3-one to prevent prednisone treated mouse developing osteoporosis and high activity suggests that these conjugates should be preferentially promising candidates for secondary osteoporosis therapies.

6. Nano-structures of RGD-peptides modified estrogen and androgen

Self-organization or self-assembly practically leads to the formation of various ordered nanostructures in solution, at bulk state, and on a solid surface [34,35]. Numerous self-assembling substances, such as highly fluorinated amphiphilic molecules[36], amphiphilic triblock copolymers with polyrotaxane as a central block [37], amphiphilic dodecyl ester derivatives from aromatic amino acids [38], dendritic molecules [39], the shape anisotropy of non-spherical colloidal building blocks [40], alkylated polycyclic aromatic hydrocarbons [41], porphyrins, graphenes and fullerenes [42], were designed. Of the self-assembling molecules, peptides have been considered a set of particular substance [43-51]. In respect of the self-assembly the formation of nano-structure is an inherent property of organic compounds. In this context, the nano-structures of **10-15** and **22-27** in aqueous are given below to explore the relationships between the nano-structure and the concentration or pH, as well as to correlate the nano-feature with the pharmacological activity.

6.1. Nano-aggregators from modification of 17β-hydroxy of estradiol with RGD-octapeptides

As explained by Figure 6, using succinyl group and RGD-octapeptides modifying the 17β-hydroxy of estradiol provides **10-12**. Figure 23 demonstrates that in water **10** forms stick like nano-aggregators of 161.1 nm in diameter and 222.2-888.9 nm in length, **11** forms maize like nano-aggregator of 388.9 nm in length, **12** forms solid pipe like nano-aggregator of 3.6 nm in diameter and 263.9 nm in length.

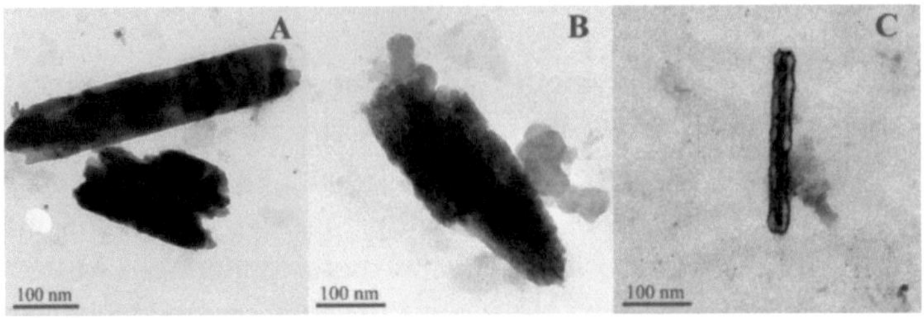

Figure 23. TEM images of **10** - **12** formed nano-aggregators. A) Stick like nano-aggregators of **10**; B) Maize like nano-aggregators of **11**; C) Solid pipe like nano-aggregator of 12.

6.2. Nano-aggregators from modification of 3-hydroxy of estradiol with RGD-octapeptides

As seen in Figure 6, carbonylmethyl and RGD-octapeptides modifying the 3-hydroxy of estradiol provides **13-15**. Figure 24 demonstrates that in water **13** forms porous nano-aggregators of 133.3-430.6 nm in length, **14** forms maize like nano-aggregator of 111.1-600.0 nm in length, **15** forms nano-globes of 66.7-237.5 nm in diameter.

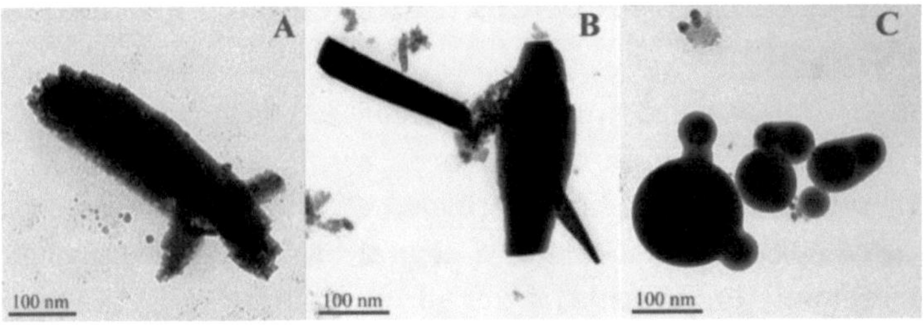

Figure 24. TEM images of **13** - **15** formed nano-aggregators. A) Porous nano-aggregators of **13**; B) Porous nano-aggregators of **14**; C) Nano-globes of **15**.

6.3. TEM image of nano-globes of androgen having RGD-tetrapeptides modified 17β-hydroxy

The nano-structures of **22-24** were explained with TEM nano-images and are shown with Figures 25-27. Figure 26 indicates that in 1.1 mM aqueous solution **22** forms numerous smaller globes aggregated nano-globe of 400 nm in diameter, dispersing globes of 55 - 200 nm in diameter, and dispersing globes of 18 - 146 nm in diameter. Figure 41 indicates that in 1.1 mM aqueous solution **23** forms nano-globe of 312.5 nm in diameter having small globes, blocks and awls on surface, nano-globes of 21.9 - 82.9 nm in diameter and nano-globes of 22.9 - 194.3 nm in diameter. Figure 27 indicates that in 1.1 mM aqueous solution **24** forms nano-globe of 183 nm in diameter having a number of nano-particles on surface, hemisphere of 275 nm in diameter having some smaller globes on incomplete surface and nano-globes of 48 - 188 nm in diameter.

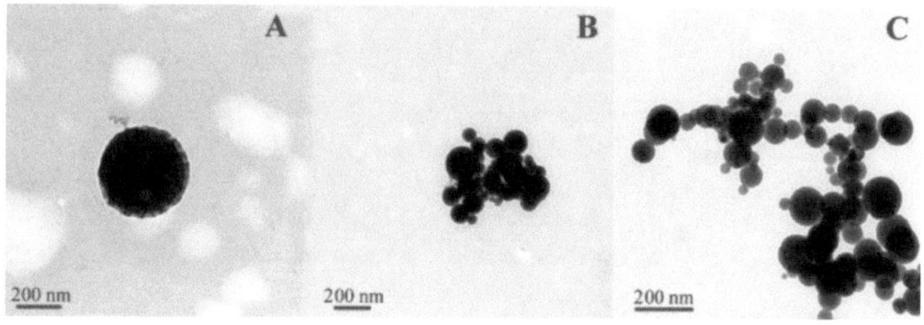

Figure 25. TEM images of 1.1 mM of **22** in ultrapure water. A) Numerous smaller globes aggregated nano-globe of 400 nm in diameter; B) Dispersing globes of 55 - 200 nm in diameter; C) Dispersing globes of 18 - 146 nm in diameter.

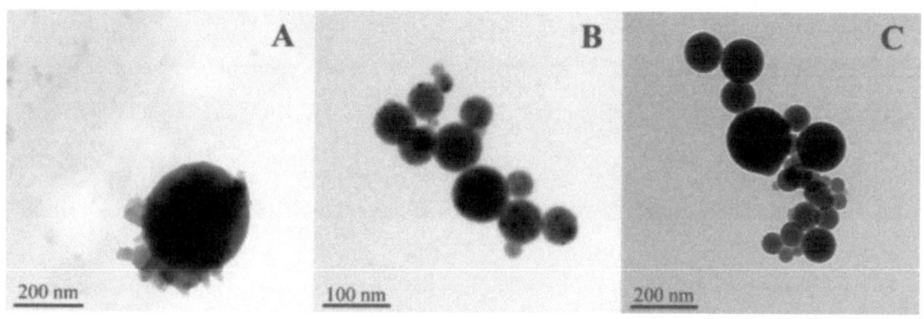

Figure 26. TEM images of 1.1 mM of **23** in ultrapure water. A) Nano-globe of 312.5 nm in diameter having small globes, blocks and awls on surface; B) Nano-globes of 21.9 - 82.9 nm in diameter; C) Nano-globes of 22.9 - 194.3 nm in diameter.

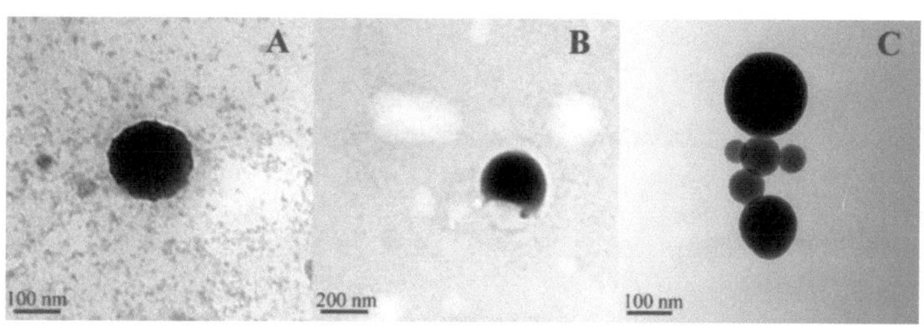

Figure 27. TEM images of 1.1 mM of **24** in ultrapure water. A) Nano-globe of 183 nm in diameter having a number of nano-particles on surface; B) A hemisphere of 275 nm in diameter having some smaller globes on incomplete surface; C) Nano-globes of 48 - 188 nm in diameter.

6.4. SEM image of nano-globes of androgen having RGD-tetrapeptides modified 17β-hydroxy

The nano-structures of **22-24** were explained with SEM nano-images and are shown with Figures 28-30. Figure 29 indicates that in solid state **22** exists as globes of 3.3 - 14.2 μm in diameter. Figure 44 indicates that in solid state **23** exists as eggs of 9.6 × 11.5 μm to 19.5 × 27.0 μm in diameter, of which surfaces have small eggs, and one egg remains its tail been incomplete. Figure 30 indicates that in solid state **24** exists as beads of 9.2 × 10.0 μm to 21.4 × 22.8 μm in diameter, and beads remain been incomplete.

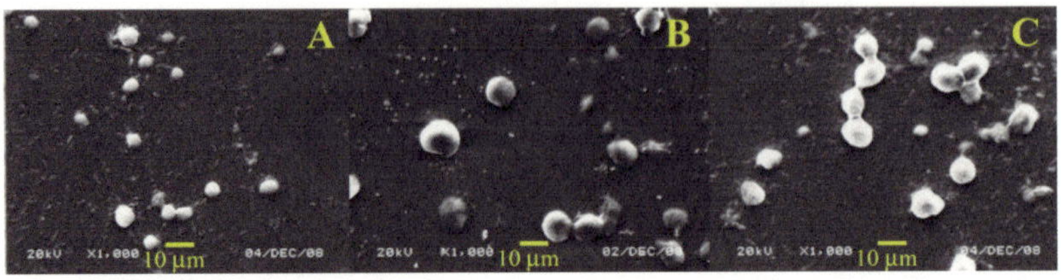

Figure 28. SEM images of **22** in solid state. A) Globes of 3.3 - 6.6 µm in diameter; B) Globes of 3.3 - 14.2 µm in diameter; C) Globes of 3.3 - 11.7 µm in diameter.

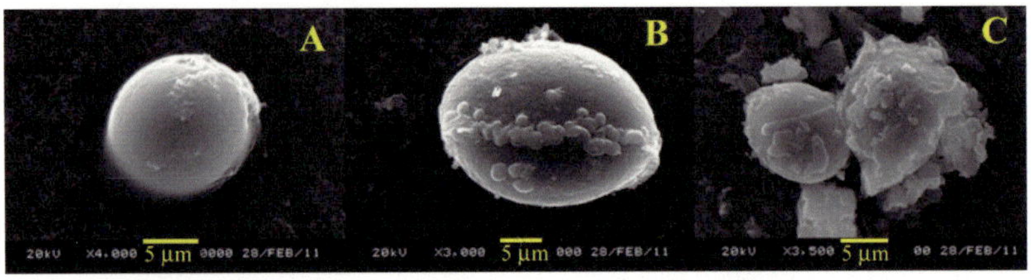

Figure 29. SEM images of **23** in solid state. A) Egg of 12.9 x 14.4 µm in diameter; B) Egg of 19.5 x 27.0 µm in diameter; C) Egg of 9.6 x 11.5 µm in diameter and egg remains its tail been incomplete.

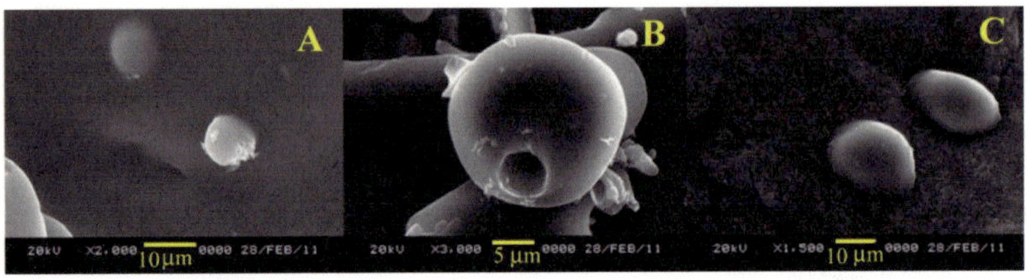

Figure 30. SEM images of **24** in solid state. A) Bead of 9.2 x 10.0 µm in diameters, and bead remains been incomplete; B) Hollow bead of 21.4 x 22.8 µm in diameters; C) Bead of 12.6 x 21.1 µm in diameter, and bead of 15.3 x 22.1 µm in diameter.

6.5. TEM image of nano-globes of androgen having RGD-tetrapeptides and succinyl modified 17β-hydroxy

The TEM images (Figures 31-33) demonstrate that in water **25-27** consistently form nano-globes with porous surface. The comparison of the nano-globes of **22-24** having no porous surface and the nano-globes of **25-27** having porous surface gave us an impression that the insertion of succinyl was a key to form the nano-globes with porous surface, 17β-ethyl-carbonylaminoandrost-1,4-diene-3-one was responsible for forming nano-globe, and RGD-tetrapeptide was responsible for characterizing the surface feature and size of the nano-globes, in particular. For instance, RGDS causes **25** to form dispersing nano-globes of 8 - 150 nm in diameter and having porous surfaces, RGDV causes **26** to form dispersing nano-globes of 29 - 150 nm in diameter and having porous surfaces, and RGDF causes **27** to form dispersing nano-globes of 76 - 343 nm in diameter and having porous surfaces.

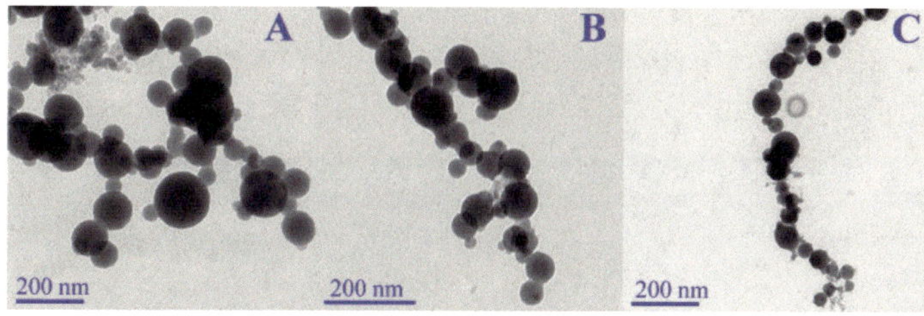

Figure 31. TEM images of 1.1 μM of **25** in ultrapure water. A) Dispersing globes of 8 - 150 nm in diameter; B) Dispersing globes of 17 - 94 nm in diameter; C) Dispersing globes of 27 - 82 nm in diameters.

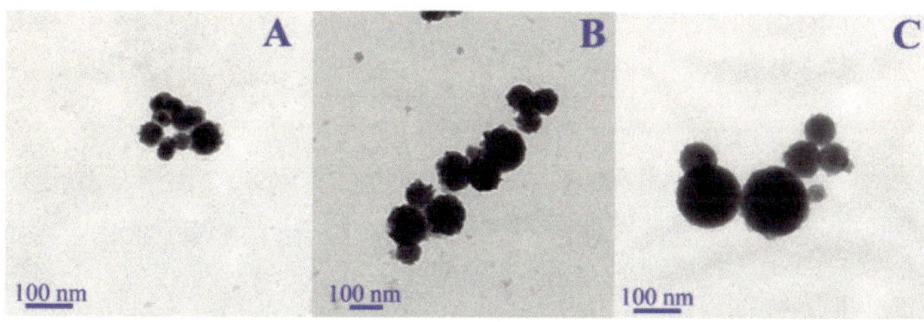

Figure 32. TEM images of 1.1 μM of **26** in ultrapure water. A)Dispersing globes of 29 - 69 nm in diameter; B) Dispersing globes of 70 - 120 nm in diameter; C) Dispersing globes of 67 - 150 nm in diameter.

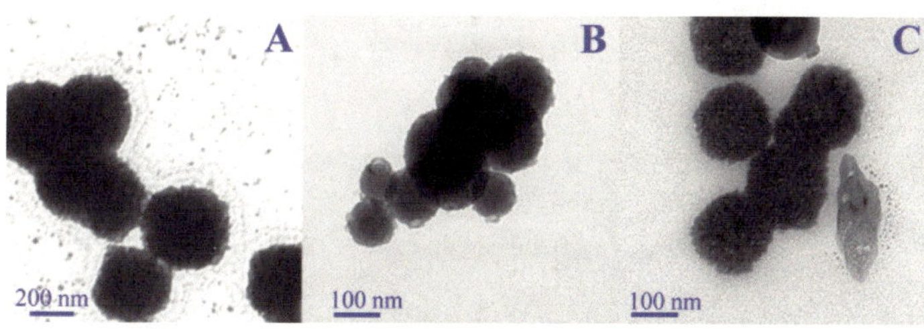

Figure 33. TEM images of 1.1 μM of **27** in ultrapure water. A) Dispersing globes of 320 - 343 nm in diameter; B) Dispersing globes of 76 - 139 nm in diameter; C) Dispersing globes of 120 - 171 nm in diameter.

6.6. SEM image of nano-globes of androgen having RGD-tetrapeptides and succinyl modified 17β-hydroxy

The SEM image (Figures 34-36) demonstrates that in solid state **25-27** exist as nano-globes of 15 nm - 6.4 μm in diameter, nano-pine seeds of 286 nm - 2.7 μm in length, nano-eggs of 1.3 - 12.9 μm in length, nano-pinecones of 5.0 - 5.6 μm in length, nano-gear of 10 μm in diameter, nano-calabash of 4 μm in length, and uncompleted nano-calabash of 11.3 μm in length. The coexistence of nano-globe having nano-egg, nano-pine seed having nano-pinecone, and uncompleted nano-calabash having nano-calabash implies that the nano-egg, nano-pinecone and nano-calabash are built by nano-globes, nano-pine seeds and uncompleted nano-calabash. The correlation of the molecular constitutions and the nano-structures gave us an impression that for **25** - **27** 17β-ethylcarbonyl-amino-androst-1,4-diene-3-one was responsible for forming a globe-like body, and RGD-tetrapeptide was responsible for characterizing globe-like body.

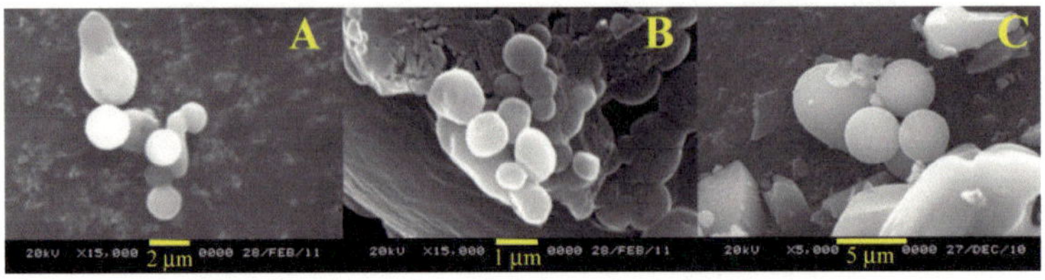

Figure 34. SEM images of **25** in solid state. A) Nano-globes of 15 nm - 2 μm in diameter and nano-calabash of 4 μm in length; B) Nano-globes of 600 nm - 1.3 μm in diameter and nano-egg of 1.3 μm in length; C) Nano-globes of 3.0 - 5.0 μm in diameter and uncompleted nano-calabash of 11.3 μm in length.

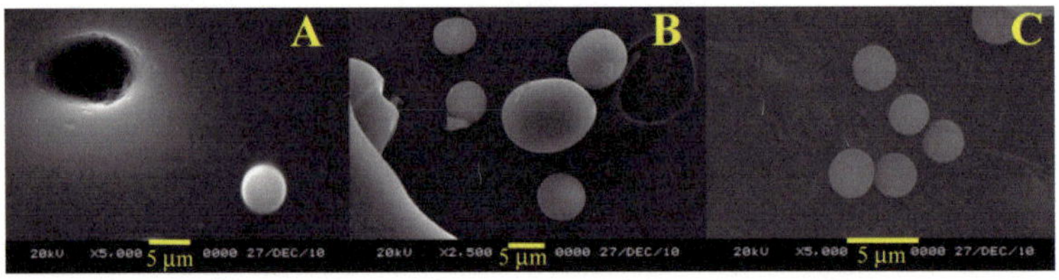

Figure 35. SEM images of **26** in solid state. A) Globe of 2.9 μm in diameter; B) Globes of 5.0 - 6.4 μm in diameter and eggs of 5.7 - 12.9 μm in length; C) Globes of 2.8 - 3.5 μm in diameter.

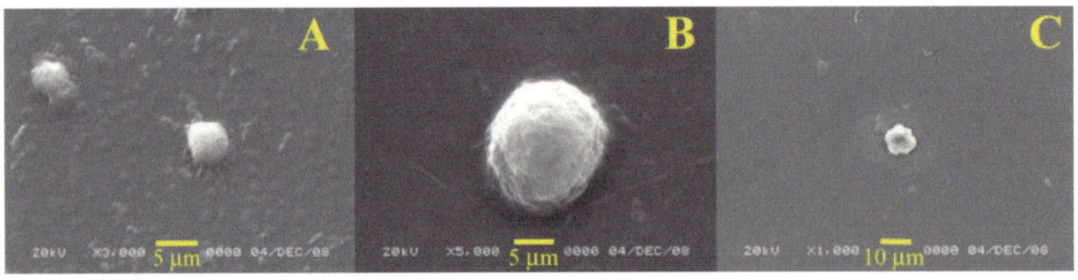

Figure 36. SEM images of **27** in solid state. A) Pine seeds of 7.1 - 9.4 μm in length; B) Globe of 8.1 μm in diameter; C) Gear of 10 μm in diameter.

6.7. Summary of the nano-structures of RGD-peptides modified sex hormones

In water RGD-peptides modified sex hormones generally formed diverse nano-species via self-assembly. Due to all non-covalent bond interactions could be involved into the self-assembly the size and the feature of the nano-species of RGD-peptides modified sex hormones clearly depend on the concentration of their aqueous solution. Similarly, due to all non-covalent bond interactions could be involved into the self-assembly the size and the feature of the nano-species usually depend on the chemical structures of the sex hormones and the sequence of the RGD-peptides. In addition, the RGD-peptides modified sex hormones possessed various anti-osteoporosis activities. Thus the feature and the size of their nano-species could be

http://dx.doi.org/10.5772/54361

correlated with their anti-osteoporosis activities. Therefore by selecting the concentration and by modifying the chemical structure we are able to optionally get the desirable nano-structure and consequently to optionally get desirable anti-osteoporosis activity.

7. Conclusions

Secondary osteoporosis is common in premenopausal women with osteoporosis and in older men, and is a major problem in clinical practice. More than one third of women with postmenopausal osteoporosis have identifiable secondary causes that contribute to bone loss. The secondary causes of osteoporosis in older men account for 50% - 80% of the cases of bone loss leading to fracture. Besides, secondary osteoporosis is common in the patients treated with glucocorticoids and in prostate cancer patients receiving ADT in particular. Glucocorticoids are ubiquitously prescribed in the fields of rheumatology, respirology, neurology, hematology, dermatology, gastroenterology, and transplant medicine. Chronic exposure to pharmacological doses of glucocorticoids causes multiple deleterious effects on osteopenia, osteoporosis and bone fracture. Prostate cancer is one of the most common diseases in the older men. After the surgery or radiation therapy the male patients with localized or metastatic prostate cancer are generally given ADT. Though male patients on ADT usually have good prognosis, osteoporosis is a very common consequence of this therapy and up to 20% of the patients will fracture within 5 years. To prevent osteoporotic fracture in premenopausal women with osteoporosis, the female patients treated with glucocorticoids and the male patients receiving ADT RGD-peptides modified sex hormones were provided. On ovariotomy and prednisone induced osteoporosis mice either ip injection or orally dosed the modified hormones were able to enhance the efficacy and minimize the adverse effects. By forming nano-species their therapy could be further improved.

Acknowledgements

This work was finished in Beijing Area Major Laboratory of Peptide and Small Molecular Drugs, supported by Innovation Platform Project of Education Committee of Beijing, Special Project (2011ZX09302-007-01), and Natural Scientific Foundation of China (81072522 and 81273379).

Author details

Ming Zhao, Yuji Wang, Jianhui Wu and Shiqi Peng*

*Address all correspondence to: sqpeng@bjmu.edu.cn

College of Pharmaceutical Sciences, Capital Medical University, Beijing, PR China

References

[1] Nagel G. Lahmann P.H. Schulz M. Boeing H. Linseisen J. Use of hormone replacement therapy (HRT) among women aged 45–64 years in the German EPIC-cohorts. Maturitas 2007; 56: 436 - 446.

[2] Brixen K. Abrahamsen B. Kassem M. Prevention and treatment of osteoporosis in women. Current Obstetrics & Gynaecology 2005; 15: 251 - 258.

[3] Keen R. Osteoporosis: strategies for prevention and management. Best Practice & Research Clinical Rheumatology 2007; 21:109-122.

[4] Compston J. Clinical and therapeutic aspects of osteoporosis. European Journal of Radiology 2009; 71: 388 - 391.

[5] López F.J. New approaches to the treatment of osteoporosis. Current Opinion in Chemical Biology 2000; 4: 383 - 393.

[6] Nimmo L.J. Alston L.A.C. McFadyen A.K. The influence of HRT on technical recall in the UK Breast Screening Programme: are pain, compression force, and compressed breast thickness contributing factors? Clinical Radiology 2007; 62: 439-446.

[7] Dietel, M. Hormone replacement therapy (HRT), breast cancer and tumor pathology. Maturitas 2010; 65: 183 - 189.

[8] Fletcher A.S. Erbas B. Kavanagh A.M. Hart S. Rodger A. Gertig D.M. Use of hormone replacement therapy (HRT) and survival following breast cancer diagnosis. The Breast 2005; 14: 192 - 200.

[9] Weaver K. Kataoka M. Murray J. Muir B. Anderson E. Warren R. Warsi I. Highnam R. Glasier A. Does a short cessation of HRT decrease mammographic density? Maturitas, 2008; 59: 315 - 322.

[10] [10] Ma L. Hofling M. Masironi B. von Schoultz B. Cline J.M. Sahlin L. Effects of tibolone and conventional HRT on the expression of estrogen and progesterone receptors in the breast. Maturitas, 2008; 61: 345 - 349.

[11] Fontanges E. Fontana A. Delmas P. Osteoporosis and breast cancer. Joint Bone Spine, 2004; 71: 102-110.

[12] Stevenson J.C. HRT and cardiovascular disease. Best Practice & Research Clinical Obstetrics and Gynaecology 2009; 23: 109 - 120.

[13] Kwee S.H. Tan H.H. Marsman A. Wauters C. The effect of Chinese herbal medicines (CHM) on menopausal symptoms compared to hormone replacement therapy (HRT) and placebo. Maturitas 2007; 58: 83 - 90.

[14] Kesim M.D. Aydin Y. Erdemir M. Atis A. Nitric oxide in postmenopausal women taking three different HRT regimens. Maturitas 2005; 50: 52 - 57.

[15] Camerona S.T. Glasier A.F. Gebbie A. Dewart H. Baird D.T. Comparison of a transdermal continuous combined and an interrupted progestogen HRT. Maturitas 2006; 53: 19 - 26.

[16] Pluchino N. Ninni F. Stomati M. Freschi L. Casarosa E. Valentino V. Luisi S. Genazzani A.D. PotìE. Genazzani A.R. One-year therapy with 10 mg/day DHEA alone or in combination with HRT in postmenopausal women: Effects on hormonal milieu. Maturitas 2008; 59: 293 - 303.

[17] Ross F.P. Interleukin 7 and estrogen-induced bone loss. Trends in Endocrinology and Metabo-lism 2003; 14: 147 - 149.

[18] Notelovitz M. Androgen effects on bone and muscle. Fertility and Sterility. 2002; 77: S34 - 41.

[19] Lammi J. Rajalin A. Huppunen J. Aarnisalo P. Cross-talk between the NR3B and NR4A families of orphan nuclear receptors. Biochemical and Biophysical Research Communications 2007; 359: 391 - 397.

[20] Ziolkowska A. Rucinski M. Pucher A. Tortorella C. Nussdorfer G.G. Malendowicz L.K. Expression of osteoblast marker genes in rat calvarial osteoblast-like cells, and effects of the endocrine disrupters diphenylolpropane, benzophenone-3, resveratrol and silymarin. Chemico-Biological Interactions 2006; 164: 147 - 156.

[21] Raboisson P. DesJarlais R.L. Reed R. Lattanze J. Chaikin M. Manthey C.L. Tomczuk B.E. Marugán J.J. Identification of novel short chain 4-substituted indoles as potent $\alpha_v\beta_3$ antagonist using structure-based drug design. European Journal of Medicinal Chemistry 2007; 42: 334 - 343.

[22] Wang C. Zhao M. Yang J. Peng S. Synthesis and analgesic effects of kyotor-phin-steroid linkers, Steroids 2001; 66: 811 - 815.

[23] Wang C. Zhao M. Peng S. The synthesis and immunosuppressive activities of steroid-urotoxin linkers, Bioorganic and Medicinal Chemistry 2004; 12: 4403 - 4421.

[24] Cui W. Wang C. Zhao M. Peng S. Effects of synthetic oligopeptides on osteoporosis, Preparative Biochemistry & Biotechnology 2002; 32: 253 - 268.

[25] Wang C. Zhao M. Cui W. Yang J. Peng S. Studies on the synthesis of estrogen-GHRPS linkers. Synthetic Communications 2003; 33: 1633 - 1641.

[26] Wang C. Cui W. Zhao M. Yang J. Peng S. Studies on the synthesis and anti-osteoporosis of estrogen-GHRPS linkers, Bioorganic and Medicinal Chemistry Letters 2003; 13: 143 - 146.

[27] Xiong Y. Zhao M. Wang C. Chang H. Peng S. Improved antiosteoporosis potency and reduced endometrial membrane hyperplasia during HRT with estrogen-RGD peptide conjugates. Journal of Medicinal Chemistry 2007; 50: 3340 - 3353.

[28] Zhao M. Peng S. Studies on hybrid peptides of fragments from fibrinogen. Journal der Praktikum Chemie 1999; 341: 668 - 676.

[29] Zhao M. Wang C. Peng S. Synthesis of RGD containing peptides and their bioactivities. Preparative Biochemistry and Biotechnology 2002; 32: 363 - 380.

[30] Liu J. Zhang X. Zhao M. Peng S. Synthesis, evaluation and 3D QSAR analysis of novel estradiol-RGD octapeptide conjugates with oral anti-osteoporosis activity. European Journal of Medicinal Chemistry 2009; 44: 1689 - 1704.

[31] Zhao M. Liu J. Zhang X. Peng L. Li C. Peng S. 3D QSAR of novel estrogen-RGD peptide conjugates: Getting insight into structural dependence of anti-osteoporosis activity and side effect of estrogen in ERT. Bioorganic and Medicinal Chemistry 2009; 17: 3680 - 3689.

[32] Wang Y. Wu J. Kang G. Zhao M. Gui L. Li N. Peng L. Zhang X. Li L. Peng S. Novel nano-materials, RGD-tetrapeptide-modified 17β-amino-11α- hydroxyl-androst-1,4-diene-3-one: Synthesis, self-assembly based nano-images and in vivo anti-osteoporosis evaluation. Journal of Material Chemistry 2012; 22: 4652 - 4659.

[33] Kang G. Wang Y. Liu J. Wu J. Zhao M. Li G, Li N. Peng L. Zhang X. Li L. Mair N. Peng S. Development of three-component conjugates: To get nano-globes with porous surface, high in vivo anti-osteoporosis activity and minimal side effects. Journal of Material Chemistry 2012; 22: 21740 – 21748.

[34] Li H. Song B. Qin L. Liu Q. Wu L. Shen J. Self-assembly and micellization of amphiphilic rod–coil block oligomer at the mica–water interface. Journal of Colloid and Interface Science 2005; 290: 557-563.

[35] Glotzer S.C. Horsch M.A. Iacovella C.R. Zhang Z. Chan E.R. Zhang X. Self- assembly of anisotropic tethered nanoparticle shape amphiphiles. Current Opinion in Colloid & Interface Science 2005; 10: 287-295.

[36] Jakobs R.T.M. van Herrikhuyzen J. Gielen J.C. Christianen P.C.M. Meskers S.C.J. Schenning A.P.H.J. Self-assembly of amphiphilic gold nanoparticles decorated with a mixed shell of oligo(p-phenylene vinylene)s and ethylenexide ligands. Journal of Material Chemistry 2008; 18: 3438-3441.

[37] Zhang X. Zhu X. Ke F. Ye L. Chen E. Zhang A. Feng Z. Preparation and self-assembly of amphiphilic triblock copolymers with polyrotaxane as a middle block and their application as carrier for the controlled release of Amphotericin B. Polymer 2009; 50: 4343-4351.

[38] Vijay R. Angayarkanny S. Baskar G. Amphiphilic dodecyl ester derivatives from aromatic amino acids: Significance of chemical architecture in interfacial adsor- ption characteristics. Colloids and Surfaces A, 2008; 317: 643-649.

[39] Mehdipoor E. Adeli M. Bavadi M. Sasanpour P. Rashidian B. A possible anti- cancer drug delivery system based on carbon nanotubedendrimer hybrid nanomaterials. Journal of Material Chemistry 2011; 21: 15456-15463.

[40] Sacanna S. Pine D.J. Shape-anisotropic colloids: Building blocks for complex assemblies. Current Opinion in Colloid & Interface Science 2011; 16: 96-105.

[41] Palermo V. Palma M. Tomović Ž. Watson M.D. Müllen K. Samorì P. Self-assembly of π-conjugated discs on heterogeneous surfaces: Effect of the micro- and nano-scale de wetting. Synthetic Metals 2004; 147: 117-121.

[42] Gadipelli S. Calizo I. Ford J. Cheng G., Walker A.R.H. Yildirim T. A highly practical route for largearea, single layer graphene from liquid carbon sources such as benzene and methanol. Journal of Material Chemistry 2011; 21: 16057-16065.

[43] Witus L.S. Rocha J.R. Yuwono V.M. Paramonov S.E. Weisman R.B. Hartgerink J.D. Peptides that non-covalently functionalize single-walled carbon nano- tubes to give controlled solubility characteristics. Journal of Material Chemistry 2007; 17: 1909-1915.

[44] Palui G. Ray S. Banerjee A. Synthesis of multiple shaped gold nanoparticles using wet chemical method by different dendritic peptides at room temperature. Journal of Material Chemistry 2009; 19: 3457-3468.

[45] Castelletto V. Hamley I.W. Self assembly of a model amphiphilic phenylalanine peptide/poly-ethylene glycol block copolymer in aqueous solution. Biophysical Chemistry 2009; 141: 169-174.

[46] Börner H.G. Strategies exploiting functions and self-assembly properties of

[47] onjugates for polymer and materials sciences. Progress in Polymer Science 2009; 34: 811-851.

[48] Carlsen A. Lecommandoux S. Self-assembly of polypeptide-based block copolymer amphiphiles. Current Opinion in Colloid & Interface Science 2009; 14, 329-339.

[49] Johnson E.K. Adams D.J. Cameron P.J. Peptide based low molecular weight gelators. Journal of Material Chemistry 2011; 21, 2024-2027.

[50] Wiradharma N. Tong Y.W. Yang Y. On-line observation of cell growth in a three- dimensional matrix on surfacemodified microelectrode arrays. Biomaterials 2009; 30: 3100-3117.

[51] Gribova V. Crouzier T. Picart C. A material's point of view on recent develop- ments of polymeric biomaterials: Control of mechanical and biochemical properties. Journal of Material Chemistry 2011; 21: 14354-14366.

Chapter 5

Oxidative Stress and Antioxidants in the Risk of Osteoporosis — Role of the Antioxidants Lycopene and Polyphenols

L.G. Rao and A.V. Rao

Additional information is available at the end of the chapter

http://dx.doi.org/10.5772/54703

1. Introduction

Osteoporosis is a metabolic bone disease known as "the silent thief" because the gradual loss of bone associated with this disease usually occurs over the years, and there are usually no noticeable symptoms until the bones are so fragile that a fracture occurs [1]. Although most statistics on the prevalence of osteoporosis quoted in the literature are from those published in 1991 to 2004 [2,3] the projection is nevertheless very consistent. Thus, osteoporosis is estimated to affect over 200 million people worldwide and 75 million people in Europe, the United States, and Japan [4]. Approximately 1 in 2 women and 1 in 5 men older than 50 years will eventually experience osteoporotic fractures [5] An increase in the worldwide incidence of hip fracture by 240% in women and 310% in men is projected by the year 2050 [6]. Osteoporosis is "a major public health threat" that is projected to results to 8.1 million fractures (78 % women, 22 % men) during the period between 2010 and 2050 [7]. The condition costs our healthcare system $18 billion per year [8]. Records show that Osteoporosis has been known to exist since the Egyptian mummies have been found with suspected dowager's hump [9]. Newer findings on all aspects of osteoporosis have increased exponentially. The more importantly ones are the introduction and improvement in more sensitive diagnostic instruments, discovering an ever increasing number of risk factors including oxidative stress, opening up new knowledge on the involvement of the bone forming cells osteoblasts and the bone resorbing cells osteoclasts in the development of osteoporosis and finding new drugs and the nutritional alternatives for the prevention and treatment of osteoporosis. Advances in knowledge on osteoporosis is not without pitfalls. Hormone Replacement Therapy (HRT), once a first line of treatment for osteoporosis has been discontinued due to side effects [10]. It is becoming more evident that the drugs known as bisphosphonates, although effective in stopping the resoption of bone and preventing osteoporosis in women, are associated with a number of side effects [11,12]. The side effects have been alarming a number of women with osteoporosis in such a way that they are now resorting to other mode of treatment, including that from natural food components. Our laboratory has carried out studies on the use of antioxidants such as lycopene and polyphenols as possible alternatives and/or complementaries to drugs in the treatment and prevention of osteoporosis. This chapter will include an overview on osteoporosis, the role of oxidative stress in bone cells osteoclasts and osteoblasts, oxidative stress as a risk factor in the development of osteoporosis and a review of studies on the use of antioxidants in counteracting oxidative stress in the prevention of osteoporosis. These topics should put our research in perspective and offer a rationale to our study approaches. Finally we will highlight our pioneering studies on the effects of the lipid-soluble antioxidant lycopene and the water-soluble antioxidant polyphenols present in a nutritional supplement in an *in vitro* cultures of osteoblasts and osteoclasts and our clinical studies in the prevention of risk for osteoporosis in postmenopausal women.

2. Osteoporosis — Overview

2.1. Bone cells involved in the development of osteoporosis

Bone as a dynamic tissue continuously renews itself throughout life by the process of bone remodeling carried out by a functional and anatomic structure known as the basic multicellular unit (BMU) that requires the coordinated action of three major types of bone cells: osteoclasts, osteoblasts and osteocytes [13,14]. The remodeling process is the result of interactions between these cells and multiple molecular agents, including hormones, growth factors, and cytokines. Bone remodeling is a physiological process that follows a time sequence lasting approximately six months wherein osteoclasts eliminate old or damaged bone which is subsequently replaced with new bone formed by osteoblasts, while the osteocytes functions in the transduction of signals necessary to sustain mechanical loads. The coupled process of bone formation and bone resorption in mature, healthy bone is tightly regulated and maintained in order to prevent a significant alterations in bone mass or mechanical strength after each remodeling cycle [14,15]. At menopause when estrogen production is decreased, the increase in resorption cavities due to increased bone resorption, but insufficient increase in bone formation, results to incomplete filling of resorption cavities with new bone leading to a permanent loss of bone mass. Disturbances in the remodeling process of this nature can lead to metabolic bone diseases. One such disturbance caused by oxidative stress, shown to control the functions of both osteoclasts and osteoblasts, may contribute to the pathogenesis of skeletal system including osteoporosis, the most prevalent metabolic bone disease [16].

2.2. Prevalence of osteoporosis

Women over the age of 50 become susceptible to osteoporosis because of the loss of estrogen at menopause [17]. As well, men's susceptibility to osteoporosis is due to low levels of the sex hormone testosterone [18-20]. In the past, a majority of men view osteoporosis as solely a "woman's disease." This is because men in their fifties do not experience the rapid loss of bone mass that women do in the years following menopause, and therefore men osteoporosis does not set in until later in life [21,22]. However, by age 65 to 70, men and women are losing bone mass at the same rate [23]. The World Health Organization (WHO) aptly defined osteoporosis as a systemic disease that is characterized by low bone mass and deterioration of the micro-architecture of bone, resulting in an increased risk of fracture. Bone mass or bone mineral density (BMD) is measured using a dual-energy x-ray absorptiometry, or DXA, at various skeletal sites, including the spine, hip and wrist [24].

2.3. Bone mineral density as predictor of osteoporosis

BMD is expressed as T-score which is a value compared to the expected value for young adults of the same sex and race. WHO has established that for normal BMD, the T-score is between standard deviation of +2.5 and -1.0; for osteopenia/low BMD, T-score is between -1.0 and -2.5, inclusive; for osteoporosis, T-score is lower than -2.5 and for severe osteoporosis,T-score is lower than -2.5 with the presence of one or more fragility fractures [25]. Thus BMD values can identify osteoporosis, determine the risk for fractures (broken bones), and measure the response to osteoporosis treatment [26]. In the case of severe osteoporosis, minimal trauma such as a minor fall or just a hug from a loved one can result to fragility fracture. Fragility fracture is defined by WHO as "a fracture caused by injury that would be insufficient to cause fracture normally. The spine, hip and distal forearm are the most common sites of fragility fracture [27]. Some doctors recommend that people be tested on a regular basis for bone loss. For women, those tests should begin after menopause. For men, they should begin after the age of sixty-five. Such tests are important since there are seldom other signs of osteoporosis. Therefore, those who have a higher rate of bone loss and are at higher risk for a fracture need a better diagnostic tool. Recently, the WHO introduced a prognostic tool to evaluate fracture risk of patients called the FRAX® [28]. The FRAX tool takes into account country, bone mineral density of the hip (when available), age, sex, and 8 clinical risk factors to calculate the 10-year probability of a major osteoporotic fracture and the 10-year probability of a hip fracture [29]. It assesses the 10-year risk of osteoporosis based on individual patient models that combines clinical risk factors (CRF) as well as BMD at the femoral neck [30].

2.4. Bone turnover markers for detecting osteoporosis

During bone remodeling in healthy young adult, bone formation by osteoblasts equals bone resorption by osteoclasts. However In postmenopausal bone loss, the remodeling process becomes significantly more active with a primary increase in bone resorption and a corresponding, but an insufficient increase in bone formation [31]. Enzymes and/or other proteins are released into the blood that are considered to reflect either bone formation or bone resorption [32] and are termed as bone turnover markers. Molecular markers of bone turnover have been developed as a product of bone remodeling [31] in the diagnostic and therapeutic assessment of metabolic bone disease [33]. They are now used for the individual monitoring of osteoporotic patients treated with antiresorptive agents [34]. Specific and sensitive assessment of the rate of bone formation and bone resorption and prediction of fracture [35] can now be possible using commercially available biochemical markers [36]. It remained to be seen whether bone turnover markers might contribute a useful independent risk factor for inclusion in FRAX [30]. The bone turnover markers we used for our clinical studies were crosslinked N-telopeptide of type I collagen (NTx) [37-39] and crosslinked C-telopeptide of type I collagen (CTx) [40,41] as bone resorption markers and bone alkaline phosphatase (BAP) [37-39] and Procollagen type I N-terminal propeptide (PINP) [40,41] for a measure of bone formation in the serum of participants.

Although BMD is considered the best parameter for determining the osteoporotic status of men and women, BMD is static and cannot predict changes that may occur post-measurement [42]. As well, changes in BMD occur slowly and can take up to one to two years to be detected during the course of therapy [43,44]. An alternative or additional parameters now measured clinically as either formation or resorption markers in the urine or serum of participants are bone turnover markers which can reveal changes much earlier in the course of therapy compared to changes in BMD [34]. When combined with BMD measurement, changes in bone turnover markers have been significantly linked to fracture risk due to a significant positive correlation between high bone turnover markers and loss of BMD [35]. Bone turnover markers are therefore very useful in assessing treatment protocol for a short duration period, e.g., 3 to 6 months. Measurement of bone turnover markers was therefore utilized in our clinical study during which postmenopausal women were given the antioxidant lycopene for 3 months [37-39] and in another study during which nutritional supplement greens+bone builder™ were administered for a period of eight weeks [40,41]. As will be reviewed in later sections, during the short period of treatment, positive changes were measured that correlated decreased bone resorption markers with decreases in oxidative stress parameters and thereby to decrease of risk for osteoporosis in postmenopausal women.

2.5. Risk factors of osteoporosis

Some of the risk factors for osteoporosis [45,46] are presented in Table 1 [47]. The risk factors that are of interest in our studies are oxidative stress-generating factors, including smoking, alcohol intake, low antioxidant status, nutrition deficiency, excessive sports activity and excessive caffeine intake. Oxidative stress will be reviewed in detail below.

2.6. Prevention and treatment of osteoporosis

Up until 10 years ago, the first line of treatment for women who have gone through menopause and was diagnosed with osteoporosis was hormone replacement therapy (HRT). However, results of the Women's Health Initiative (WHI) warned women that HRT leads to higher risks for breast cancer, cardiovascular events, blood clots, cognitive decline, and more [10]. This treatment for osteoporosis has since been discontinued and is prescribed only for a short period of time to alleviate hot flashes in menopausal women [48]. A wide range of pharmaceuticals are available for the treatment of osteoporosis. The current antiresorptive treatments approved by the Food and Drug Administration (FDA) include a number of bisphosphonates under specific trademarks which inhibit bone resorption [49]. Some are taken daily while others are formulated for weekly, monthly or intermittent oral use [50,51]. The newer bisphophonates are injectables such as ibandronate and Zoledronate [51] Other drugs available include calcitonin, strontium renalate and the Selective Estrogen Receptor Modulator (SERM), Raloxifene (Evista) [52]. Parathyroid hormone, PTH1-34 or teriparatide (Forteo), is the only anabolic agent currently approved for use by the FDA [24,53]. The new class of osteoporosis medications now approved for use is a fully human monoclonal antibody (Denosumab) which bind to RANKL, imitating the effects of OPG and acting as an inhibitor of RANKL [54]. A number of other drugs are being tested clinically for osteoporotic treatment and prevention.[24].

Unmodifiable	Modifiable
Race	Chronic inactivity
Sex	Low body weight
Age	Low lifetime calcium intake
Genetics	Medication used
Body size	Oxidative stress-related factors
Family History	Smoking
Previous Fractures	Alcohol intake
	Low antioxidant status
	Nutrition deficiency
	Excessive sports activity
	Excessive caffeine intake

Table 1. Risk Factors for Osteoporosis

None of the drugs are without side effects. Side effects that emerged in clinical trials include esophageal irritation with oral administration and acute phase response with iv treatment or high-dose oral therapy. Uncommon side effects that have been noted with wide clinical use include osteonecrosis of the jaw, musculoskeletal complaints, and atypical fractures. The numbers of events are small, and a clear cause-and-effect relationship between these events and bisphosphonate treatment has not been established. Because Bisphosphonates accumulate in the bone, they create a reservoir leading to continued release from bone for months or years and provide some residual antifracture reduction when treatment is stopped. For this reason, there is a recommendation for a drug holiday after 5 –10 yr of bisphosphonate treatment [12,55]. The length of the holiday is based on fracture risk and previous duration of treatment and BMD status. Studies with risedronate and alendronate suggest that if treatment is stopped after 3–5 yr, there is persisting antifracture efficacy, at least for 1–2 yr. For those who are not on holiday, the consensus from expert panels [12] suggest not stopping the use of drug since the side effects are often rare, and that the benefits outweigh the side effects. In the balance, most individuals who have osteoporosis are much better taking an osteoporosis medication [11].

2.7. Alternative approach to prevention and treatment of osteoporosis

Considering the possible adverse side effects of HRT and the ever increasing reports on the side effects of bisphosphonates in the management of postmenopausal osteoporosis, there is an increasing demand for complementary and alternative medicine (CAM) for the prevention and treatment of osteoporosis [56]. CAM is the term for medical practices, services and products that are not a part of standard care. Some of the approaches include exercise, acupuncture, diet, herbs rich in polyphenols and nutritional supplements including calcium, zinc, magnesium boron and other vitamins and minerals. Recent dietary guidelines for the prevention of chronic diseases have recommended an increase in the consumption of fruits and vegetables worldwide [57] that are good sources of dietary antioxidants [58]. The beneficial effects of antioxidants in bone health and osteoporosis are demonstrated epidemiologically and through clinical intervention. Given that many nutrients have been identified as being beneficial to bone health [59,60], there is strong scientific support for the potential benefits of incorporating therapeutic nutritional interventions with contemporary pharmaceutical treatments [61]. Diet is now recognized as an important life-style factor in the management of bone health [62]. As will be reviewed in this chapter, our clinical studies on lycopene treatment and nutritional supplements containing polyphenols and other nutritional components showed positive results on bone health.

3. Oxidative stress

Oxidative stress is caused by reactive oxygen species (ROS) which are the main by-products formed in the cells of aerobic organisms that can initiate autocatalytic reactions in such a way that the target molecules gets converted into free radicals causing a chain of damage [63]. There is ample evidence to show that oxidative stress induced by ROS increases the rate of bone loss and is therefore a risk factor for osteoporosis. Epidemiological evidence in humans and studies in animals indicate that aging and the associated increase in ROS are responsible for bone loss [64]. As will be reviewed in later sections, oxidative stress is associated with the activity and function of both the osteoblasts and osteoclasts cells, the two major bone cells involved in the pathogenesis of osteoporosis.

Oxidative stress results from the weakening of antioxidant defense or an over production of ROS in the body. ROS contains one or more unpaired electrons, a state that makes them highly reactive as they seek out another electron to fill their orbital and stabilize their electron balance [65]. Therefore, ROS are a family of highly reactive, oxygen-containing molecules and free radicals, including hydroxyl (OH –), superoxide radicals (O2 –), hydrogen peroxide (H_2O_2), singlet oxygen, and lipid peroxides [66]. ROS have an extremely short half-life and are difficult to measure in humans, but it is possible to measure the damage they cause to protein, lipids, and DNA and the damage is manifested as chronic diseases including osteoporosis [67]. This can occur by the induction of apoptosis, reduction of cellular proliferation, cell cycle arrest and modulation of cellular differentiation [68]. The major intracellular sites for the generation of ROS are via electron transport chains in the mitochondria, endoplasmic reticulum and nuclear membranes [69]. Oxidative stress may result from normal metabolic activity [70]; during acute or chronic immune responses [71]; lifestyle factors such as cigarette smoke [72,73], high alcohol intake [74,75], low antioxidant status [76], nutrition deficiency [74] excessive sports activity [77], excessive caffeine [78]; and environmental factors such as ultraviolet radiation, chemicals, pollution and toxins [79]. ROS production increases with age [80,81] and is associated with several chronic diseases including osteoporosis.

4. Antioxidants

Under normal physiological conditions, the cells can fight free radical attack or oxidative stress by promoting antioxidant defenses. A number of endogenous defense mechanisms are present in the body, including the metal chelating proteins and the endogenous antioxidant enzymes catalase (CAT), glutathione peroxidase (GPx) and superoxide dismutase (SOD). [82]. Exogenous antioxidants come from dietary sources present in fruits and vegetables containing several phytonutrient antioxidants such as the carotinoids potent antioxidant lipid-soluble lycopene; the water-soluble antioxidant polyphenols; and vitamins such as C and E [83]. In cases where the endogenous antioxidants or antioxidants from diet fail to prevent oxidative damage, the repair antioxidants come into play which include DNA repair enzymes, lipase, protease and transferase [69]. When antioxidants loses its fight with oxidative stress, diseases associated with oxidative stress develop, which include cardiovascular disease, cancer, diabetes, neurological diseases and osteoporosis [84].

The phytochemical antioxidants that are naturally present in plant- and animal-derived foods include the carotenoids, which are lipid-soluble, to which the potent antioxidant lycopene belongs and the water-soluble antioxidants such as polyphenols [85]. Figure 1 is a cartoon depicting the production of oxidative stress from ROS, the damaging effects they exert on DNA, lipid and protein which subsequently leads to chronic diseases and the protection afforded by antioxidants.

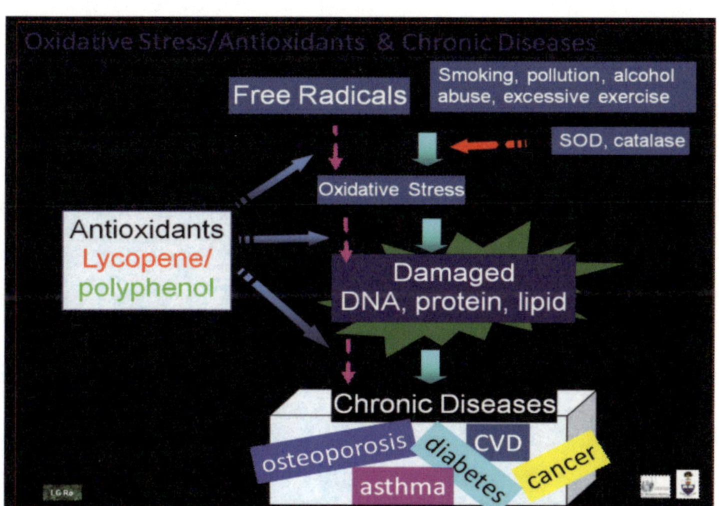

Figure 1. Oxidative Stress/Antioxidants & Chronic Diseases

4.1. Lycopene, a carotinoid lipid-soluble antioxidant

Lycopene is a potent antioxidant that is not synthesized in the body. It is a carotenoid acyclic isomer of ß-carotene, with no vitamin A activity [86]. It is a highly unsaturated, straight-chained hydrocarbon containing a total of 13 double bonds, of which 11 are conjugated, making it one of the most potent antioxidants [84,87]. The singlet oxygen-quenching ability of lycopene is twice that of ß-carotene and 10 times that of α-tocopherol [88]. The chemistry and antioxidant properties of lycopene have been comprehensively reviewed [87]. Other than from tomatoes and processed tomato, the dietary lycopene source of 85% of North Americans, lycopene can also be obtained from watermelon, pink guavas, and pink grapefruit [85]. Lycopene in an all-trans configuration such as that found in raw tomatoes, is not readily absorbed. Lycopene is absorbed more efficiently from processed tomato products than from raw tomatoes because it is converted from the all-trans to the cis-isomeric configuration with heat processing [89,90]. Since lycopene is a lipid-soluble compound that is absorbed via a chylomicron-mediated mechanism [91], the presence of small amounts of lipids further enhance its absorption [92]. The health benefits of lycopene may be due to its potent antioxidant property, although there is evidence for other mechanisms such as its effects on gap junction communication [93] and cell cycling [94]. The reported average daily intake levels of lycopene vary considerably from country to country, from 0.7 mg per day in Finland to 25 mg per day in Canada. However, a generally accepted universal level of daily intake is 2.5 mg. There is no official recommended daily intake of lycopene, but based on published research, a daily intake of 7 mg is suggested [95].

The role of lycopene in the prevention of human diseases is supported by a number of evidence [96]. Giovannicci was the first to publish the initial epidemiological observations suggesting an inverse relationship between the intake of tomatoes and lycopene and the incidence of prostate cancer [97]. Since then, there have been several epidemiological as well as clinical intervention studies showing the relationship between lycopene intake and the prevention of cancers at other sites, as well as coronary heart disease, hypertension, diabetes, macular degenerative disease, male infertility, and neurodegenerative disease [84]. The role of lycopene in bone health has so far been based on its potent antioxidant properties, the well known role of oxidative stress in bone health, and the limited studies on the effects of lycopene in bone cells in culture (see below) and more recently, the results of epidemiological studies [39,98]. To date our clinical intervention studies at St. Michael's Hospital on the role of lycopene and elucidation of its mechanism in lowering the risk for osteoporosis in postmenopausal women (aged 50 to 60 years) are so far the only studies reported in the literature.

4.2. Polyphenols, the water-soluble antioxidant

Polyphenols are a class of water-soluble molecules naturally found in plants. They are defined as compounds having molecular masses ranging from 500 to 3000–4000 Da and possessing 12 to 16 phenolic hydroxy groups on five to seven aromatic rings per 1000 Da of relative molecular mass [99]. It is estimated that there are 10,000 different phytonutrients (phyto, meaning from plants). To date, over 8000 polyphenols have been identified [100]. Polyphenols can be divided into 2 main groups: flavonoids and non-flavonoids [101-103]. The health benefits associated with fruits, vegetables, red wine, tea, and Mediterranean diets are probably linked to the

http://dx.doi.org/10.5772/54703

polyphenol antioxidants they contain [59,104,105]. The polyphenols of interest in our study are a mixture of flavonoids such as quercetin, apigenin, kaempferol and luteolin present in the supplement greens+™ [106]. greens+™ in combination with another supplement, bone builder™, were used in our study on osteoblasts cells and in clinical intervention studies on the prevention of risk of osteoporosis in postmenopausal women. Studies on polyphenols and bone will be reviewed in later sections.

5. Studies on the damaging effects of oxidative stress and the beneficial effects of antioxidants

(Studies involving lycopene and polyphenols will be reviewed at a later section)

5.1. Studies on osteoblasts

The evidence being reported on the role of oxidative stress in osteoblasts has increased exponentially. Up until 2002, only a few studies were reported. Thus, it was reported that treatment of rat osteosarcoma ROS 17/2.8 cells with tumor necrosis factor-alpha (TNF-a) suppressed bone sialoprotein (BSP) gene transcription through a tyrosine kinase-dependent pathway that generates ROS [107]. Osteoblasts can be induced to produce intracellular ROS [108,109], which can cause a decrease in alkaline phosphatase (ALP) activity that is partially inhibited by vitamin E and cause cell death [108,109]. The intracellular calcium (Ca++) activity in osteoblasts is modulated by H_2O_2 by increasing Ca++ release from the intracellular Ca++ stores [110]. High concentrations of ROS can damage osteoblast cells to prevent normal growth and development [111] and have been shown to induce osteoblast death [112]. In osteoblasts, H_2O_2 has been shown to decrease cell growth, ALP activity, calcification, mineralization and gene expression of osteogenic markers such as ALP, bone sailoprotein (BSP) and runt-related transcription factor 2 (Runx2) [113,114]. More recently, Ueno et al induced oxidative stress by adding 100 microM H_2O_2 to osteoblasts cultured from rat bone marrow, and showed that this treatment substantially impaired the proliferation, differentiation, and mineralization and that addition of the antioxidant N-acetyl cysteine into the culture restored these damages to a near normal level [115]]. With their study on hydrogen sulphide, Xu et al concluded that hydrogen sulfide (H_2S) protected MC3T3-E1 osteoblastic cells via a MAPK (p38 and ERK1/2)-dependent mechanism against hydrogen peroxide (H_2O_2)-induced oxidative injury that cause the suppression of proliferation and differentiation of the cells [116].

More recently reported inducers of oxidative stress include Arsenic trioxide [117], Cobalt and Chromium ion [118] and Vanadium Compounds [119].

In vitro studies suggest an important role for antioxidants in abrogating the effects of oxidative stress on bone. Trolox, a water soluble vitamin E analogue, was shown to enhance ALP activity in MC3T3-E1 osteoblast-like cells, thus enhancing osteoblast differentiation by decreasing the generation of ROS [111]. The addition of metallothionein, a metal-chelating preventative anti-oxidant, to primary mouse bone marrow stromal cells impaired H_2O_2-stimulated NfκB signalling, consequently preventing any inhibition of osteoblast differentiation [114]. Osteoblasts have been shown to produce antioxidants such as GPx which can protect against the damaging effects of ROS [120]. In MC3T3-E1 osteoblast-like cells, treatment with H_2O_2 to induce oxidative stress was associated with the prolonged up-regulation in gene expression of the transcription factor nuclear factor E2 p45-related factor 2 (Nrf2), which regulates antioxidant enzymes by assisting with recognition of the antioxidant-response element [113]. Using xanthine/xanthine oxidase to generate ROS, Fatokun *et al.*[120] showed that damage induced by ROS, as evidenced by decreased cell viability, was prevented by CAT in MC3T3-E1 osteoblast-like cells. This effect is attributed to the ability of CAT to neutralize H_2O_2 [120]. Newer mechanism of action of ROS is beginning to come to light. It has been shown that increased ROS production diverts the limited pool of β-catenin from TCF/LEF to FOXO-mediated transcription, converting the beneficial effects of Wnt/β-catenin on bone, eventually leading to decrease osteoblasts number and activity and eventually leading to osteoporosis [121-124].

In recent years, the number of antioxidants reported to prevent oxidative stress in osteoblasts are as follows: Tetrahydrostibene [125,126], Curculigoside [127], Green tea [128], Simvastatin [129], N-acetylcysteine [115], flavonoids from parsimmon [130], prevastatin [131], Linarin [132], Panaxnotaginseng saponin [133], crysoeriol from surya cilliata leaves [134], quercetin [135] Drynaria fortunei [136], cathamus tinctorium flower extract [137], estrogen [138], diazoxide, atractylodes japonica root extract [139]. and Myrcetin, a naturally occurring flavonoid [140]. The mechanism of osteblastic defense against oxidative stress was shown to involve β-Catenin which serves as a cofactor of the forkhead box O (FOXO) transcription factors [121].

5.2. Studies on osteoclasts

The mechanisms involved in the differentiation of osteoclasts and their ability to resorb bone is beginning to be unraveled, and evidence shows that ROS may be involved in this process [141]. Superoxide was detected both at the osteoclast-bone interface and intracellularly using nitroblue tetrazolium (NBT), which is reduced to purple-colored formazan by ROS, suggesting the participation of superoxide in bone resorption [142]. Both the H_2O_2 produced by endothelial cells [143] intimately associated with osteoclasts and the H_2O_2 that is produced by osteoclasts [144] increase osteoclastic activity and bone resorption. H_2O_2 may also be involved in osteoclast motility [144], differentiation of osteoclast precursors [145] and the regulation of osteoclast formation [146]. Osteoclastic superoxide is produced by NADPH oxidase [147]. The degradation of collagen and other proteins is caused by highly destructive ROS as a result of the reaction of H_2O_2 with tartrate-resistant acid phosphatase (TRAP), found on the surface of osteoclasts [148]. 1,25-Dihydroxyvitamin D3 had a direct nongenomic effect on the generation of superoxide anion (O2_), which was inhibited by estrogen [149]. Estrogen has been reported to have an antioxidant property [150]. Hormones known to stimulate bone resorption, such as parathyroid hormone (PTH) [151] and 1,25(OH)2D3, have stimulatory effects on ROS production in osteoclasts [149] and hormones known to have inhibitory effects on bone resorption, such as calcitonin, inhibit ROS production [151].

Antioxidants also play a role in osteoclast activity. Osteoclasts produce the antioxidant enzyme SOD in the plasma membrane [152]. ROS production in osteoclasts was inhibited after treating the cells with antioxidant enzymes such as SOD [142] and catalase [146]. ROS production in osteoclasts was also inhibited by estrogen [149], the superoxide scavenger deferoxamine mesylatemanganese complex [153], pyrrolidine dithiocarbamate (PDTC), and N-acetyl cysteine (NAC) [154].

Other more recent antioxidant shown to affect osteoclasts include polyphenol extracts from dried plums [155], curcumerin [156], ascorbic acid [157], salvia miltorrhiza [158], coffee diterpene Kahweol [159], delthametrin [160], to name a few. The use of antioxidants from natural sources, such as fruits and vegetables, could be another way of inhibiting ROS. The use of lycopene and polyphenols in this regard is reviewed in a later section.

5.3. Studies of on animal

OVXed rats were treated with Strontium ranelate and at the end of the treatment, oxidative parameters including malondialdehyde (MDA) level, superoxide dismutase (SOD), glutathione peroxidase (GSH-Px) and catalase (CAT) activities were determined by biochemical analysis methods. Their results showed that Sr has preventive effect on oxidative damage in ovariectomized rats [161]. Yin et al showed that protection against osteoporosis by statins is linked to a reduction of oxidative stress and restoration of NO formation in aged and ovariectomized rats [162]. To investigate the anti-osteoporosis effect of Rhizoma Drynariae (RD), an effectively traditional Chinese medicine and its action mechanism, Liu et al administered with or without RD extract at a therapeutic dose to a group of rats for 12 weeks and showed that the anti-osteoporosis effect of RD has been reliably confirmed by the metabonomics method and that the osteoporosis might be prevented by RD via, among other things, through intervening antioxidant-oxidation balance in vivo in rats [163]. Treatment of OVXed rats with Salvia miltiorrhiza ethanol extract significantly ameliorated the decrease in BMD and trabecular bone mass according to DEXA and trabecular bone architecture analysis of trabecular bone structural parameters by μ-CT scanning. As well, SM decreased the released TRAP-5b, an osteoclast activation marker and oxidative stress parameters including MDA and NO induced by OVX [164]. Oxidative stress (OS) was assessed 100 days postovariectomy by measuring the activity of several enzymes, including catalase (CAT), superoxide dismutase (SOD), and glutathione peroxidase, as well as the concentrations of malondialdehyde (MDA), nitric oxide (NO), and total sulfhydryl groups in plasma and bone homogenates of OVXed rats treated with or without vitamin C. Their results suggest that ovariectomy may produce osteoporosis and oxidative stress in females, and vitamin C supplementation may provide alterations regarding improvement in OS and BMD values [165]. Curcumin was shown to inhibit OVX-induced bone loss, at least in part by reducing osteoclastogenesis as a result of increased antioxidant activity and impaired RANKL signaling [166]. In order to investigate the pathologic significance of oxidative stress in bones, Nojiri et al showed that mice deficient in cytoplasmic copper/zinc superoxide dismutase exhibited a distinct weakness in bone stiffness and decreased BMD, aging-like changes in collagen cross-linking, and transcriptional alterations in the genes associated with osteogenesis. They further demonstrated that intracellular oxidative resulted in the decrease in osteoblast number and accompanied by suppression of RANKL/M-CSF osteoclastogenic signaling in bone; treatment with an antioxidant, vitamin C, effectively improved bone fragility and osteoblastic survival [167].

5.4. Epidemiological and clinical studies on osteoporosis

The detrimental effect of oxidative stress and the beneficial role of antioxidant in osteoporosis have been reviewed [58,83,168,169]. There is now ample evidence to suggest that ROS-induced oxidative stress is associated with the pathogenesis of osteoporosis. Thus, epidemiological studies demonstrated the adverse effect on bone of oxidative stress produced during strenuous exercise [170]; among heavy smokers [171] and that antioxidants including vitamin C, E and β-carotene may counteract these adverse effects and reduce the risk of osteoporosis [170-173]. A study of severe osteoporotic syndrome in relatively young males showed evidence linking osteoporosis to an increase in oxidative stress [174]. Maggio et al [175] demonstrated that women with osteoporosis had markedly decreased plasma antioxidants. A biochemical link between reduced bone density and increased oxidative stress biomarker 8-iso-prostaglandin F alpha (8-iso-PGF) has been reported [176,177]. Positive correlation was found between the severity of osteoporosis and the level of oxidative stress marker lactic acid in 2 men with mitochondrial deletion (mtDNA) [178].

Evidence points to the fact that Postmenopausal women are more prone to osteoporosis due to reduction in estrogen, but there is also ample evidence to support the theory that oxidative stress which accompanies the reduction in estrogen level may be the cause of osteoporosis [179]. Indeed, estrogen has been shown to have antioxidant properties [150]. Earlier reports on the association of oxidative stress with osteoporosis were confined mainly to epidemiological studies. Vitamins C, E, and A, uric acid, the antioxidant enzymes SOD in plasma and erythrocytes and GPx in plasma were consistently lower in osteoporotic than in control subjects. An epidemiological study by Hahn *et al* [180] found that GPx activity was significantly higher in postmenopausal women with osteopenia than that of postmenopausal women with a normal BMD, likely as a primary defense against the high levels of H_2O_2 in osteopenic women [180]. Osteoporotic women were found to have significantly depressed activities of CAT, GPx and SOD, compared to those found in healthy control women [177,181,182]. Furthermore, concentrations of the antioxidant enzymes SOD and CAT have been positively correlated with BMD which demonstrates a link between antioxidant status and BMD in postmenopausal women[182]. Surprisingly, a cross sectional analysis in healthy postmenopausal women aged 60-78 years revealed a negative association between 8-OH-dG levels and BMD of the lumbar spine, total hip, femoral neck, and trochanter and positive association with type I collagen C-telopeptide (ICTP) levels, showing that oxidative stress is associated with increased bone resorption and low bone mass even in otherwise healthy women. Medications used to treat postmenopausal osteoporosis such as HRT and Raloxifene [183] may act in part to decrease oxidative stress by acting in part as antioxidants. A 3-month course of Raloxifene therapy significantly decreased the lipid peroxidation and increased the CAT activity in women with postmenopausal osteoporosis [177,181,182]. Raloxifene treatment for 12 months significantly decreased protein oxidation in osteoporotic participants compared to matched, non-osteoporotic controls [183]. Supplementation of ascorbic acid and alpha-tocopherol was found useful in preventing bone loss linked to oxidative stress in elderly [181].

Postmenopausal women with osteoporosis have been shown to have markedly reduced serum concentrations of retinol, β-cryptoxanthin, zeaxanthin and α- and β-carotene, compared to healthy postmenopausal women [175]. Overall carotenoid intake has been found to be inversely associated with risk of fracture [184]. Sadly, the effect of β-carotene on the risk of osteoporosis is still controversial. There are studies which suggest that β-carotene has beneficial effect on bone [98,185,186], while other studies suggest a null or even detrimental effect, most probably due to its association with vitamin A [187].

In summary, the studies presented above provide evidence of the detrimental effects of oxidative stress and beneficial effects of antioxidants on the risk of osteoporosis.

6. Studies on lycopene

The direct role of lycopene in osteoblasts and osteoclasts, the cells involved in the pathogenesis of osteoporosis is now being unraveled. This involvement is further supported by both epidemiological and clinical intervention with lycopene in postmenopausal women men who are at risk of osteoporosis.

6.1. *In vitro* studies of lycopene in osteoblasts

Only few studies on the effects of lycopene in osteoblasts have been reported. This is most likely because lycopene is not soluble in the culture medium and needed to be solubilized in organic solvent before it can be added to the cell culture. In our study, we used lyc-o-mato preparation that is partially dispersed in micelle form in water. When added to the human osteoblast-like SaOS-2 cells, lycopene had a stimulatory effect on cell proliferation as well as a stimulatory effect on alkaline phosphatase activity, a marker of osteoblastic differentiation in more mature cells but, depending on the time of addition, it had an inhibitory or no effect on younger SaOS-Dex cells. These findings comprised the first report on the effect of lycopene on human osteoblasts [188]. In another study, the effect of lycopene on MC3T3 cells (the osteoblastic cells of mice) was contrary to the findings of Kim et al. [188] in that lycopene had an inhibitory effect on cell proliferation [189]. The discrepancy in the effects of lycopene on cell proliferation could be a result of species differences, age of the cells when lycopene was added or experimental conditions. Both studies, however, reported an effect of lycopene on the differentiation of the cells by stimulating the alkaline phosphatase activity [188,189] and gene expression of BSP [189]. The lycopene used in our study is the trans-configuration (95% trans, 5% cis). Subsequently, we studied which configuration of lycopene will prevent the damaging effect of oxidative stress as well as repair this damage in human osteoblast cultures. Lycopene with varying content of cis- and trans- configuration (45:55, 28:72 or 5:95 *cis:trans* lycopene) were added to cell cultures before and after challenging with H_2O_2 and the effect on the generation of ROS and stimulation of mineralized bone nodule were assessed. Our results demonstrated that the addition of H_2O_2 resulted in significant increase in generation of ROS

($p<0.001$), which long-term resulted in a decreased number and area of mineralized bone nodules (both: $p<0.001$). Pre- and post-treatment with 45:55 or 28:72 *cis:trans* lycopene resulted in significantly lower ROS generation ($p<0.001$) and higher mineralized bone nodule area ($p<0.05$), compared to treatment with H_2O_2 alone, vehicle or 5:95 *cis:trans* lycopene. These findings support the hypothesis that the *cis* isomers of lycopene are capable of preventing and repairing the damaging effects of H_2O_2-induced oxidative stress on the formation of mineralized bone nodules (unpublished observation) [169,190].

6.2. *In vitro* studies of lycopene in osteoclasts

To date, there have been only 2 studies on the effects of lycopene in osteoclasts [191,192]. Rao et al. cultured cells from bone marrow prepared from rat femur in 16 well, calcium phosphate-coated Osteologic™ multi-test slides. Lycopene was added to the cells in the absence or presence of the resorbing agent parathyroid hormone (PTH) (1-34) and mineral resorption, TRAP+ multinucleated osteoclast formation, and NBT-staining were measured. Lycopene inhibited TRAP+ multinucleated cell formation in both vehicle- and PTH-treated cultures. The cells that were stained with the NBT reduction product formazan were decreased in number after treatment with lycopene, indicating that lycopene inhibited the formation of ROS-secreting osteoclasts [192]. The effect of lycopene on osteoclast formation and bone resorption was also reported by Ishimi et al in murine osteoclasts formed in co-culture with calvarial osteoblasts [191]. Their results differed from those of Rao et al [192] in that they found that lycopene inhibited PTH-induced, but not basal, TRAP+ multinucleated cell formation. Furthermore, they could not demonstrate any effect of lycopene on bone resorption. They also did not study the effect of lycopene on ROS production.

6.3. Lycopene intervention studies in animals

Other than our intervention studies to be discussed in the next section, most of the intervention studies with lycopene were carried out in animals. Liang et al investigated the beneficial effect of lycopene on bone biomarkers in ovariectomized (OVX) rats. Their results showed that administration of lycopene (20, 30 and 40 mg/kg b.w.) for 8 weeks to OVXed rats significantly enhanced BMD, concluding that the consumption of lycopene may have the most protective effect on bone in OVX [193]. Ke et al fed OVXed rats for 3 months with EM-X, an antioxidant beverage derived from ferment of unpolished rice, sea weeds and papaya with combinations of microorganisms and contains, among other things, lycopene. Results showed that rats receiving EM-X for 3 months after sham operation or ovariectomy had increased bone density of the middle of femur that was statistically significantly different from unreated rats [194].

6.4. Epidemiological studies on lycopene

A systematic review of the experimental studies on Mediterranean diet and disease prevention was made and analyzed [195]. Although the Mediterrenean diet comprised of many different food components, it is striking that one of the components is abundance of plant foods including fruits, vegetables [195]. The two possible active components in its properties to prevent diseases are lycopene [196] and polypenols [197]. Epidemiological evidence support the beneficial effects of tomatoes and tomato products in the prevention of osteoporosis in the Mediterranean population [104].

The role of lycopene in the prevention of risk for osteoporosis has recently been reviewed [58, 83,168,169]. Maggio et al [175] and Yang et al [198] both demonstrated that serum lycopene concentrations are lower in women with osteoporosis than in healthy women of the same age. The antioxidant mechanistic effect of lycopene is demonstrated by Misra *et al.* who have shown that HRT has the same antioxidant effects as lycopene in postmenopausal women by demonstrating that lipid peroxidation was significantly decreased while GSH significantly increased by both [199]. Epidemiological studies revealed the relationship between lycopene and BMD [185,186,200]. A cross-sectional and longitudinal analyses in men and women were carried out to evaluate the associations between total and individual carotenoid intakes (a-carotene, β-carotene, β-cryptoxanthin, lycopene, lutein and zeaxanthin) with BMD at the hip, spine, and radial shaft and the 4-y change in BMD. Their analyses showed significant associations between lycopene intake and 4-y change in lumbar spine BMD for women [200] protective associations by total carotenoids against 4-y loss in trochanter BMD in men and in lumbar spine in women [98]. On the other hand, radial BMD was not correlated with serum lycopene in postmenopausal Japanese participants, while there was a weak correlation between radial BMD and β-cryptoxanthin and β-carotene [185]. These discrepancy maybe resolved by further in-depth study into the effect of lycopene on BMD. On the positive note, lycopene was shown to contribute to a decrease in the risk of fragility fracture related to osteoporosis.

We carried out a cross-sectional study in which 33 postmenopausal women aged 50–60 years provided seven-day dietary records and blood samples for analysis of oxidative stress parameters and bone turnover markers. Our results showed that postmenopausal women who consumed an average of 7.4 mg of lycopene per day had significantly higher serum lycopene. Our finding that the estimated dietary lycopene had a significant and direct correlation with serum lycopene suggests that lycopene from the diet is bioavailable. Our finding that a higher serum lycopene was associated with a low NTx ($p<0.005$) and lower protein oxidation ($p<0.05$). supports the antioxidative properties of lycopene involvement in its mechanisms of action in bone [39].

The overrall conclusions from the epidemiological studies support the beneficial role of lycopene in the prevention of risk for osteoporosis. Further clinical studies described below support this conclusion.

6.5. Clinical intervention studies on lycopene

Since our laboratory is the only one to this date that reported clinical intervention studies with lycopene, this section will focus on reviewing our studies on the role of lycopene in the prevention of risk for osteoporosis in postmenopausal women.

We carried out 4 different clinical studies. In the first study, the objective was to determine the effects of a lycopene-restricted diet on oxidative stress parameters and bone turnover markers in postmenopausal women [38]. To avoid the effects of compounding factors with antioxidants, women who smoked or were on medications which may affect bone metabolism or have antioxidant properties were excluded from participating. Twenty-three healthy postmenopausal women, 50-60 years old, provided blood samples at baseline and after a one-month lycopene-depletion period. Serum samples were analyzed for carotenoids; the oxidative stress parameters protein thiols and lipid peroxidation TBARS; the antioxidant enzymes SOD, CAT and GPx, and the bone turnover markers BAP and NTX. Results revealed that lycopene restriction resulted in significant decrease in serum lycopene, lutein/zeaxanthin and α-/β-carotene as shown in Table 2, However, the overall percent change in these serum carotenoids was not as high as that seen for lycopene. Figure 2 demonstrates that all configurations of lycopene (all trans, 5-cis- and other cis lycopene) were all decreased after lycopene restriction. The antioxidant enzymes CAT and SOD were significantly depressed (data not shown). These changes were accompanied by a significant increase in the bone resorption marker NTx [Figure 3].

Carotenoid	Concentration in serum (nM)		Results of paired t-test[1]	Average % change (mean ± SEM)
	Baseline (mean ± SEM)	lycopene restricted , (mean ± SEM)		
α-carotene	408.4 ± 131.4	334.4 ± 110.6	p<0.05	-13.03 ± 6.88
β-carotene	1443.0 ± 278.9	1035.0 ± 221.7	p<0.0005	-22.84 ± 5.09
β-cryptoxanthin	403.2 ± 58.4	367.6 ± 47.3	p = 0.229	-1.29 ± 8.21
Lycopene	1171.0 ± 111.1	494.9 ± 48.46	p<0.0001	-54.86 ± 3.59[a]
Lutein/zeaxanthin	516.4 ± 49.57	443.0 ± 47.04	p<0.01	-12.77 ± 5.03

[1] Wilcoxon matched pairs test used for these non-normally distributed data sets.

[a] Average percent change in lycopene was significantly higher than that seen for all the other carotenoids (p<0.0001), as determined by unpaired t-test or Mann-Whitney test.

Table 2. Change in serum carotenoid concentrations after postmenopausal women were assigned to Lycopene-restricted diet for a period of 1 month.

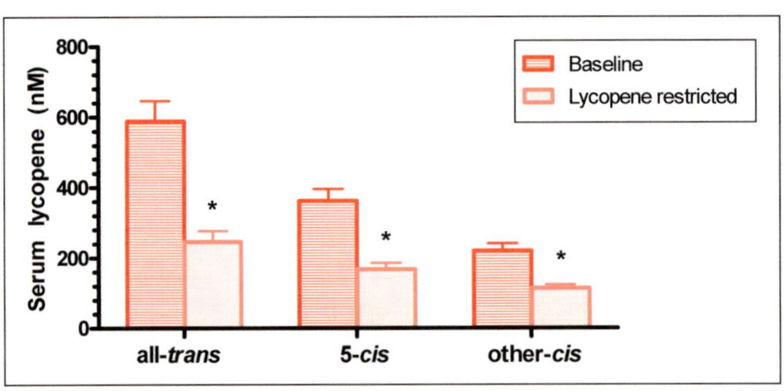

Figure 2. Decrease in all configurations of lycopene (all trans, 5-cis- and other cis lycopene) in the serum of postmenopausal women after lycopene restriction.

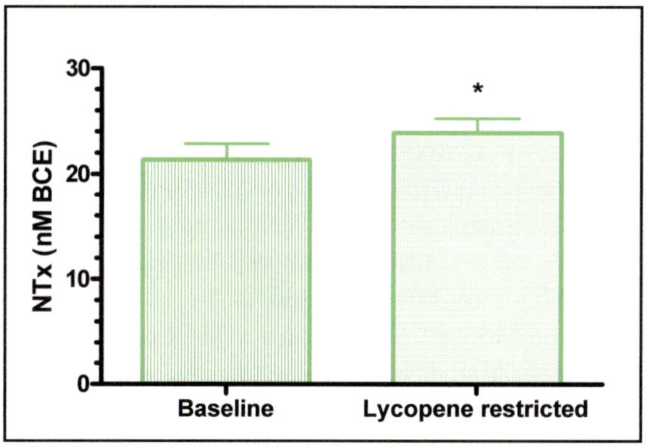

Figure 3. Increase in the concentrations of the bone resorption marker, NTx, in the serum of postmenopausal women after lycopene restriction.

To our knowledge, this is the first study on the effects of dietary lycopene restriction on increasing the risk for osteoporosis in postmenopausal women which proves that lycopene may be beneficial in reducing this risk. It can be speculated that this significant increase in the bone resorption marker NTx may lead to a long-term decrease in BMD and increased fracture risk as was observed by Brown et al [42], and that a longer restriction period may be detrimental to a group of postmenopausal women who were already at high risk for osteoporosis. It can also mean that shorter wash-out periods of no lycopene consumption is all that is needed in clinical trials examining the effects of lycopene on bone health. In addition, lycopene is present in a select number of foods; therefore not consuming these products as a part of the regular daily diet may result in negative health consequences to bone health.

In a second study [37], clinical intervention was carried out to investigate directly the effects of supplementation with lycopene on decreasing the risk for osteoporosis. Sixty postmenopausal women, 50-60 years old, were recruited for a fully randomized controlled intervention. Following a one-month washout without lycopene consumption, participants consumed either (N=15/group): (1) regular tomato juice, (2) lycopene-rich tomato juice, (3) tomato lycopene capsules or (4) placebo capsules, twice daily for total lycopene intakes of 30, 70, 30 and 0 mg/day, respectively for 4 months. Serum collected was assayed for oxidative stress parameters and bone turnover markers. Lycopene-supplementation for 4 months significantly increased serum lycopene compared to placebo ($p<0.001$). Since the increase in serum lycopene was similar for all three supplements, the participants were pooled into a "LYCOPENE-supplemented" and PLACEBO-supplement group for further statistical analyses. LYCOPENE-supplementation for 4 months resulted in significant increase in total antioxidant capacity as shown in Figure 4, decreased in oxidative stress parameters protein oxidation [Figure 5] and lipid peroxidation [Figure 6] which correlated to a decrease in NTx [Figure 7] in the LYCOPENE-supplemented group; all changes were significantly different from the PLACEBO group. These findings suggest that it did not matter whether lycopene was in the form of tomato juice or capsule to exert its potent antioxidant properties beneficial in reducing the risk of osteoporosis in postmenopausal women [37].

In a third study [169]. Serum lycopene, bone turnover markers and oxidative stress parameter data were compared between postmenopausal women who were supplemented with lycopene and those who obtained lycopene from both a low and high daily food intake of lycopene to determine whether the elevated dose obtained through supplementation was more beneficial in reducing bone turnover markers than intakes typically obtained from the usual daily diet. Table 3 showed that women supplemented with lycopene had significantly lower TBARS and marginally significant lower NTx values than participants who obtained a low intake (or high intake lycopene, data not show) through their usual daily diets. These differences in NTx and TBARS may be attributed to a significantly higher concentration of serum 5-*cis* in lycopene-supplemented participants compared to low or high usual daily intake participants. This suggests that it is the 5-*cis* isomer, with the most potent antioxidant capacity which, at higher concentrations, decreases bone turnover markers due to its ability to provide the greatest protection against oxidative stress. It also appears to show that supplementation with lycopene may be necessary in spite of the daily intake of lycopene.

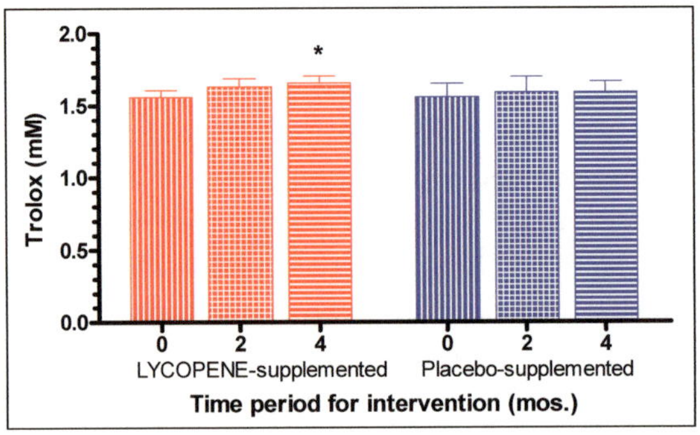

Figure 4. Increase in the serum total antioxidant capacity of postmenopausal women supplemented with LYCOPENE compared to placebo capsules for 4 months. Values are mean ± SEM. Values compared within supplement group was determined to be statistically significant using repeated-measures ANOVA (*p<0.05).

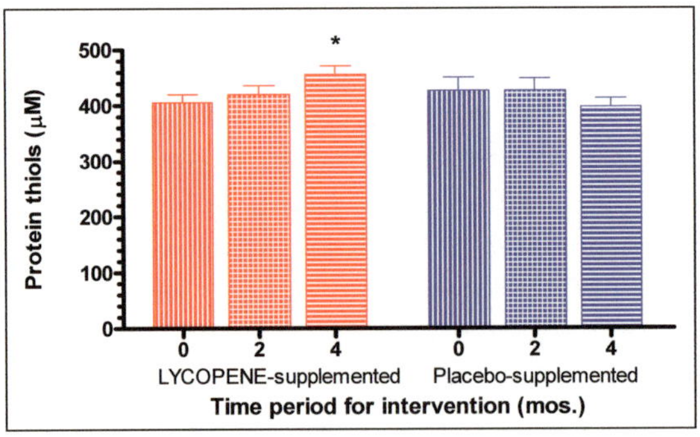

Figure 5. Increase the serum concentration of thiol (meaning decreased protein oxidation) in postmenopausal women supplemented with LYCOPENE compared to placebo capsules for a period of 4 months. Values are mean ± SEM. Values compared within supplement group was determined to be statistically significant using repeated-measures ANOVA (*p<0.001).

http://dx.doi.org/10.5772/54703

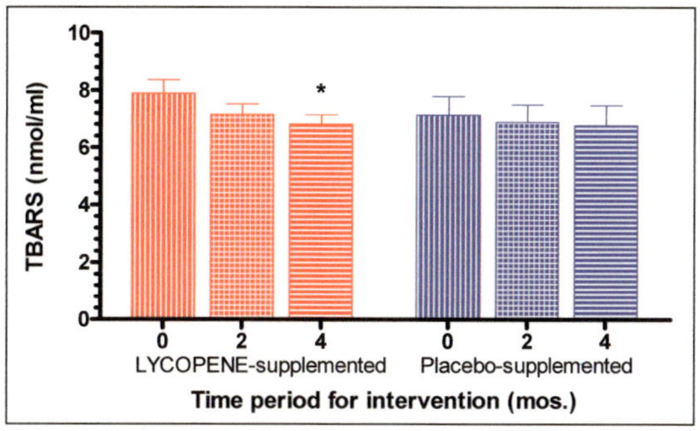

Figure 6. Decrease in the serum concentration of TBARS or lipid peroxidation in postmenopausal women supplemented with LYCOPENE compared to placebo capsules for a period of 4 months. Values are mean ± SEM. Values compared within supplement group was determined to be statistically significant using repeated-measures ANOVA (*p<0.001).

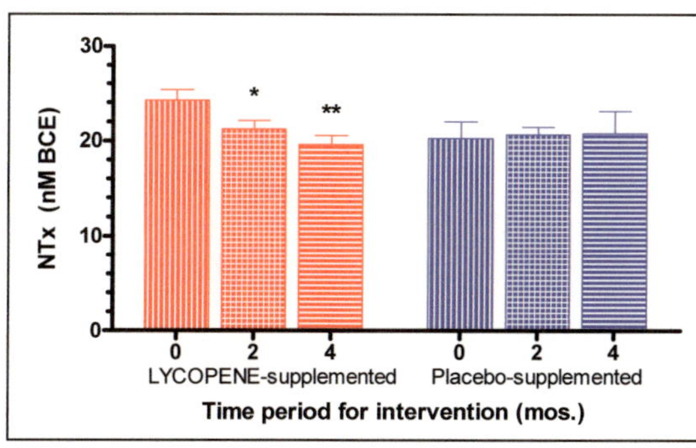

Figure 7. Decrease in the serum concentration of bone resorption marker NTx in postmenopausal women supplemented with LYCOPENE compared to placebo capsules for a period of 4 months. Values are mean ± SEM. Values compared within supplement group was determined to be statistically significant at 2 and 4 months using repeated-measures ANOVA (*p<0.01 and **p<0.001).

In a fourth study, we investigated whether the 172T→A or 584A→G polymorphisms of the paraoxonase 1 (PON 1) modulated the effects of serum lycopene on bone turnover markers, oxidative stress parameters and antioxidant capacity in women between the ages of 25-70 years. We showed that the PON1 polymorphism modified the association between lycopene and NTx and BAP ($p<0.02$ and $p<0.05$ for interaction). In the combined 172TT and 584G genotype, high serum lycopene was associated with decreased BAP ($p<0.01$) and NTx ($p<0.05$). Among those with the combined 172A and 584G genotype, however, increased serum lycopene was associated with increased BAP ($p<0.05$) and NTx ($p<0.05$). These findings show that PON1 polymorphisms modified the association between serum concentrations of lycopene and oxidative stress parameters and bone turnover markers and may, therefore, moderate the risk of osteoporosis [201].

		Mean ± SEM		
		Low usual daily intake group (N=48)	Lycopene-supplemented group (N=45)	p value[1]
Lycopene intake (mg/day)		2.59 ± 0.32[a]	43.33 ± 2.84	<0.0001
Serum lycopene (nM)	Total	1094 ± 80.24	2012 ± 88.56	<0.0001
	all-*trans*	539.0 ± 40.07	979.0 ± 48.48	<0.0001
	5-*cis*	342.4 ± 26.13	685.0 ± 30.22	<0.0001
	other-*cis*	212.6 ± 15.96	347.7 ± 17.36	<0.0001
Total antioxidant capacity (mM)		1.65 ± 0.03	1.66 ± 0.05	0.190
Bone turnover markers	NTx (nM BCE)	21.97 ± 1.11	19.19 ± 0.79	0.047
	BAP (U/L)	24.42 ± 1.40	23.56 ± 1.02	0.900
Oxidative stress parameters	Protein thiols (μM)	454.7 ± 15.37	455.2 ± 15.50	0.982
	TBARS (nmol/mL)	9.06 ± 0.35	6.80 ± 0.35	<0.0001
Antioxidant enzymes	CAT (K/g Hb)	81.50 ± 4.13	58.59 ± 2.06	<0.0001
	SOD (U/mg Hb)	47.60 ± 2.44	39.22 ± 4.72	0.001
	GPx (U/g Hb)	15.44 ± 1.40	32.82 ± 2.85	<0.0001

[1] Data that were not normally distributed were compared using the Mann-Whitney test

[a] The range of lycopene intake for the low usual daily intake group is 0.0-6.07 mg/day.

Table 3. Comparison of lycopene values, oxidative stress parameters and bone turnover markers between women who were supplemented with lycopene with those who obtained a low lycopene (not shown) intake from their usual daily diet (unpaired t-test).

A similar investigation was carried out in a fifth study to assesses whether the PON1 172T→A polymorphism affects the response to dietary intervention with lycopene. We showed that supplementation in the TT genotype and carriers of the A allele significantly increased serum lycopene (both: $p<0.0001$) while decreasing protein oxidation ($p<0.005$ and $p<0.05$, respectively) and lipid peroxidation ($p<0.005$ and $p<0.0005$). However, participants with the TT genotype responded more favourably to lycopene, with corresponding significant increase in total antioxidant capacity (TAC) ($p<0.01$) and significant decrease in NTx ($p<0.001$); this effect was not significant in carriers of the A allele. Further analyses showed that there was a significant interaction between PON1 genotype and change in TBARS ($p<0.05$) suggesting that supplementation with lycopene resulted in decreased lipid peroxidation, which interacted with the PON1 genotype to decrease bone resorption markers in postmenopausal women. These findings provide mechanistic evidence of how intervention with lycopene may act to decrease lipid peroxidation and thus the risk of osteoporosis in postmenopausal women [169,202].

http://dx.doi.org/10.5772/54703

6.6. Concluding remark

There is now ample evidence to show that oxidative stress brought about by the accumulation of ROS in the body is one of the causes of the development of several chronic diseases including osteoporosis and that antioxidants such as lycopene can counteract this damaging effect. The evidence includes studies on their role in osteoclastic resorption and osteoblastic bone formation, animal intervention studies, epidemiological studies and, more recently, clinical intervention studies. Considering the possible adverse side effects of the conventional therapy (eg, HRT and bisphosphonates) in the management of postmenopausal osteoporosis, there is an increasing demand for the use of antioxidants naturally present in foods. The results of these studies indicate that lycopene maybe useful either as a dietary alternative to drug therapy or as a complement to the drugs presently used by women at risk for osteoporosis.

7. Studies on polyphenols

Polyphenols have long been known to have a role in the prevention of chronic diseases such as cardiovascular diseases, cancers, neurodegenerative diseases, diabetes, or osteoporosis. Only in the last 10 years has there been an increase in the interest on polyphenols and bone health [203-206]. Horcajada [204] has recently reviewed the anabolic role of phytonutrients and especially polyphenols in bone while Trzeciakiewicz [205] reviewed the mechanisms of action of polyphenol in osteoblast function and its interaction with osteoclasts. The beneficial effects of green tea polyphenols has been reviewed [207,208].

Currently, most of the research on polyphenols and their effects have emerged from *in vitro* and *in vivo* animal studies with only a few clinical studies available. In our recent review, we have included tables listing all the studies on polyphenols *in vitro* bone cell culture and the epidemiologic studies on the protective effects of polyphenol consumption against osteoporosis [209] and only a few studies will be reviewed here.

7.1. *In vitro* studies on polyphenols in bone cells

The most commonly studied polyphenol abundant in green tea is epigallocatechin-3-Gallate (EGCG). We have shown that epigallocathechin-3-gallate (EGCG) increased the formation of mineralized bone nodules by human osteoblast-like cells [210]. EGCG has been shown to inhibit the expression of matrix metalloproteinase 9 (MMP-9) and the formation of osteoclasts [211]. H_2O_2-induced alterations of osteoblast viability and reduction in alkaline phosphatase activity were prevented by pre-incubating the osteoblasts with green tea polyphenol [212]. Green tea was shown to protect human osteoblasts from cigarette smoke-induced injury [128]. EGCG was shown to inhibit thyroid hormone-stimulated osteocalcin synthesis in osteoblasts [213], suppressed the differentiation of murine osteoblastic MC3T3-E1 cells [214], inhibit rat osteoclast formation and differentiation [215] and induces apoptosis via caspase activation in osteoclasts differentiated from RAW 264.7 cells [216]. Horcajada suggested that most studies investigating the effects of polyphenols on osteoblast cells have reported involvement of complex networks of anabolic signaling pathways such as BMPs or estrogen receptor mediated pathways [204]. Trzeciakiewicz describing a more detailed mechanisms, suggested that polyphenols modulate the expression of transcription factors in osteoblasts such as runt-related transcription factor-2 (Runx2) and Osterix, NFkappaB and activator protein-1 (AP-1) [205]. In agreement with Hocajada (2012), Trzeciakiewicz (2009) stated in his review that polyphenol may act on cellular signaling such as mitogen-activated protein kinase (MAPK), bone morphogenetic protein (BMP), oestrogen receptor and osteoprotegerin/receptor activator of NF-kappaB ligand (OPG/RANKL) and thus may affect osteoblast functions. The two reviews complement each other and paint a better understanding of the mechanisms of action of polyphenols in bone cells, with the warning that it is also important to take into account the possible interaction of these compounds on osteoblasts metabolism.

Other polyphenols/sources of polyphenols which were found to have beneficial effects on bone cells include the dried plum polyphenols found to attenuate the detrimental effects of TNFalpha on osteoblast function coincident with up-regulation of Runx2, Osterix and IGF-I and increasing lysyl oxidase expression, and at the same time attenuate osteoclastogenesis signalling [217]; black tea polyphenol which affects the MMP activity and osteoclast formation and differentiation in vitro [215]; phenolic leaf extract of Heimia myrtifolia (Lythraceae) found to stimulate mineralization of SaOS-2 osteosarcoma cells) [218]; Oleuropein which enhances osteoblastogenesis and inhibits adipogenesis and the effects on differentiation in stem cells derived from bone marrow [219] and the polyphenol component of red wine resveratrol which promotes osteogenic differentiation and protects against dexamethasone damage in murine-induced pluripotent stem cells [220] and facilitates in vitro mineralization and in vivo bone regeneration [221]. A number of animal studies have been reported and this was reviewed by Rao et al [209].

Other good sources of polyphenols that are frequently studied are extracts containing combinations of polyphenols. One such source is the nutritional supplement greens+™, a blend of several herbal and botanical products containing a substantial amount of polyphenols including quercetin, apigenin and luteolin [106] which act as antioxidants and therefore should be able to counteract oxidative stress. Our laboratory has shown that the polyphenolic extracts from greens+™ have stimulatory effect on mineralized bone nodule formation in human osteoblast cells in a dose- and time- dependent manner and is more effective than epicatechin (EC) as shown in Figure 8 [222]. We have further shown that this stimulatory effect is accompanied by decreases in the reactive oxygen species H_2O_2 shown in Figure 9 [223], thus proving that greens+™ is able to counteract oxidative stress in human osteoblastic cells and may therefore be a good candidate as a nutritional supplement to prevent the risk of osteoporosis.

Two additional nutritional supplements have since been formulated which may prove to be good for bone health. These are the bone builder™ and the greens+bone builder™ ; the latter is the original greens+™ product that has been supplemented with the bone builder™ formula containing several compounds including vitamins, minerals, and antioxidants. These various components have been separately shown to have some beneficial effect on bone [224]. Using the human osteoblast SaOS-2 cells, we showed that similarly to the greens+™, the water-soluble bone-builder™ extract had a significant dose-dependent stimulatory effect on bone nodules formation (Figure 10) [225]. Figure 11 shows that when the two supplements, greens

+TM and bone builderTM, were tested as combination, the effects were six times more effective than either one alone in stimulating bone formation in osteoblast culture [226].

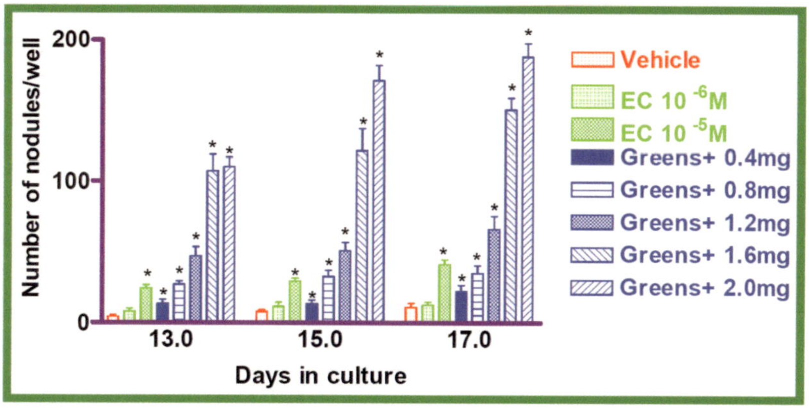

Figure 8. Effect of continuous addition of greens+TM extract on the number of SaOS-2 cells cultured in the presence of EC, or varying dilutions of greens+TM at an early time points and number of nodules analyzed at the indicated time points. An asterix, *, on a bar indicates statistical significance ($p < .05$) between a treatment and the control.

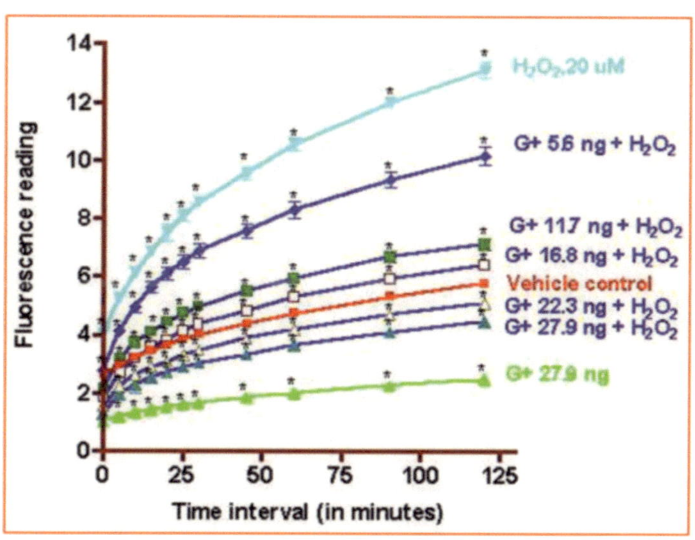

Figure 9. Dose-dependent inhibitory effects of phenolic extracts of greens+TM on intracellular ROS levels stimulated by 20 uM H_2O_2 in SaOS-2 cells. Data are mean ± SEM of 6 replicates. *p = < 0.05.

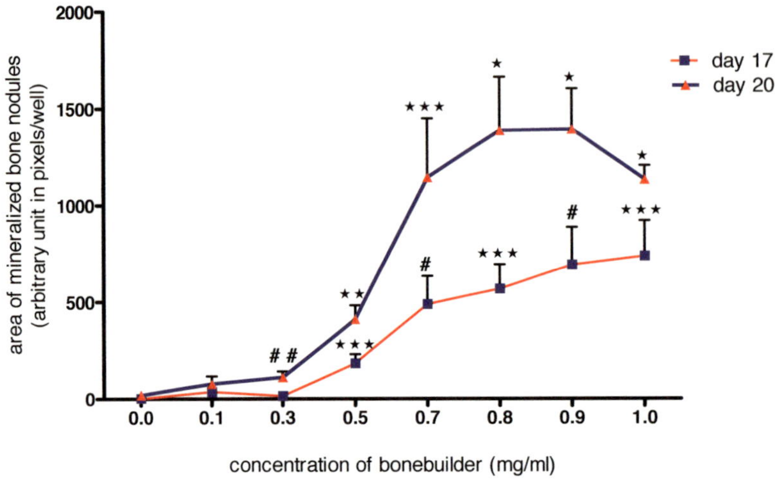

Figure 10. Time and Dose-dependent Effects of bone builder™ on mineralized bone nodule area in SaOS-2 cells. indicates significant difference from vehicle: p<0.0001; p<0.0005; p<0.005, #, p<0.01 and ##, p< 0.05. There is a significant dose-dependent effect both at day 17 and day 20, according to One-way ANOVA; p<0.0001.

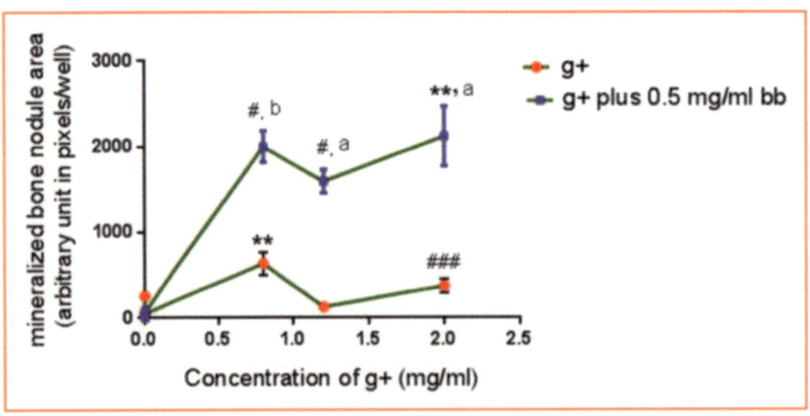

Figure 11. Dose dependent effect of greens + (g+) with and without 0.5 mg/ml of bone builder (bb) on the area of mineralized bone nodules in osteoblasts SaOS-2 Cells. Significant differences were found compared to respective controls. g+bb was more effective than either g+ or bb alone.

7.2. Clinical intervention studies of polyphenol

We have recently reviewed earlier clinical studies on polyphenols and osteoporosis [209]. Only the more recent reports, as well as our own clinical studies will be reviewed here. Shen et al [227] have extended their studies in osteopenic women and showed that dietary supplement in the form of green tea combined with tai-chi, a mind-body exercise, can alleviating bone loss in osteopenic women. The effect of catechin was studied in perimenopausal Scottish women

http://dx.doi.org/10.5772/54703

and it was found that catechin was negatively associated with bone-resorption markers, association between energy-adjusted total flavonoid intakes and BMD at the femoreal neck and lumbar spine while annual percent change in BMD was associated with intakes of procyanidins and catechins [228].

Other than these clinical studies in the last two years, there has not been not been anymore reported clinical studies on polyphenols in human subjects except our studies.

Our results on the in vitro effects of greens+™, bone builder™ and greens+bone builder™ on bone formation in osteoblasts encouraged us formed the rationale for our clinical studies to test whether these products can prevent the risk of osteoporosis in postmenopausal women. We chose to study the greens+bone builder™ since of the three products, it gave the greatest stimulatory effect on bone formation, being six times more effective than the other two. The first randomized cross-sectional clinical intervention study was carried out to test whether a daily supplementation with greens+ bone builderTM may be important in reducing oxidative damage in postmenopausal women at risk for osteoporosis. [40]. Forty-seven postmenopausal women, 50-60 years old were randomized to either Treatment group consuming 1 scoop (equivalent to ¼ cup) daily of greens+ bone builder*™* (N=23) or Placebo (N=24) group for a period of 8 weeks. Blood samples were collected at 0, 4 and 8 weeks of supplementation, processed and assayed for serum total antioxidant capacity (TAC), lipid peroxidation and protein oxidation as markers of oxidative stress. Results revealed that there was an increase in total antioxidant capacity (Figure 12, as well as a decrease in both protein oxidation (Figure 13) and lipid peroxidation (Figure 14) over a 4 and 8-weeks of intervention with greens+ bone builder*™* compared to placebo. This suggests that the nutritional supplement may have a beneficial effect on bone health by counteracting the effects of oxidative stress [40].

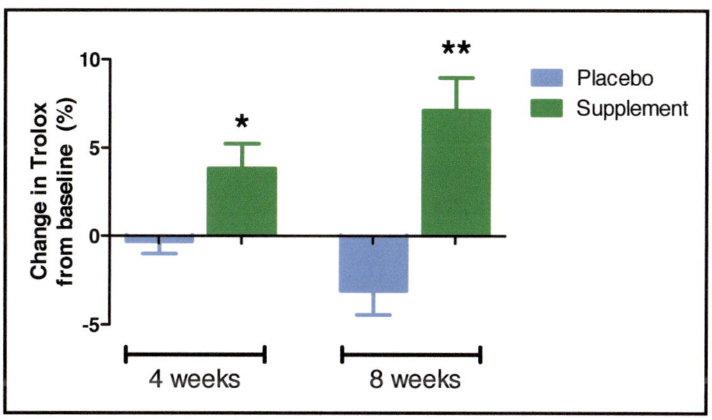

Figure 12. Change relative to baseline in serum concentrations of trolox, a measure of total antioxidant capacity, in greens+bone builder™-treated postmenopausal women was significantly increased after 4 and 8 weeks while that in the placebo-treated control was marginally decreased. Treated values were also higher than the placebo [unpaired t-test (*p<0.01, **p<0.0001)]. Values are mean ± SEM.

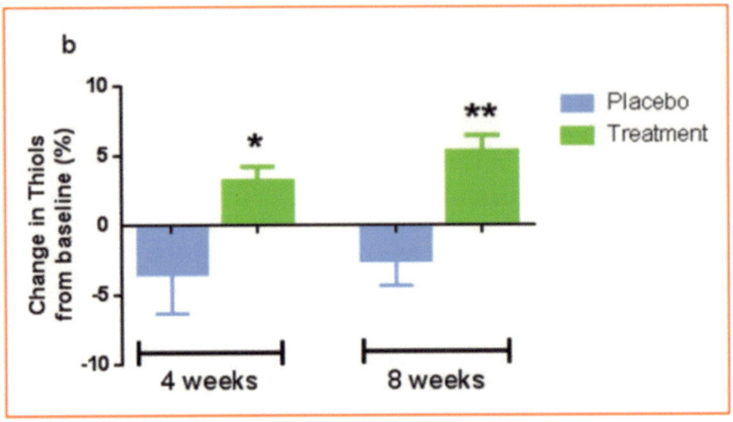

Figure 13. Change relative to baseline in serum concentrations of thiol in greens+bone builder-treated postmenopausal women was significantly increased after 4 and 8 weeks (meaning decreased protein oxidation) while that in the placebo-treated control was unchanged; treated values were also higher than the placebo. Mann-Whitney test (*p<0.05, **p<0.001). Values are mean ± SEM.

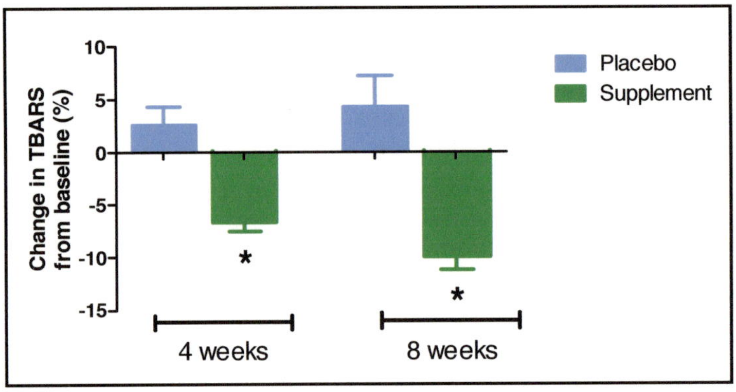

Figure 14. Change relative to baseline in serum concentrations of TBARS in greens+bone builder™-treated postmenopausal women was significantly decreased after 4 and 8 weeks (meaning decreased lipid peroxidation) while that in the placebo-treated control was unchanged; treated values were also lower than the placebo. Mann-Whitney test (*p<0.05, **p<0.001). Values are mean ± SEM.

In order to test whether the antioxidant properties of greens+bone builder™ can prevent the risk of osteoporosis in postmenopausal women, we also measured the serum bone turnover markers, C-terminal telopeptide of type I collagen (CTX) as indicator of bone resorption, and procollagen type I N-terminal propeptide (PINP) as indicator of bone formation, in addition to the serum antioxidant capacity, and the oxidative stress parameters lipid peroxidation, protein oxidation. As shown in Figure 15, statistical analysis showed that at 8 weeks, the greens +bone builderTM supplement group significantly decreased the bone resorption marker CTX, while the Placebo group showed no significant changes. The supplement group was also significantly different from that of the Placebo group in all parameters measured. This decrease in CTX correlated to the increase in their serum total antioxidant capacity [Figure 12] and decreases in oxidative parameters protein oxidation [Figure 13] lipid peroxidation [Figure 14]. These results suggest that a daily supplementation with polyphenols and micronutrients may be important in reducing oxidative damage by reducing bone resorption, thereby reducing the risk of osteoporosis in postmenopausal women [41].

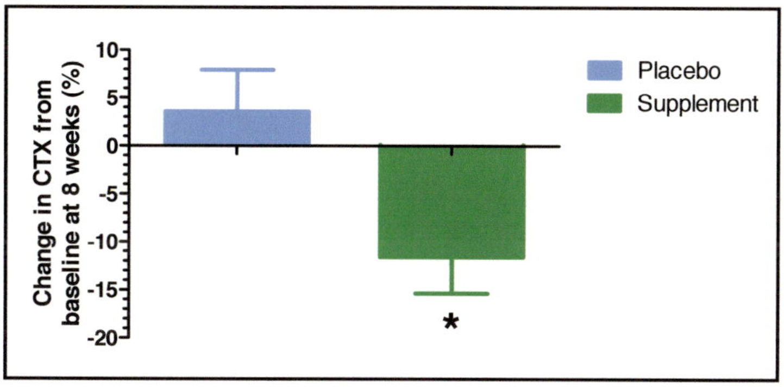

Figure 15. Change relative to baseline in serum concentrations of CTX in greens+bone builder™-treated postmenopausal women was significantly decreased after 8 weeks (meaning decreased bone resorption marker) compared to that of the placebo-treated control (a paired t-test (*$p<0.05$).. Values are mean ± SEM.

7.3. Concluding remarks

Studies reported in the literature on the role of polyphenols in bone health have exploded in the last 10 years, but most of the reports involved in vitro studies in osteoclasts and osteoblasts, animal studies and epidemiologicai studies. There is little doubt from the excellent studies reported that oxidative stress is one of the primary culprits responsible for the pathogenesis of osteoporosis via its role in osteoclastic resoption and the detrimental effects on the bone-forming osteoblasts. To date, only four clinical intervention studies have been reported, including ours. It is easy to see why it is very difficult to evaluate the role of polyphenols since, as we learned from this review, there are at least 8,000 different polyphenols identified to date, and each one probably having different effects on humans. Additionally, polyphenols are present in food with other constituents that may also be beneficial to bone health. In our clinical study, we combined the effects of a combination of polyphenols present in the nutritional supplement from greens+™ with the nutritional components present in bone builder™ such as minerals, vitamins and other nutrients. It is possible that the effects of greens+bone builder^{tm} in increasing total antioxidant capacity, decreasing the oxidative stress markers protein oxidation and lipid peroxidation which correlated to the decrease in bone turnover marker for bone resorption is a result of the combined effects of the different polyphenols it contained with those of the other nutritional components present in the bone builder™. It remained for future studies to zero in on specific component that is responsible for its beneficial effect.

8. General summary and conclusion

In conclusion, we showed that oxidative stress due to ROS that are shown to cause the development of osteoporosis may be prevented by supplementation with the antioxidants lycopene and polyphenols. Results of in vitro studies in osteoblasts and osteoclasts, animal intervention studies, epidemiological studies and clinical intervention studies on lycopene and polyphenols are evidence for their potential use as alternative or complementary agent with other established drugs approved for the prevention or treatment of osteoporosis in postmenopausal women.

Acknowledgements

Funding for this research into Oxidative Stress, Antioxidants and Bone Health is shared by Genuine Health Ltd (Canada), the H.J. Heinz Co (Canada), Millenium Biologix Inc. (Canada), Kagome Co. (Japan) and LycoRed Natural Product Industries, Ltd. (Israel) and matched by the Canadian Institutes of Health Research (CIHR). We sincerely thanked the valuable contributions to this research by the following students/graduate students and staff at the Calcium Research Laboratory, Department of Medicine at St Michael's Hospital and the University of Toronto and Department of Nutritional Sciences, University of Toronto: Dr. Bala Balachandran, Jaclyn Beca, Dawn Snyder, Loren Chan, Honglei Shen, Salva Sadeghi, Ayesha Quireshi, Dr. Erin Mackinnon and Nancy Kang. Their contributions were based on their experimental data, written reports published/in press manuscripts. We would also like to thank to Dr. R.G. Josse for providing us with his medical expertice as well as allowing us access to his list of patients we were able to recruit. Special thanks to Dr. H. Vandenberghe for carrying out the CTX assay and for her valuable suggestions.

Author details

L.G. Rao[1*] and A.V. Rao[2]

*Address all correspondence to: leticia.rao@utoronto.ca

1 Department of Medicine, St Michael's Hospital and University of Toronto, Canada

2 Department of Nutritional Sciences, University of Toronto, Canada

References

[1] Ahmed, S, & Elmantaser, M. Secondary osteoporosis. Endocr Dev. (2009). , 16, 170-90.

[2] Hopkins, R, Pullenayegum, E, Goeree, R, Adachi, J, Papaioannou, A, Leslie, W, et al. Estimation of the lifetime risk of hip fracture for women and men in Canada. Osteoporos Int (2012). , 23(3), 921-7.

[3] Tarride, J, Hopkins, R, Leslie, W, Morin, S, & Adachi, J. Papaioannou Aea. The burden of illness of osteoporosis in Canada. Osteoporos Int 2012. (2012). Epub Mar 8. [Epub ahead of print].

[4] Cooper, C, & Campion, G. Melton Lr. Hip fractures in the elderly: a world-wide projection. Osteoporos International. (1992).

[5] Coxam, V. New advances in osteoporosis nutritional prevention. Med Sci (Paris). (2005). , 21(3), 297-301.

[6] Gullberg, B, Johnell, O, & Kanis, J. World-wide projections for hip fracture. Osteoporos International. (1997).

[7] Bleibler, F, Konnopka, A, Benzinger, P, Rapp, K, & König, H. The health burden and costs of incident fractures attributable to osteoporosis from 2010 to 2050 in Germany-a demographic simulation model. Osteoporos Int. (2012). Epub July 14 2012[Epub ahead of print].

[8] Lindsay, R, Burge, R, & Strauss, D. One year outcomes and costs following a vertebral fracture. Osteoporosis Int. (2005). , 16, 78-85.

[9] wwwfountia.com/history-osteoporosis.

[10] [10] Rossouw, J, Anderson, G, & Prentice, R. LaCroix A, Kooperberg C, Stefanick M, et al. Risks and Benefits of Estrogen Plus Progestin in Healthy Postmenopausal Women Principal Results From the Women's Health Initiative Randomized Controlled Trial. JAMA. (2002).

[11] Schmidt, G, Horner, K, Mcdanel, D, Ross, M, & Moores, K. Risks and benefits of long-term bisphosphonate therapy. Am J Health Syst Pharm. (2010).

[12] Diab, D, & Watts, N. Bisphosphonates in the treatment of osteoporosis. Endocrinol Metab Clin North Am. 2012((3)):487-506. Epub 41 Epub (2012). Jun 9.

[13] Feng, X, & Mcdonald, J. Disorders of bone remodeling. Annu Rev Pathol. (2011). , 6, 121-45.

[14] Baron, R, & Hesse, E. Update on Bone Anabolics in Osteoporosis Treatment: Rationale, Current Status, and Perspectives J Clin Endocrinol Metab (2012).

[15] Gallagher, J, & Sai, A. Molecular biology of bone remodeling: implications for new therapeutic targets for osteoporosis. Maturitas. (2010). , 65(4), 301-7.

[16] Riggs, B, & Melton, L. I. The worldwide problem of osteoporosis: Insights afforded by epidemiology. Bone. (1995). Suppl):505S-11S.

[17] Christenson, E, Jiang, X, Kagan, R, & Schnatz, P. Osteoporosis management in post-menopausal women. Minerva Ginecol. (2012).

[18] Watts, N, Adler, R, Bilezikian, J, Drake, M, Eastell, R, Orwoll, E, et al. Osteoporosis in men: an Endocrine Society clinical practice guideline Clin Endocrinol Metab. (2012)., 97(6), 1802-22.

[19] Legrand, E, Hoppé, E, Bouvard, B, & Audran, M. Osteoporosis in men (Review). Rev Prat (2012)., 62(2), 193-7.

[20] Drake, M, & Khosla, A. Male osteoporosis Endocrinol Metab. Clin North Am. 2012;41((3)):629-41. Epub (2012). June 17.

[21] Szulc, P. Biochemical Bone TurnoverMarkers and Osteoporosis in OlderMen:Where AreWe? (Review). Journal of Osteoporosis. 2011;Epub Epub (2011). Dec 15., 2011, 1-5.

[22] Szulc, P, Garnero, P, Munoz, F, Marchand, F. D, & Cross-sectional, P. D. evaluation of bone metabolism in men. Journal of Bone and Mineral Research. (2001)., 16(9), 1642-50.

[23] Dennison, E, Eastell, R, Fall, C, Kellingray, S, Wood, P, & Cooper, C. Determinants of bone loss in elderly men and women: a prospective population-based study. Osteoporosis International. (1999)., 10(5), 384-91.

[24] Hegge, K, Fornoff, A, Gutierres, S, & Haack, S. New therapies for osteoporosis. Journal of Pharmacy Practice (2009)., 22, 53-64.

[25] Czerwinski, E, Badurski, J, & Osieleniec, E M-S. J. Current understanding of osteoporosis according to the position of the World Health Organization (WHO) and International Osteoporosis Foundation.. Ortop Traumatol Rehabil. (2007).

[26] Nelson, H, Haney, E, Chou, R, Dana, T, Fu, R, & Bougatsos, C. Screening for Osteoporosis: Systematic Review to Update the 2002 U.S. Preventive Services Task Force Recommendation. Evidence Synthesis AHRQ Publication No. 10-05145-EF-1. Agency for Healthcare Research and Quality. (2010). (77)

[27] Wright, N, & Saag, K. From fracture risk prediction to evaluating fracture patterns: recent advances in the epidemiology of osteoporosis. Curr Rheumatol Rep. (2012).

[28] Leslie, W, Majumdar, S, Lix, L, Johansson, H, Oden, A, Mccloskey, E, et al. High fracture probability with FRAX usually indicates densitometric osteoporosis: implications for clinical practice. Osteoporos Int. 2012;Epub (2011). Mar, 23(1), 391-7.

[29] Shuler, F, Conjeski, J, Kendall, D, & Salava, J. Understanding the Burden of Osteoporosis and Use of the World Health Organization FRAX. Orthopedics. (2012)., 35(9), 798-805.

[30] Mccloskey, E, & Kanis, J. FRAX updates. Curr Opin Rheumatol. (2012)., 24(5), 554-60.

[31] Kular, J, Tickner, J, Chim, S, & Xu, J. An overview of the regulation of bone remodelling at the cellular level. Clin Biochem. 2012;45(12):12. Epub (2012). Mar 23.

[32] Lee, J, & Vasikaran, S. Current recommendations for laboratory testing and use of bone turnover markers in management of osteoporosis. Annual Lab Med. (2012)., 32, 105-12.

[33] Kim, N, & Eastell, R. Bone turnover markers: use in osteoporosis. Nature Reviews Rheumatology (2012). , 8, 379-89.

[34] Silverman, S, Nasser, K, & Nattrass, S. B D. Impact of bone turnover markers and/or educational information on persistence to oral bisphosphonate therapy: a community setting-based trial. Osteoporos Int. 2011;Epub (2011). Jul 14., 23(3), 1069-74.

[35] Vasikaran, S, Eastell, R, Bruyère, O, Foldes, A, Garnero, P, Griesmacher, A, et al. Markers of bone turnover for the prediction of fracture risk and monitoring of osteoporosis treatment: a need for international reference standards. Osteoporos Int ((2011).

[36] Seibel, M. J. Biochemical Markers of Bone Turnover Part I: Biochemistry and Variability. Clin Biochem Rev (2005). , 26(4), 97-122.

[37] Mackinnon, E, Rao, A, Josse, R, & Rao, L. Supplementation with the antioxidant lycopene significantly decreases oxidative stress parameters and the bone resorption marker N-telopeptide of type I collagen in postmenopausal women. Osteoporosis International. (2011). , 22(4), 1091-101.

[38] Mackinnon, E, Rao, A, & Rao, L. Dietary restriction of lycopene for a period of one month resulted in significantly increased biomarkers of oxidative stress and bone resorption in postmenopausal women. Journal of Nutrition, Health & Aging. (2011). , 15(2), 133-8.

[39] Rao, L, Mackinnon, E, Josse, R, Murray, T, Strauss, A, & Rao, A. Lycopene consumption decreases oxidative stress and bone resorption markers in postmenopausal women. Osteoporosis International. (2007).

[40] Kang, N, Rao, A, De Asis, K, Chan, L, & Rao, L. Antioxidant effects of a nutritional supplement containing polyphenols in postmenopausal women: a randomized controlled study. Journal of Aging: Research and Clinical Practice. (2012).

[41] Kang, N, Rao, A, Josse, R, Vandenberghe, H, De Asis, K, Chan, L, et al. Dietary polyphenols and nutritional supplements significantly decreased oxidative stress parameters and the bone resorption marker collagen type 1 cross-linked C-telopeptide in postmenopausal women. Osteoporosis International (Submitted for publication). (2012).

[42] Brown, J, Albert, C, Nassar, B, Adachi, J, Cole, D, Davison, K, et al. Bone turnover markers in the management of postmenopausal osteoporosis (review). Clin Biochem :. 2009; 42(10-11):929-42. Epub (2009). Apr 10.

[43] Bergmann, P, & Al, e. Evidence-based guidelines for the use of biochemical markers of bone turnover in the selection and monitoring of bisphosphonate treatment in osteoporosis: a consensus document of the Belgian Bone Club. Int J Clin Pract (2009). , 63, 19-26.

[44] Glover, S, Garnero, P, Naylor, K, Rogers, A, & Eastell, R. Establishing a reference range for bone turnover markers in young, healthy women. Bone. (2008). , 42, 623-30.

[45] Monti, J. Osteoporosis Risk Factors http://askhealthlinecom/health/osteoporosis-risk-factors.(2010).

[46] Stetzer, E. Identifying Risk Factors for Osteoporosis in Young Women. The Internet Journal of Allied Health Sciences and Practice. (2011). , 9(4), 1-8.

[47] Rao, L. Will tomatoes prevent osteoporosis. Snell Endocrine Rounds. (2005). , 5(2), 1-6.

[48] Furness, S, Roberts, H, Marjoribanks, J, & Lethaby, A. Hormone therapy in postmenopausal women and risk of endometrial hyperplasia. Cochrane Database of Systematic Reviews. 2012(8). Epub 15 AUG (2012).

[49] Bell, N. H, & Johnson, R. H. Bisphosphonates in the treatment of osteoporosis: virtual symposium on osteoporosis. Endocrine. (1997). , 6(2), 203-6.

[50] Dempster, D. W, & Bolognese, M. A. Ibandronate: The Evolution of a Once-a-Month Oral Therapy for Postmenopausal Osteoporosis. Journal of Clinical Densitometry. (2006). , 9(1), 58-65.

[51] Sunyecz, J. Optimizing dosing frequencies for bisphosphonates in the management of postmenopausal osteoporosis: patient considerations. Clin Interv Aging. 2008;Epub (2008). December., 3(4), 611-27.

[52] Lyritis, G. P. Fracture healing and antiosteoporotic treatments. Medicographia 2010; (2010). , 32, 79-85.

[53] Han, S, & Wan, S. Effect of teriparatide on bone mineral density and fracture in postmenopausal osteoporosis: meta-analysis of randomised controlled trials. International Journal of Clinical Practice. (2012). , 66(2), 199-209.

[54] Adler, R. A, & Gill, R. S. Clinical utility of denosumab for treatment of bone loss in men and women. Clin Interv Aging. 2011;Epub (2011). May 24., 6, 119-24.

[55] Watts, N, & Long-term, D. L D. Use of Bisphosphonates in Osteoporosis. The Journal of Clinical Endocrinology & Metabolism. 2010;Epub February 19, (2010). , 95(4), 1555-65.

[56] Rees, M. Management of the menopause: integrated health-care pathway for the menopausal woman. Menopause Int. (2011).

[57] Pomerleau, J, Lock, K, Knai, C, & Mckee, M. Effectiveness of intervention and programmes promoting fruit and vegeta ble intake. WHO. (2005).

[58] Rao, A, & Carotenoids, L. G R. and human health (Review) Pharmacological Research. (2007). , 55(3), 207-16.

[59] New, S. Intake of fruit and vegetables: Implications for bone health. The Proceedings of the Nutrition Society. (2003). , 62(4), 889-99.

[60] Lister, C, Skinner, M, & Hunter, D. Fruits, vegetables and their phytochemicals for bone and joint health. Curr Top Nutraceut Res. (2007). , 5, 67-82.

[61] Tucker, K, Hannan, M, Chen, H, Cupples, L, Wilson, P, & Kiel, D. Potassium, magnesium, and fruit and vegetable intakes are associated with greater bone mineral density in elderly men and women. The American Journal of Clinical Nutrition. (1999). , 69(4), 727-36.

[62] Palacious, C. The role of nutrients in bone health, from A to Z. Critical Reviews in Food Science & Nutrition. (2006). , 46, 621-8.

[63] Raman, W, & Khalid, A. right Nin. Studies on free radicals, antioxidants, and co-factors. Clinical Interventions in Aging. (2007). , 2(2), 219-36.

[64] Manolagas, S, & Parfitt, A. What old means to bone. Trends Endocrinol Metab. 2010;Epub (2010). Mar 11., 21(6), 369-3744.

[65] Sahnoun, Z, Jamoussi, K, & Zeghal, K. Free radicals and antioxidants: human physiology, pathology and therapeutic aspects. Therapie. (1997). , 52, 251-0.

[66] Juránek, I, & Bezek, Š. S. Controversy of Free Radical Hypothesis: Reactive Oxygen Species- Cause or Consequence of Tissue Injury? Gen Physiol Biophys (2005), 24, 263-278 263. (2005). , 24, 2263-278.

[67] Semba, R. D, Ferrucci, L, Sun, K, Walston, J, Varadhan, R, Guralnik, J. M, et al. Oxidative Stress Is Associated with Greater Mortality in Older Women Living in the Community. J Am Geriatr Soc 2007. (2007). , 55(9), 1421-5.

[68] Lee, D, Lim, B, Lee, Y. K, & Yang, H. C. Effects of hydrogen peroxide (H2O2) on alkaline phosphatase activity and matrix mineralization of odontoblast and osteoblast cell lines. Cell Biol Toxicol 22. (2006). , 22, 39-46.

[69] Willcox, J, Ash, S, & Catignani, G. Antioxidants and prevention of chronic disease. Crit Rev Food Sci Nutr. (2004). , 44, 275-95.

[70] Griffiths HReaBiomarkers. Mol Aspects Med. (2002). , 23, 101-8.

[71] Videra, J, Lehtmaab, J, Kullisaarc, T, Vihalemmc, T, Zilmerc, K, Kairanec, Č, et al. Acute immuneresponse in respect to exercise-induced oxidativestress. Pathophysiology. (2001). , 7(4), 263-70.

[72] Turan, V, Mizrak, S, Yurekli, B, Yilmaz, C, & Ercan, G. The effect of long-term nicotine exposure on bone mineral density and oxidative stress in female Swiss Albino rats. Arch Gynecol Obstet (2012). Epub Sep 7. [Epub ahead of print].

[73] Tanriverdi, H, Evrengul, H, Kuru, O, Tanriverdi, S, Seleci, D, Enli, Y, et al. Cigarette smoking induced oxidative stress may impair endothelial function and coronary blood flow in angiographically normal coronary arteries. Official Journal of the Japanese Circulation Society. (2006). , 70(5), 593-9.

[74] Ronis, M, Mercer, K, & Chen, J. Effects of nutrition and alcohol consumption on bone loss (Review). Curr Osteoporos Rep. (2011). , 9(2), 53-9.

[75] Maurel, D, Boisseau, N, Benhamou, C, & Jaffre, C. Alcohol and bone: review of dose effects and mechanisms. Osteoporos Int. 2012;Epub Epub (2011). Sep 17. Review., 23(1), 1-16.

[76] Altindag, O, Erel, O, Soran, N, Celik, H, & Selek, S. Total oxidative/anti-oxidative status and relation to bone mineral density in osteoporosis. Rheumatol Int. 2008;Epub Epub (2007). Sep 6., 28(4), 317-21.

[77] Baur, A, Henkel, J, Bloch, W, Treiber, N, Scharffetter-kochanek, K, Brüggemann, G, et al. Effect of exercise on bone and articular cartilage in heterozygous manganese superoxide dismutase (SOD2) deficient mice. Free Radic Res. 2011;Epub Epub (2011). Feb 4., 5(45), 550-80.

[78] Lu, P, Lai, C, & Chan, W. Caffeine induces cell death via activation of apoptotic signal and inactivation of survival signal in human osteoblasts. Int J Mol Sci. 2008;Epub Epub (2008). May 8., 9(5), 698-718.

[79] Schröder, P, & Krutmann, J. Environmental Oxidative Stress- Environmental Sources of ROS. Heidelberg: Springer Verlag; (2005).

[80] Schoneich, C. Reactive oxygen species and biological aging: a mechanistic approach. Experimental Gerontology. (1999)., 34, 19-34.

[81] Zhang, Y, Zhong, Z, Hou, G, Jiang, H, & Chen, J. Involvement of oxidative stress in age-related bone loss. J Surg Res. 2011;169(1):eEpub Epub (2011). Mar 21., 37-42.

[82] Mate, J. M, & Perez-gomez, C. Nunez de Castro I. Antioxidant Enzymes and Human Diseases. Clinical Biochemistry. (1999)., 32(8), 595-603.

[83] Rao, L. Lycopene and the Prevention of Osteoporosis. AV R, editor. Scotland: Caledonia Science; (2006).

[84] Rao, A, & Carotenoids, L. G R. and human health (Review). Pharmacological Research. (2007)., 55(3), 207-16.

[85] Rao, A, Ray, M, & Rao, L. Lycopene. In: SL T, editor. Advances in Food and Nutrition Research. New York,: Academic Press Publication; (2006)., 99-164.

[86] Agarwal, S. AV R. Tomato lycopene and its role in human health and chronic diseases. CMAJ. (2000)., 163(6), 739-44.

[87] Khachik, F, Carvallo, L, Bernstein, P, Muir, G, Zhao, D, & Katz, N. Chemistry, distribution and metabolism of tomato carotenoids and their impact on human health. Exp Biol Med. (2002)., 227(10), 845-51.

[88] Di Mascio PKaiser S, Sies H. Lycopene as the most effcient biological carotenoid singlet oxygen quencher. Arch Biochem Biophys. (1989)., 274, 532-8.

[89] Stahl, W, & Sies, H. Uptake of lycopene and its geometrical isomers is greater from heat-processed than from unprocessed tomato juice in humans. J Nutr. (1992)., 122, 2161-6.

[90] Stahl, W, Schwarz, W, Sundquist, A, & Sies, H. cis-trans Isomers of lycopene and b-carotene in human serum and tissues. Arch Biochem Biophys. (1992). , 294, 173-7.

[91] Parker, R. Absorption, metabolism and transport of carotenoids.. FASEB J. (1996). , 10, 542-51.

[92] Ahuja, K, Pittaway, J, & Ball, M. Effects of olive oil and tomato lycopene combination on serum lycopene, lipid profile, and lipid oxidation. Nutrition. (2006). , 22, 259-65.

[93] Zhang, L, Cooney, R, & Bertram, J. Carotenoids enhance gap junctional communication and inhibit lipid peroxidation in C3H/10T1/2 cells: relationship to their cancer chemo-preventive action. Carcinogenesis. (1991). , 12, 2109-14.

[94] Amir, H K. M, Giat, J, et al. Lycopene and 1,25(OH)2D3 cooperate in the inhibition of cell cycle progression and induction of HL-60 leukemic cells. Nutr Cancer. (1999). , 33, 105-12.

[95] Rao, A. Lycopene and the prevention of chronic diseases: major findings from five international conferences. In: Rao A, Heber D, editors. Lycopene, tomatoes and health: new perspectives. Scotland: Caledonian Science Press; (2002).

[96] Rao, A, & Rao, L. Lycopene and human Health. Current Topics in Nutraceutical Research. (2004). , 2, 127-36.

[97] Giovannucci, E. Tomatoes, tomato-based products, lycopene, and cancer: Review of the epidemiologic literature. J Natl Cancer Inst. (1999). , 91, 317-31.

[98] Sahni, S, Hannan, M, Blumberg, J, Cupples, L, Kiel, D, & Tucker, K. Protective effect of total carotenoid and lycopene intake on the risk of hip fracture: a 17-year follow-up from the Framingham Osteoporosis Study. Journal of Bone & Mineral Research (2009). , 24(6), 1086-94.

[99] Quideau, S, Deffieux, D, Douat-casassus, C, & Pouysegu, L. Plant polyphenols: chemical properties, biological activities, and synthesis. Angew Chem Int Ed Engl. (2011). Epub 2011/01/13., 50(3), 586-21.

[100] Hendrich, A. Flavonoid-membrane interactions: Possible consequences for biological effects of some polyphenolic compounds. Acta Pharmacologica Sinica. (2006). , 27(1), 27-40.

[101] Woo, J, Yonezawa, T, & Nagai, K. Phytochemicals that stimulate osteoblastic differentiation and bone formation. Journal of Oral Bioscience. (2010). , 52(1), 15-21.

[102] Manach, C, Scalbert, A, Morand, C, Rémésy, C, & Jimenez, L. Polyphenols: food sources and bioavailability. American Journal of Clinical Nutrition. (2004). , 79, 727-47.

[103] Tsao, R. Chemistry and biochemistry of dietary polyphenols. Nutrients. (2010). Epub 2010/01/19., 2(12), 1231-46.

[104] Puel, C, Coxam, V, & Davicco, M. Mediterranean diet and osteoporosis prevention. Med Sci (Paris). (2007). , 23, 756-60.

[105] Urquiaga, I, Strobel, P, Perez, D, Martinez, C, Cuevas, A, Castillo, O, et al. Mediterranean diet and red wine protect against oxidative damage in young volunteers. Atherosclerosis. (2010). Epub 2010 Apr 21., 211(2), 694-9.

[106] Rao, A, Balachandran, B, Shen, H, Logan, A, & Rao, L. In Vitro and in Vivo Antioxidant Properties of the Plant-Based Supplement Greens+. Int J Mol Sci. (2011). , 12, 4896-908.

[107] Samoto, H, Shimizu, E, Matsuda-honjo, Y, & Al, e. TNF-alpha suppresses bone sialoprotein (BSP) expression in ROS17/2.8 cells. J Cellular Biochemistry. (2002). , 87(3), 313-23.

[108] Cortizo, A, Bruzzone, L, Molinuevo, S, & Etcheverry, S. A possible role of oxidative stress in the vanadium-induced cytotoxicity in the MC3T3E1 osteoblast and UMR106 osteosarcoma cell lines. Toxicology. (2000). , 147, 89-99.

[109] Liu, H-C, Cheng, R-M, Lin, F-H, & Fang, H-W. Sintered beta-dicalcium phosphate particles induce intracellular reactive oxygen species in rat osteoblasts. Biomed Eng Appl Basis Commun. (1999). , 11, 259-64.

[110] Nam, S, Jung, S, Yoo, C, Ahn, E, & Suh, C. H. O2 enhances Ca2+ release from osteoblast internal stores. Yonsei Medical Journal. (2002). , 43(2), 229-35.

[111] Mody, N, Parhami, F, Sarafian, T, & Demer, L. Oxidative stress modulates osteoblastic differentiation of vascular and bone cells. Free Radic Biol Med. (2001). , 31, 509-19.

[112] Park, B, Yoo, C, Kim, H, Kwon, C, & Kim, Y. Role of mitogen-activated protein kinases in hydrogen peroxide-induced cell death in osteoblastic cells. Toxicology. (2005).

[113] Arai, M, Shibata, Y, Pugdee, K, Abiko, Y, & Ogata, Y. Effects of reactive oxygen species (ROS) on antioxidant system and osteoblastic differentiation in MC3T3-E1 cells. IUBMB Life. (2007). , 59, 27-33.

[114] Liu, A, Zhang, Z, Zhu, B, Liao, Z, & Liu, Z. Metallothionein protects bone marrow stromal cells against hydrogen peroxide-induced inhibition of osteoblastic differentiation. Cell Biol Int. (2004). , 28, 905-11.

[115] Ueno, T, Yamada, M, & Igarashi, Y. Ogawa T. N-acetyl cysteine protects osteoblastic function from oxidative stress. J Biomed Mater Res A. (2011). Epub 2011 Sep 13., 99(4), 523-31.

[116] Xu, Z, Wang, X, Xiao, D, Hu, L, Lu, M, Wu, Z, et al. Hydrogen sulphide protects MC3T3-E1 osteoblastic cells against H2O2-induced oxidative damage-implications for the treatment of osteoporosis. Free Radical Biology & Medicine. (2011). , 50(10), 1314-23.

[117] Hu, Y, Cheng, H, Hsieh, B, Huang, L, & Huang, T. KL C. Arsenic trioxide affects bone remodeling by effects on osteoblast differentiation and function. Bone. (2012). Epub 2012 Mar 19., 50(6), 1406-15.

[118] Zijlstra, W, Bulstra, S, Van Raay, J, Van Leeuwen, B, & Kuijer, R. Cobalt and chromium ions reduce human osteoblast-like cell activity in vitro, reduce the OPG to RANKL ratio, and induce oxidative stress. J Orthop Res. (2012). Epub 2011 Oct 24., 30(5), 740-7.

[119] Rivadeneira, J. Di Virgilio A, Barrio D, Muglia C, Bruzzone L, Etcheverry S. Cytotoxicity of a Vanadyl(IV) Complex with a Multidentate Oxygen Donor in Osteoblast Cell Lines in Culture. Med Chem (2010). Epub 2010 Feb 16. [Epub ahead of print].

[120] Fatokun, A, Stone, T, & Smith, R. Responses of differentiated MC3T3-E1 osteoblast-like cells to reactive oxygen species. Eur J Pharmacol. (2008). , 587, 35-41.

[121] Manolagas, S. C, & Almeida, M. Gone with the Wnts: β-Catenin, T-Cell Factor, Forkhead Box O, and Oxidative Stress in Age-Dependent Diseases of Bone, Lipid, and Glucose Metabolism. Molecular Endocrinology. (2007). , 21(11), 2605-14.

[122] Almeida, M, Han, L, Martin-millan, M, Brien, O, & Manolagas, C. S. Oxidative stress antagonizes Wnt signaling in osteoblast precursors by diverting beta-catenin from T cell factor- to forkhead box O-mediated transcription. J Biol Chem. (2007). Epub 2007 Jul 10., 282(37), 298-305.

[123] Rached, M, Kode, A, Xu, L, Yoshikawa, Y, Paik, J, Depinho, R, et al. FoxO1 is a positive regulator of bone formation by favoring protein synthesis and resistance to oxidative stress in osteoblasts. Cell Metab. (2010). , 11(2), 147-60.

[124] Ambrogini, E, Almeida, M, Martin-millan, M, Paik, J, Depinho, R, Han, L, et al. FoxO-mediated defense against oxidative stress in osteoblasts is indispensable for skeletal homeostasis in mice. Cell Metab. (2010). , 11(2), 136-46.

[125] Zhang, J, Yang, L, Meng, G, Fan, J, & Al, e. Protective effect of tetrahydroxystilbene glucoside against hydrogen peroxide-induced dysfunction and oxidative stress in osteoblastic MC3TE1 cells. Eur J Pharmacol. (2012). Epub 2012 Jun 7, 3.

[126] Liang, D, Yang, M, Guo, B, Cao, J, Yang, L, Guo, X, et al. Zinc inhibits H(2)O(2)-induced MC3T3-E1 cells apoptosis via MAPK and PI3K/AKT pathways. Biol Trace Elem Res. (2012). Epub 2012 Mar 21., 148(3), 420-9.

[127] Wang, Y, Zhao, L, Wang, Y, Xu, J, Nie, Y, Guo, Y, et al. Curculigoside isolated from Curculigo orchioides prevents hydrogen peroxide-induced dysfunction and oxidative damage in calvarial osteoblasts. Acta Biochim Biophys Sin (Shanghai). (2012). Epub 2012 Mar 16., 44(5), 431-41.

[128] Holzer, N, Braun, K, Ehnert, S, Egaña, J, Schenck, T, Buchholz, A, et al. Green tea protects human osteoblasts from cigarette smoke-induced injury: possible clinical implication. Langenbecks Arch Surg (2012). Epub 2011 Dec 8., 397(3), 467-74.

[129] Zhao, X, Xu, Z, Zhang, Q, & Yang, Y. Simvastatin protects human osteosarcoma cells from oxidative stress-induced apoptosis through mitochondrial-mediated signaling. Mol Med Report. (2012). Epub 2011 Oct 19., 5(2), 483-8.

[130] Sun, L, Zhang, J, Lu, X, Zhang, L, & Zhang, Y. Evaluation to the antioxidant activity of total flavonoids extract from persimmon (Diospyros kaki L.) leaves. Food Chem Toxicol. (2011). Epub 2011 Jul 23.

[131] Iwasaki, Y, Yamato, H, & Fukagawa, M. Treatment with pravastatin attenuates oxidative stress and protects osteoblast cell viability from indoxyl sulfate. Ther Apher Dial. (2011). Epub 2011 Feb 20., 15(2), 151-5.

[132] Kim, Y, Lee, Y, & Choi, E. Linarin isolated from Buddleja officinalis prevents hydrogen peroxide-induced dysfunction in osteoblastic MC3T3-E1 cells. Cell Immunol. (2011). Epub 2011 Feb 19., 268(2), 112-6.

[133] Qiang, H, Zhang, C, Shi, Z, Yang, H, & Wang, K. Protective effects and mechanism of Panax Notoginseng saponins on oxidative stress-induced damage and apoptosis of rabbit bone marrow stromal cells. Chin J Integr Med. (2010). Epub 2010 Nov 26., 16(6), 525-30.

[134] Kim, Y, Lee, Y, & Choi, E. Chrysoeriol isolated from Eurya cilliata leaves protects MC3T3-E1 cells against hydrogen peroxide-induced inhibition of osteoblastic differentiation. J Appl Toxicol. (2010). , 30(7), 666-73.

[135] Choi, E. Protective effect of quercitrin against hydrogen peroxide-induced dysfunction in osteoblastic MC3T3-E1 cells. Exp Toxicol Pathol. (2012). Epub 2010 Sep 6., 64(3), 211-6.

[136] Hung, T, Chen, T, Liao, M, Ho, W, Liu, D, Chuang, W, et al. Drynaria fortunei J. Sm. promotes osteoblast maturation by inducing differentiation-related gene expression and protecting against oxidative stress-induced apoptotic insults. J Ethnopharmacol. (2010). Epub 2010 Jun 8.

[137] Choi, E, Kim, G, & Lee, Y. Carthamus tinctorius flower extract prevents H2O2-induced dysfunction and oxidative damage in osteoblastic MC3T3-E1 cells. Phytother Res. (2010). , 24(7), 1037-41.

[138] Almeida, M, Martin-millan, M, & Ambrogini, E. Bradsher Rr, Han L, Chen X, et al. Estrogens attenuate oxidative stress and the differentiation and apoptosis of osteoblasts by DNA-binding-independent actions of the ERalpha. J Bone Miner Res. (2010). , 25(4), 769-81.

[139] Choi, E, Kim, G, & Lee, Y. Atractylodes japonica root extract protects osteoblastic MC3T3-E1 cells against hydrogen peroxide-induced inhibition of osteoblastic differentiation. Phytother Res. (2009). , 23(11), 1537-42.

[140] Lee, K, & Choi, E. Myricetin, a naturally occurring flavonoid, prevents deoxy-D-ribose induced dysfunction and oxidative damage in osteoblastic MC3T3-E1 cells. Eur J Pharmacol. (2008). Epub 2008 Jun 7., 2.

[141] Silverton, S. Osteoclast radicals. J Cellular Biochemistry. (1994). , 56(3), 367-73.

[142] Key, L, Ries, W, Taylor, R, Hays, B, & Pitzer, B. Oxygen derived free radicals in osteoclasts: the specificity and location of the nitroblue tetrazolium reaction. Bone. (1990).

[143] Zaidi, M, Alam, A, Bax, B, et al. Role of the endothelial cell in osteoclast control: new perspectives. Bone. (1993). , 14, 97-102.

[144] Bax, B, Alam, A, Banerji, B, et al. Stimulation of osteoclastic bone resorption by hydrogen peroxide. Biochemical & Biophysical Research Communications. (1992). , 183, 1153-8.

[145] Steinbeck, M, Kim, J, Trudeau, M, Hauschka, P, & Karnovsky, M. Involvement of hydrogen peroxide in the differentiation of clonal HD-11EM cells into osteoclast-like cells. J Cell Physiology. (1998). , 176(3), 574-87.

[146] Suda, N, Morita, I, Kuroda, T, & Murota, S. Participation of oxidative stress in the process of osteoclast differentiation Biochimica et Biophysica Acta. (1993). , 1157, 318-23.

[147] Darden, A, Ries, W, Rodriguiz, R, & Key, J. L. Osteoclastic superoxide production and bone resorption: stimulation and inhibition by modulators ofn NADPH oxidase. J Bon Min Res 671-75. (1996). , 11(5), 671-5.

[148] Halleen, J, Raisanen, S, Salo, J, et al. Intracellular fragmentation of bone resorption products by reactive oxygen species generated by osteoclastic tartrate-resistant acid phosphatase. J Biological Chem. (1999). , 22907-10.

[149] Berger, C, Horrocks, B, & Datta, H. Direct non-genomic effect of steroid hormones on superoxide generation in the bone resorbing osteoclasts. Molecular and Cellular Endocrinology. (1999). , 149, 53-9.

[150] Wagner, A, Schroeter, M, & Hecker, M. b-estradiol inhibition of NADPH oxidase expression in human endothelial cells. FASEB J. (2001). , 15, 2121-30.

[151] Datta, H, Rathod, H, Manning, P, Turnbull, Y, & Mcneil, C. Parathyroid hormone induces superoxide anion burst in the osteoclasts: evidence of the direct instantaneous activation of the osteoclast by the hormone. J Endocrinology. (1996). , 149, 269-75.

[152] Oursler, M, Collin-osdoby, P, Li, L, Schmitt, E, & Osdoby, P. Evidence for an immunological and functional relationship between superoxide dismutase and a high molecular weight osteoclast plasma membrane glycoprotein. J Cellular Biochemistry. (1991). , 46(4), 331-44.

[153] Key, L, Wolf, W, Gundberg, C, & Ries, W. Superoxide and bone resorption. Bone. (1994). , 15, 431-6.

[154] Hall, T, Schaeublin, M, Fuller, K, & Chambers, T. The role of oxygen intermediates in osteoclastic bone resorption. Biochem Biophys Res Commun. (1995). , 207, 280-7.

[155] Bu, S, Lerner, M, Stoecker, B, Boldrin, E, Brackett, D, Lucas, E, et al. Dried plum polyphenols inhibit osteoclastogenesis by downregulating NFATc1 and inflammatory mediators. Calcif Tissue Int. (2008). , 82(6), 475-88.

[156] Oh, S, Kyung, T, & Choi, H. Curcumin inhibits osteoclastogenesis by decreasing receptor activator of nuclear factor-kappaB ligand (RANKL) in bone marrow stromal cells. Mol Cells. (2008). , 26(5), 486-9.

[157] Le Nihouannen DBarralet J, Fong J, Komarova S. Ascorbic acid accelerates osteoclast formation and death. Bone. (2010). Epub 2009 Nov 20., 46(5), 1336-43.

[158] Cui, Y, Bhandary, B, Marahatta, A, Lee, G, Li, B, Kim, D, et al. Characterization of Salvia miltiorrhiza ethanol extract as an antiosteoporotic agent. BMC Complement Altern Med. (2011).

[159] Fumimoto, R, Sakai, E, Yamaguchi, Y, Sakamoto, H, Fukuma, Y, Nishishita, K, et al. The coffee diterpene kahweol prevents osteoclastogenesis via impairment of NFATc1 expression and blocking of Erk phosphorylation. J Pharmacol Sci. (2012). Epub 2012 Mar 23., 118(4), 479-86.

[160] Sakamoto, H, Sakai, E, Fumimoto, R, Yamaguchi, Y, Fukuma, Y, Nishishita, K, et al. Deltamethrin inhibits osteoclast differentiation via regulation of heme oxygenase-1 and NFATc1. Toxicol In Vitro. (2012). Epub 2012 May 23., 26(6), 817-22.

[161] Yalin, S, Sagír, O, Comelekoglu, U, Berköz, M, & Eroglu, P. Strontium ranelate treatment improves oxidative damage in osteoporotic rat model. Pharmacol Rep. (2012). , 64(2), 396-402.

[162] Yin, H, Shi, Z, Yu, Y, Hu, J, Wang, R, Luan, Z, et al. Protection against osteoporosis by statins is linked to a reduction of oxidative stress and restoration of nitric oxide formation in aged and ovariectomized rats. Eur J Pharmacol. (2012). Epub 2011 Nov 23.

[163] Liu, X, Zhang, S, Lu, X, Zheng, S, & Xiong, F L. Z. Metabonomic study on the anti-osteoporosis effect of Rhizoma Drynariae and its action mechanism using ultraperformance liquid chromatography-tandem mass spectrometry. J Ethnopharmacol. (2011). Epub 2011 Nov 20., 139(1), 311-7.

[164] Cui, Y, Bhandary, B, Marahatta, A, Lee, G, Li, B, Kim, D, et al. Characterization of Salvia miltiorrhiza ethanol extract as an anti-osteoporotic agent. BMC Complement Altern Med. (2011). , 11, 120.

[165] Arslan, A, Orkun, S, Aydin, G, Keles, I, Tosun, A, Arslan, M, et al. Effects of ovariectomy and ascorbic acid supplement on oxidative stress parameters and bone mineral density in rats. Libyan J Med. (2011). Epub 2011 Oct 3.

[166] Kim, W. K K. K, Sul, O. J, Kim, H. J, Kim, S. H, Lee, M. H, Kim, H. J, Kim, S. Y, Chung, H. T, & Choi, H. S. Curcumin protects against ovariectomy-induced bone loss and decreases osteoclastogenesis. J Cell Biochem. (2011). , 112(11), 159-66.

[167] Nojiri, H, Saita, Y, Morikawa, D, Kobayashi, K, Tsuda, C, Miyazaki, T, et al. Cytoplasmic superoxide causes bone fragility owing to low-turnover osteoporosis and impaired collagen cross-linking. Journal of Bone & Mineral Research. Journal of Bone & Mineral Research (2011). , 26(11), 2682-94.

[168] Rao, L, Guns, M, & Rao, A. The role of lycopene in the prevention of chronic diseases. Agro Food Industry Hi Tech (Invited review). (2003).

[169] MacKinnon EThe Role of the Carotenoid Lycopene as an Antioxidant to Decrease Osteoporosis Risk in Women: Clinical and in vitro Studies [PHD desertation, Insitute of Medical Science]. Toronto, Ontario: University of Toronto; (2010).

[170] Singh, V. A current perspective on nutrition and exercise. J Nutr (1992)., 122, 760-65.

[171] Melhus, H, Michaelsson, K, Holmberg, L, Wolk, A, & Ljunghall, S. Smoking, antioxidant vitamins, and the risk of hip fracture. J Bone Min Res. (1999)., 14, 129-35.

[172] Morton, D, Barrett-connor, E, & Schneider, D. Vitamin C supplement and bone mineral density in postmenopausal women. J Bone Min Res. (2001)., 16, 135-40.

[173] Leveille, S. LaCroix A, Koepsell T, Beresford S, VanBelle G, Buchner D. Dietary vitamin C and bone mineral density in postmenopausal women in Washington State, USA. J Epidemiol Community Health. (1997).

[174] Polidori, M, Stahl, W, Eichler, O, Niestroj, I, & Sies, H. Free Rad Biol Med. (2001).

[175] Maggio, D, Barabani, M, Pierandrei, M, et al. Marked decrease in plasma antioxidants in aged osteoporotic women: results of a crosssectional study. J Clin Endocrin & Metabol. (2003)., 88(4), 1523-7.

[176] Basu, S, Michaelsson, K, Olofsson, H, Johansson, S, & Melhus, H. Association between oxidative stress and bone mineral density. Biochem Biophys Res Commun. (2001)., 288, 275-9.

[177] Sontakke, A, & Tare, R. A duality in the roles of reactive oxygen species with respect to bone metabolism. Clinica Chimica Acta. (2002)., 318, 145-8.

[178] Varanasi, S, Francis, R, Berger, C, Papiha, S, & Datta, H. Mitochondrial DNA deletion associated oxidative stress and severe male osteoporosis. Osteoporosis International. (1999).

[179] Telci AeaPostmenopausal hormone replacement therapy use decreases oxidative protein damage. Gynecol Obstet Invest. (2002)., 54, 88-93.

[180] Hahn MeaEffects of bone disease and calcium supplementation on antioxidant enzymes in postmenopausal women. Clin Biochem. (2008)., 41, 69-74.

[181] Sanchez-rodriguez, M, Ruiz-ramos, M, Correa-munoz, E, & Mendoza-nunez, V. Oxidative stress as a risk factor for osteoporosis in elderly Mexicans as characterized by antioxidant enzymes. BMC Musculoskelet Disord. (2007).

[182] Ozgocmen, S, Kaya, H, Fadillioglu, E, & Yilmaz, Z. Effects of calcitonin, risedronate, and raloxifene on erythrocyte antioxidant enzyme activity, lipid peroxidation, and nitric oxide in postmenopausal osteoporosis. Arch Med Res. (2007)., 38, 196-205.

[183] Korucuoglu UeaAssessment of protein oxidation in women using raloxifene. Mol Cell Biochem. (2006)., 290, 97-101.

[184] Sahni SeaProtective effect of total and supplemental vitamin C intake on the risk of hip fracture-a 17-year follow-up from the Framingham Osteoporosis Study. Osteoporos Int. (2009). , 20, 1853-61.

[185] Sugiura MeaBone mineral density in post-menopausal female subjects is associated with serum antioxidant carotenoids. Osteoporos Int. (2008). Epub 2011 Jul 16., 19, 211-9.

[186] Wattanapenpaiboon, N, Lukito, W, Wahlqvist, M, & Strauss, B. Dietary carotenoid intake as a predictor of bone mineral density. Asia Pac J Clin Nutr. (2003). , 12, 467-73.

[187] Wolf ReaLack of relation between vitamin and mineral antioxidants and bone mineral density: results from the Women's Health Initiative. Am J Clin Nutr. (2005). , 82, 581-8.

[188] Kim, L, Rao, A, Rao, L, & Lycopene, I. I. Effect on osteoblasts: The carotenoid lycopene stimulates cell proliferation and alkaline phosphatase activity of SaOS-2 cells. Journal of Medicinal Food. (2003). , 6, 79-88.

[189] Park, C. K, Ishimi, Y, Ohmura, M, Yamaguchi, M, Ikegami, S, & Vitamin, A. and carotenoids stimulate differentiation of mouse osteoblastic cells. J Nutr Sci and Vitaminol. (1997). , 43, 281-96.

[190] Rao, L, & Mackinnon, E. Cis lycopene isomers found in high concentrations in human serum, and which possess the greatest antioxidant capacity, were capable of preventing and repairing the damaging effects of reactive oxygen species in human osteoblast cells. May (2013). Lisbon, Portugal2013., 18-21.

[191] Ishimi, Y, Ohmura, M, Wang, X, Yamaguchi, M, & Ikegami, S. Inhibition by carotenoids and retinoic acid of osteoclast-like cell formation induced by bone resorbing agents in vitro. J Clin Biochem Nutr. (1999). , 27, 113-22.

[192] Rao, L, Krishnadev, N, Banasikowska, K, Rao, A, & Lycopene, I. Effect on Osteoclasts; Lycopene inhibits basal and parathyroid hormone (PTH)-stimulated osteoclast formation and mineral resorption mediated by reactive oxygen species (ROS) in rat bone marrow cultures. Journal of Medicinal Food. (2003). , 6, 69-78.

[193] Liang, H, Yu, F, Tong, Z, & Zeng, W. Lycopene effects on serum mineral elements and bone strength in rats. Molecules. (2012). , 17(6), 7093-102.

[194] Ke, B, & Xu, Z. Ling Yea. Modulation of experimental osteoporosis in rats by the antioxidant beverage effective microorganism-X (EM-X). Biomedicine & Pharmacotherapy. (2009). , 63(2), 114-9.

[195] Serra-majem, L, Roman, B, & Estruch, R. Scientific Evidence of Interventions Using the Mediterranean Diet: A Systematic Review. Nutrition Reviews. (2006). SS47., 27.

[196] Hagfors, L, Leanderson, P, Skoldstam, L, et al. Antioxidant intake, plasma antioxidants and oxidative stress in a randomized, controlled, parallel, Mediterranean dietary intervention study on patients with rheumatoid arthritis. Nutr J. (2003).

[197] Leighton, F, Cuevas, A, Guasch, V, et al. Plasma polyphenols and antioxidants, oxidative DNA damage and endothelial function in a diet and wine intervention study in humans. Drugs Exp Clin Res. (1999). , 25, 133-41.

[198] Yang, Z, Zhang, Z, Penniston, K, Binkley, N, & Tanumihardjo, S. Serum carotenoid concentrations in postmenopausal women from the United States with and without osteoporosis. International Journal for Vitamin & Nutrition Research. (2008).

[199] Misra, R, Mangi, S, Joshi, S, Mittal, S, Gupta, S, & Pandey, R. LycoRed as an alternative to hormone replacement therapy in lowering serum lipids and oxidative stress markers: a randomized controlled clinical trial. J Obstet Gynaecol Res. (2006). , 32, 299-304.

[200] Sahni, S, Hannan, M, Blumberg, J, Cupples, L, Kiel, D, & Tucker, K. Inverse association of carotenoid intakes with 4-y change in bone mineral density in elderly men and women: the Framingham Osteoporosis Study. American Journal of Clinical Nutrition. (2009). , 89(1), 416-24.

[201] Mackinnon, E, Sohemy, A, Rao, A, & Rao, L. Paraoxonase 1 polymorphisms 172T->A and 584A->G modify the association between serum concentrations of the antioxidant lycopene and bone turnover markers and oxidative stress parameters in women years of age. Journal of Nutrigenetics & Nutrigenomics. (2010). , 25-70.

[202] Rao, L, Mackinnon, E, Sohemy, A, & Rao, V. Postmenopausal Women with PON1 172TT Genotype Respond to Lycopene Intervention With a Decrease in Oxidative Stress Parameters and Bone Resorption Marker NTx Annual Meeting of the American Society for Bone and Mineral Research (ASBMR); October Toronto, Ontario(2010). , 13-16.

[203] Everitt, A, Hilmer, S, Brand-miller, J, Jamieson, H, Truswell, A, Sharma, A, et al. Dietary approaches that delay age-related diseases. Clin Interv Aging. (2006). , 1(1), 11-31.

[204] Horcajada, M, & Offord, E. Naturally plant-derived compounds: role in bone anabolism. Curr Mol Pharmacol. (2012). , 5(2), 205-18.

[205] Trzeciakiewicz, A, Habauzit, V, & Horcajada, M. When nutrition interacts with osteoblast function: molecular mechanisms of polyphenols. Nutr Res Rev. (2009). Epub 2009 Feb 26., 22(1), 68-81.

[206] Scalbert, A, Manach, C, Morand, C, Rémésy, C, & Jiménez, L. Dietary polyphenols and the prevention of diseases. Crit Rev Food Sci Nutr. (2005). , 45(4), 287-306.

[207] Cabrera, C, & Giménez, R A. R. Beneficial effects of green tea--a review. J Am Coll Nutr. (2006). , 25(2), 79-99.

[208] Yang, C, & Landau, J. Effects of tea consumption on nutrition and health. J Nutr. (2000). , 130(10), 2409-12.

[209] Rao, L, Kang, N, & Rao, A. Polyphenols and bone health: A review. In: Rao A, editor. Phytochemicals. Rijeka, Croatia: In Tech Open Access Publisher; (2012). , 958-973.

[210] Vali, B, Rao, L, & Sohemy, A. Epigallocathechin-3-gallate (EGCG) increases the formation of mineralized bone nodules by human osteoblast-like cells. J Nutr Biochem. (2007). Epub 2006 Sep 8., 18(5), 341-7.

[211] Yun, J, Pang, E, Kim, C, Yoo, Y, Cho, K, Chai, J, et al. Inhibitory effects of green tea polyphenol (-)-epigallocatechin gallate on the expression of matrix metalloproteinase-9 and on the formation of osteoclasts. J Periodontal Res. (2004). , 39(5), 300-7.

[212] Park, Y, Han, D, Suh, H, Ryu, G, Hyon, S, Cho, B, et al. Protective effects of green tea polyphenol against reactive oxygen species-induced oxidative stress in cultured rat calvarial osteoblast. Cell Biol Toxicol (2003). , 19(5), 325-37.

[213] Kato, K, Otsuka, T, Adachi, S, Matsushima-nishiwaki, R, Natsume, H, Kozawa, O, et al. Green tea polyphenol (-)-Epigallocatechin gallate inhibits thyroid hormone-stimulated osteocalcin synthesis in osteoblasts. Mol Med Report (2011). Epub 2011 Jan 11., 4(2), 297-300.

[214] Kamon, M, Zhao, R, & Sakamoto, K. Green tea polyphenol (-)-epigallocatechin gallate suppressed the differentiation of murine osteoblastic MC3T3-E1 cells. Cell Biol Int. (2009). , 34(1), 109-16.

[215] Oka, Y, Iwai, S, Amano, H, Irie, Y, Yatomi, K, Ryu, K, et al. Tea polyphenols inhibit rat osteoclast formation and differentiation. J Pharmacol Sci. (2012). Epub 2011 Dec 21., 118(1), 55-64.

[216] Yun, J, Kim, C, Cho, K, Chai, J, Kim, C, & Choi, S. Epigallocatechin gallate induces apoptosis, via caspase activation, in osteoclasts differentiated from RAW 264.7 cells. J Periodontal Res. (2007). , 42(3), 212-8.

[217] Bu, S, Hunt, T, & Smith, B. Dried plum polyphenols attenuate the detrimental effects of TNFalpha on osteoblast function coincident with up-regulation of Runx2, Osterix and IGF-I. J Nutr Biochem. (2009). Epub 2008 May 20.., 20(1), 35-44.

[218] Ayoub, N, Singab, A, Naggar, M, & Lindequist, U. Investigation of phenolic leaf extract of Heimia myrtifolia (Lythraceae): Pharmacological properties (stimulation of mineralization of SaOS-2 osteosarcoma cells) and identification of polyphenols. Drug Discov Ther. (2010). , 4(5), 341-8.

[219] Santiago-mora, R, Casado-díaz, A, De Castro, M, & Quesada-gómez, J. Oleuropein enhances osteoblastogenesis and inhibits ad pogenesis: the effect on differentiation in stem cells derived from bone marrow. Osteoporos Int. (2011). Epub 2010 May 21., 22(2), 675-84.

[220] Kao, C, Tai, L, Chiou, S, Chen, Y, Lee, K, Chou, S, et al. Resveratrol promotes osteogenic differentiation and protects against dexamethasone damage in murine induced pluripotent stem cells. Stem Cells Dev. (2010). , 19(2), 247-58.

[221] Li, Y, Edlund, S D, Finne-wistrand, U, He, A, & Norgård, X. M, et al. Resveratrol-conjugated poly-e-caprolactone facilitates in vitro mineralization and in vivo bone regeneration. Acta Biomater. (2011). Epub 2010 Sep 16., 7(2), 751-8.

[222] Rao, L, Balachandran, B, & Rao, A. Polyphenol Extract of Greens+™ Nutritional Supplement Stimulates Bone Formation in Cultures of Human Osteoblast-like SaOS-2 Cells. J Diet Suppl. (2008). , 5(3), 264-82.

[223] Rao, L, Balachandran, B, & Rao, A. The stimulatory effect of the polyphenols in the extract of Greens+TM herbal preparation on the mineralized bone nodule formation (MBNF) of SaOS-2 cells is mediated via its inhibitory effect on the intracellular reactive oxygen species (iROS). 27th Annual Meeting of the American Society of Bone and Mineral Research; September (2005). Nashville, Tennesse2005., 23-27.

[224] Graci, S. The Bone Building Solution. Graci S, DeMarco C, Rao L, editors. Mississauga, Ontario: John Wylie And Sons Canada, Ltd; (2006). p.

[225] Rao, L, Snyder, D, Balachandran, B, Beca, B, Shen, H, Sedeghi, S, et al. Herbal extract and nutritional bone-building supplement synergistically stimulate bone formation in human osteoblast cells in vitro. IOF Regionals- 1st Asia-Pacific Osteoporosis Meeting; December (2010). Singapore,2010., 10-13.

[226] Snyder, D, Rao, A, Balachandran, B, Beca, J, Shen, H, Sadeghi, S, et al. Extracts of the Nutritional Supplement, bone builderTM, and the Herbal Supplement, greens+TM, Synergistically Stimulate Bone Formation by Human Osteoblast Cells in Vitro. Annual Meeting of the American Society for Bone and Mineral Research (ASBMR); October (2010). Toronto, Ontario2010., 13-16.

[227] Shen, C, Chyu, M, Yeh, J, Zhang, Y, Pence, B, Felton, C, et al. Effect of green tea and Tai Chi on bone health in postmenopausal osteopenic women: a 6-month randomized placebo-controlled trial. Osteoporos Int. (2012). Epub 2011 Jul 16., 23(5), 1541-52.

[228] Hardcastle, A, Aucott, L, Reid, D, & Macdonald, H. Associations between dietary flavonoid intakes and bone health in a scottish population. Journal of Bone and Mineral Research Journal of the American Society for Bone and Mineral Research. (2011). , 26(5), 941-7.

Chapter 6

Pathogenesis, Clinical Diagnosis and Treatment, and Animal Models for Ckd-Mbd

Yan Zhang and Yoseph Asmelash Gebru

Additional information is available at the end of the chapter

http://dx.doi.org/10.5772/54238

1. Introduction

People with chronic kidney disease (CKD) develop changes in circulating blood levels of calcium and phosphorus. The kidney gradually loses the ability to remove phosphorus from the blood and cannot produce adequate amounts of active vitamin D to maintain normal levels of calcium. This occurs mainly because of decreased renal excretion of phosphate and diminished renal hydroxylation of 25-hydroxyvitamin D to calcitriol due to low expression of alpha-1-hydroxylase in the failed kidneys [1]. Further compensation to maintain normal serum calcium and phosphorus homeostasis includes increased production and release of parathyroid hormone (PTH) and potentially other phosphaturic factors, such as fibroblast growth factor-23 (FGF23) [2].

Two main complications follow to the above mentioned molecular responses namely secondary hyperparathyroidism (sHPT) and vascular calcification (VC), which occur in a high percentage of CKD patients [1]. These molecular disorders alter bone metabolism which leads to bone abnormalities including altered bone production and resorption. In turn, bony changes may result in bone deformation, bone pain, and more risks of fracture [3]. All of the above biochemical abnormalities (calcium, phosphorus, vitamin D and PTH disturbances) and vascular calcification as well as changes in bone metabolism such as variation in turnover and bone mineralization can be included under the descriptions for CKD-associated mineral and bone disorders (CKD-MBD) [4].

This review explains the main pathological causes and mechanisms of CKD-MBD and the possible animal models for basic research on this disease. It also describes some clinically applicable diagnosis techniques and treatment methods with their advantages and side effects for CKD-MBD.

2. Potential pathological mechanisms

2.1. sHPT-related bone disorders

The first changes that usually occur with the decline of renal function involve the deficiency of active vitamin D and decrease in phosphorus excretion by the remaining functional nephrons [5]. In CKD, the failed kidney is inefficient in alpha-1-hydroxylase expression resulting in low synthesis of calcitriol. Simultaneously the kidney with lower function has reduced ability to reabsorb calcium from urine [6]. Therefore, low serum calcium level, high serum phosphorus level and impaired renal 1, 25-dihydroxyvitamin D synthesis with attendant reduction in serum calcitriol concentration and decrease in vitamin D receptor expression in the parathyroid glands contribute to excess PTH secretion in patients with CKD [7].

PTH strongly influences the exchange of calcium to and from bone through its involvement in bone cell apoptosis mechanisms and effects on the receptor activator of NF-kappa B (RANK)/receptor activator of NF-kappa B ligand (RANKL)/osteoprotegerin (OPG) axis. Continuously elevated PTH could upregulate RANKL expression, leading to an increase in the formation rate and survival time of bone-resorbing osteoclasts and net bone loss [8, 9]. Excess PTH also leads to high bone turnover, a condition characterized by accelerated rates of bone formation and bone resorption [1]. The high bone turnover due to sHPT is accompanied by about 5% (up to 10%) lower bone mass, which is partly reversible (low mineral bone, increased remodeling space) and partly irreversible (cortical thinning) [10]. The new formed bone in the course of sHPT is structurally inferior and fragile, and carries an increased risk of fractures.

Another main molecular mechanism underlying sHPT is attributed to Klotho-fibroblast growth factor-23 (FGF-23) system. Humans with CKD experience decreased Klotho expression as early as stage 1 CKD. Klotho continues to decline as CKD progresses, causing FGF-23 resistance and provoking large FGF-23 and parathyroid hormone increases [11]. FGF-23 is a novel bone-derived hormone, in conjunction with its co-receptor, Klotho, activates FGF receptor 1 (FGFR1) and acts on the kidney to induce renal phosphate wasting and to suppress 1,25-dihydroxyvitamin D synthesis [12]. In patients with CKD, circulating FGF23 levels are progressively increased to compensate for persistent phosphate retention, but this result in reduced renal production of 1, 25-dihydroxyvitamin D through suppressing 1α-hydroxylase activity, which leads to sHPT [13].

2.2. VC-related bone disorders

Vascular calcification is very common in patients with CKD, appearing in 30-65% of patients with stage 3-5 CKD, 50-80% of patients with stage 5 CKD [14]. Calcium, a divalent cation, and phosphate, a trivalent anion, have a high binding affinity for one another and as the concentration of one or both ions increases in serum, there is an increased risk for an ionic bond to form, creating an insoluble complex which leads to vascular calcification [5]. Clinically, when the serum calcium-phosphate product exceeds 60 mg^2/dl^2, widespread tissue deposition of amorphous calcium phosphate occurs [15].

There are a large number of promoters and inhibitors involved in vascular calcification and there are more vascular calcification inhibitors circulating in the blood under normal conditions [1]. Phosphorus is the most significant studied vascular calcification promoter which is available at higher level in patients with low renal function. Hyperphosphatemia reverses the normal process in which calcification inhibitors are down-regulated, while promoters are up-regulated [1].

On the other hand, many bone-associated proteins including osteocalcin, osteopontin and osteoprotegerin, and many bone morphogenetic proteins are involved in the process of VC [16]. Previous studies have proven that active mineralization mechanisms clearly resembling those of skeletal endochondral and membranous ossification participate in vascular calcium accumulation [17]. The findings of bone-related factors in the vasculature and the vascular calcification observed in several gene-knockout mouse models imply that CKD-MBD is an actively regulated process that may be preventable or even reversed [18]. The most striking among these mouse models is the matrix gamma-carboxyglutamic acid (Gla) protein (MGP) knockout mouse, which exhibits extensive and lethal calcification and cartilaginous metaplasia of the media of all elastic arteries as early as 2 weeks after birth [19, 20], indicating that this protein may be of primary importance in human vascular calcification [18].

3. Clinical diagnosis

3.1. Biomarkers

According to the standardized diagnostic criteria for CKD-MBD developed and published by the international expert consensus group, kidney disease improving global outcomes (KDIGO), monitoring serum levels of calcium, phosphorus, PTH, and alkaline phosphatase is strongly recommended, and the frequency of monitoring is based on the occurrence and extent of abnormalities as well as the rate of CKD progression [21]. Phosphorus level equal to the upper phosphorus level of 5.5 mg/dL and calcium level more than 9.5 mg/dL have been suggested to be associated with increased mortality in CKD patients [22]. The combined use of second- and third-generation PTH assays allows to measure PTH (1–84) and PTH (7–84) as PTH (7-84) interacts with distinct receptors and thereby may have important roles in the regulation of bone resorption and serum calcium concentration [23]. The frequency of measurement on alkaline phosphatases is very similar to that of PTH and can provide additional information on bone turnover. The recent more KDIGO guidelines recommend that the measurement on alkaline phosphatase levels should commence in stage 3 of CKD, and that in patients with stage 4-5 of CKD, alkaline phosphatase should be measured at least every 12 months [24].

The first measurable biomarker in urine is the decline of secreted Klotho expression (as detected by western blotting of concentrated urine samples, normalized to the same creatinine content) occurs as early as stage 1 of CKD [25], therefore, Kuro-O contends that decreased Klotho expression is the initiator of CKD-MBD pathophysiology and is potentially an early clinical marker of CKD [11]. The study, performed on sixty pre-dialysis patients with CKD 1-5, showed that the changing of serum OPG level happened at the earliest time (CKD 3) and its correlation coefficient with estimated glomerular filtration rate (eGFR) and BMD of Ward's triangle was statistically high, suggesting serum OPG may be a useful biomarker for early diagnosis of CKD-MBD [26], additionally, the multivariate analysis demonstrated that OPG was associated with aortic stiffness in patients with CKD stages 3-4, indicating OPG is also a marker to evaluate the cardiomyocyte dysfunction of CKD-MBD [27].

3.2. Imaging

Histomorphometry remains the gold standard to evaluate bone, but it is rarely performed in clinical practice. Areal measurement of bone mineral density by dual-energy x-ray absorptiometry (DEXA) is routinely performed to evaluate bone mass. However, this technique presents some limitations. In 2000, the United States National Institutes of Health defined new "quality" criteria for the diagnosis of osteoporosis in addition to decreased bone mass. Bone strength actually integrates two concepts: bone quantity and bone quality (i.e., microarchitectural organization, bone turnover, bone material properties such as mineralization, collagen traits, and micro-damage) that cannot be evaluated by DEXA. New three-dimensional, noninvasive bone-imaging techniques have thus been developed, e.g., high-resolution peripheral quantitative computed tomography (HR-pQCT). HR-pQCT allows evaluation of both volumetric density and microarchitecture in different compartments of bone [28]. Bacchetta reported for the first time an early impairment of trabecular microarchitecture in stage 2-4 CKD patients using a noninvasive bone-imaging device, HR-pQCT [29].

Physicians usually use a variety of noninvasive imaging tools to identify VC, some with merely qualitative and others with both qualitative and quantitative capabilities. Plain x-rays and ultra-sonography can be used to identify macroscopic calcification of aorta and peripheral arteries, and computed tomography technologies constitute the gold standard for quantification of cardiovascular calcification [30].

4. Clinical treatment strategy

The clinical treatment for CKD-MBD targets the possible pathological mechanisms of mainly sHPT and VC in patients with kidney failure as treating these abnormalities will have a direct positive impact on preventing the metabolic bone disease. However, the heterogeneity of CKD-MBD makes strict protocol-driven therapeutic approaches difficult. Accordingly, considerable individualized therapy is required [31]. The followings are currently the most common and effective intervening methods.

4.1. Phosphate binders

In patients at stage 3-5 of CKD, multiple studies from different parts of the world have shown that higher levels of serum phosphorus have been associated with an increased relative risk of mortality [24]. Many clinical trials show that phosphate binders are effective in reducing serum phosphorus and PTH levels [32]. Therefore, the use of phosphate binders might be a promising and most practical strategy for the prevention of VC and sHPT which are the main pathological manifestations of the metabolic bone disease in CKD patients. The following categories of phosphate binders are being applied clinically so far:

1. Aluminum-based phosphate binders are the first type of phosphate binders to be used. They are very effective at controlling phosphorus. The most common binder of this type is aluminum hydroxide. However, aluminum has toxic effects on bone and nervous system. For this reason, aluminum-based phosphate binders are not often used much anymore [33].

2. Calcium-based phosphate binders are effective in binding phosphates and can be source of calcium. Common types of calcium-based binders include calcium acetate and calcium carbonate, both of which could cause the elevation of free calcium cation level in the gastrointestinal tract and the subsequent increase of intestinal calcium absorption [34]. The Japanese Society of Dialysis Therapy (JSDT) clinical practice guideline has recommended a higher level of these oral phosphate binders as the upper limit for clinical use [35]. These binders can also serve as calcium supplements if the calcium is low. However, if the patient is taking vitamin D supplements, he/she may already have high calcium levels, and these types of phosphate binders may provide more calcium than the normal level (i.e., excess calcium load). Therefore using calcium based phosphate binders should be accompanied with monitoring calcium levels and it should be prescribed while limiting total calcium intake.

3. Aluminum-free, calcium-free phosphate binders are newer binders that are effective at controlling phosphorus. Because they do not contain aluminum or calcium, they do not cause problems with excess aluminum or calcium load. Lanthanum carbonate is a novel non-calcium, non-aluminum phosphate-binding agent, and has been approved for clinical use in patients on hemodialysis in Japan on March in 2009 [33]. Sevelamer is a polymeric amine, which is the only non-absorbed, non-calcium-based phosphate binder currently indicated for phosphate control. The first formulation of sevelamer to be approved was sevelamer hydrochloride, while a newer formulation, sevelamer carbonate, has more recently become available [36]. Sevelamer carbonate was developed to offer phosphorus lowering while eliminating the risk of worsening metabolic acidosis associated with sevelamer hydrochloride and the consequent need to monitor for changes in serum chloride or bicarbonate levels [37].

4.2. Vitamin D compounds

Vitamin D analogues suppress PTH synthesis and secretion in patients with sHPT. Repletion with native vitamin D may lead to improved control of secondary hyperparathyroidism in patients with CKD which reduces the risk of bone mineral disease. It has been demonstrated that treatment with vitamin D analogues can decrease mortality in dialysis patients [38]. There might be some differences in clinical outcomes among vitamin D compounds with fewer calcemic and phosphatemic effects [39], such as paricalcitol, doxercalciferol, and maxacalcitol. Therefore, it is important for desirable active vitamin D compounds to achieve optimal vitamin D receptor (VDR) activation without inducing hypercalcemia. It is likely that the elevated calcium levels caused by calcitriol may be directly and/or indirectly responsible for the relative risk of the cardiovascular diseases that are aggravated by hypercalcemia in patient populations.

4.3. Calcimimetics

Calcimimetics bind to the calcium sensing receptor (CaSR) in parathyroid gland and mimic the effect of an elevated extracellular ionized calcium concentration. These molecules reduce serum levels of PTH and calcium, with a leftward shift in the set-point for calcium-regulated PTH secretion [40]. Cinacalcet is the only clinically available calcimimetic and has been shown to be a very effective therapeutic compound in the metabolic bone disease associated with CKD. Many clinical trials with cinacalcet in hemodialysis patients have shown a reduction in parathyroid hormone, calcium, phosphate and calcium × phosphate product levels, allowing far greater success in reaching therapeutic goals as recommended by international guidelines [41]. In addition to effective control of secondary hyperparathyroidism, treatment with cinacalcet may improve the mineral balance in patients with dialysis who have serum phosphate/calcium disequilibrium, and furthermore helps treating the vascular calcification as well. While, calcimimetics are not approved for use in paediatric patients with CKD and long-term data on their effects on bone, growth and biochemical parameters in children are lacking. Thus, further studies are warranted to determine the optimal strategy for controlling secondary hyperparathyroidism in the paediatric CKD population [42].

4.4. Administering BMP-7

One of the bone morphogenetic proteins, BMP-7, also known as osteogenic protein 1, is highly expressed in the adult kidney, and circulates in the bloodstream [43]. Therefore, it is apparent that the decrease of renal mass results in the decreased production of BMP-7, causing mineral bone disease in CKD patients [44]. One may expect an accumulation of osteoblast precursors as stimulated by PTH in CKD. While, these progenitors may be unable to differentiate mature osteoblasts because of BMP-7 deficiency considering it is important in osteoblast development and function. In this situation, the subsequent accumulation of fibrous cells could then offer an explanation for the marrow fibrosis observed in secondary hyperparathyroidism in the setting of CKD and applying BMP-7 externally can heal the disorder. There are an increasing number of recent clinical trials that provide supportive evidence for the use of BMP-7 in the treatment of fractures and bone nonunions [45]. It is not yet started to use BMP-7 as a routine clinical treatment tool except for trials in patients even though many of the studies have shown the bone healing efficacy of this molecule.

4.5. Surgery on thyroid gland

A surgical correction in the parathyroid gland is the final, symptomatic therapy for the most severe forms of sHPT which cannot be controlled by the above medical treatments.

http://dx.doi.org/10.5772/54238

The 2009 KDIGO guideline suggested parathyroidectomy to patients who are at CKD stages 3-5 with severe hyperparathyroidism and fail to respond to medical/pharmacological therapy [46]. There are two main surgical procedures which are generally used, namely subtotal parathyroidectomy and total parathyroidectomy with immediate autotransplantation. The number and size of affected parathyroid glands are the most important factors for selecting the treatment procedure [47, 48]. Clinical studies proved that parathyroidectomy with autotransplantation from forearm was significantly effective and safe in patients in whom medical treatment had failed, particularly in terms of improving calcium and phosphate control [49, 50]. The procedure need to be performed as early as possible to avoid the adverse, irreversible effects of prolonged hyperparathyroidism, and to improve osteoarticular symptoms. Future strategies may focus on the stimulation of apoptotic activity of hyperplastic parathyroid cells [51].

5. Animal models

5.1. 5/6 nephrectomy model

Experimental model of 5/6 nephrectomy or the remnant kidney model represents one of the most used animal models of progressive renal failure by reducing nephron number, best-characterized in rats [52]. The reduction of renal mass is achieved by either infarction or surgical excision of both poles, with removal of the contra-lateral kidney. The 5/6 nephroctomy model has been found to produce serum creatinine level which is on average 2.2-fold higher than control animals, and thereafter, if without the concurrent use of vitamin D, the phosphorus level after 8 weeks of surgery would range up to 2.6-fold higher than control animals [53]. Increased fibrosis, increased number of osteoblasts and osteoclasts as well as a mineralization defect (increased osteoid volumes and osteoid surface), those of which are typical bone changes upon sHPT, have been observed in 5/6 nephrectomy animal models [14].

The operation of 5/6 nephrectomy, combining with a diet containing 1.2% P plus 0.6% Ca, could effectively induce sHPT in rats [54]. Additionally, the progressive partial nephrectomy with thyroparathyroidectomy (TPTx-Nx) reduced the storage modulus, which is a mechanical factor, in CKD model rats as compared with controls that underwent thyroparathyroidectomy alone (TPTx). Moreover, the TPTx-Nx rats exerted different cortical bone chemical composition and increased enzymatic crosslinks ratio and pentosidine to matrix ratio [55].

As concerned as VC associated with CKD-MBD, it can be induced in 5/6 nephrectomy rat model by feeding a high-phosphorus, high-lactose diet (1.2% P, 1% Ca, and 20% lactose) after 10 weeks follow up for the reason that lactose increases calcium and phosphorus absorption in intestine [56].

5.2. Electrocautery models

In the mouse electrocautery model, CKD is induced by surgical ablation of the kidneys. This is a two-step procedure. Initially the cortex of one kidney is electrocauterized paying careful attention to avoid destroying the adrenals and the hilum of kidney. One week later, once the animals have recovered, the second kidney is nephrectomized [44]. This procedure appears to produce variable severity of CKD with blood urea levels ranging from 1.5- to 4.8-fold higher than normal animals [53]. This murine model displayed an increase in osteoblast surface and osteoid accumulation as well as increased activation frequency and increased osteoclast surface consistent with high turnover renal osteodystrophy [44]. Lund developed a standard CKD rat models by involving electrocauthery of the right kidney followed by nephroctomy of the left kidney, and found that there was a significant hyperosteoidosis produced in this model as a result of the secondary hyperparathyroidism [57].

5.3. Adenine-contained diet

Normally, adenine is efficiently salvaged by adenine phosphoribosyltransferase (APRT) and is present at very low level in blood and urine. APRT is involved in the conversion of adenine to adenosine monophosphate. When adenine is administered in high level, APRT activity is saturated and adenine is oxidized to 2,8-dihydroxyadenine. Adenine and 2,8-dihydroxyadenine are excreted in the urine. However, the very low solubility of 2,8-dihydroxyadenine results in its precipitation in the kidney. The accumulation of insoluble 2,8-dihydroxyadenine results in nephrolithiasis and renal failure with permanent kidney damage. Induction of chronic renal failure (CRF) in mice by dietary administration of 0.75% adenine for 4 weeks results in irreversible renal dysfunction and then CKD [53]. High-adenine feeding in rats results in the formation of crystals in the renal tubules, with subsequent tubular injury and inflammation, obstruction, and marked fibrosis [56]. Future investigations of the biochemical basis for the link between vascular calcification and bone resorption will be facilitated by the present discovery that a synthetic, 2.5% protein diet containing 0.75% adenine produces consistent and dramatic medial calcification in adult rats within just 4 weeks [58].

5.4. Gene knockout mice

JCK mouse is a genetic model of polycystic kidney disease. At 6 weeks of age, the mice have normal renal function and no evidence of bone disease but exhibit continual decline in renal function and death by 20 weeks of age, when approximately 40% to 60% of them have vascular calcification. Temporal changes in serum parameters of JCK mice relative to wild-type mice from 6 through 18 weeks of age were shown to largely mirror serum changes commonly associated with clinical CKD-MBD. Bone histomorphometry revealed progressive changes associated with increased osteoclast activity and elevated bone formation [59].

Klotho null mice display premature aging and CKD-MBD-like phenotypes mediated by hyperphosphatemia and remediated by phosphate-lowering interventions (diets low in phosphate or vitamin D; knockouts of 1α-hydroxylase, vitamin D receptor, or NaPi cotransporter) [11].

http://dx.doi.org/10.5772/54238

5.5. Obstructive nephropathy

The mouse with unilateral ureteral obstruction (UUO) is a well-established model of tubulointerstitial fibrosis of the kidney as the interstitial fibrosis is a hallmark of chronic renal failure [60]. We previously reported the vitamin D signaling attenuates renal fibrosis in obstructive nephropathy by suppressing the renin-angiotensin system (RAS) [61], furthermore, we found the mice developed hypocalcaemia and hyperparathyroidism after 7 days of ureteric obstruction [62], and the down-regulation of *Cbfa1* and *Col* mRNA expression (Fig. 1) and the up-regulation of *Tgf-β*, *CtsK*, *CaII*, *Opg* and *Rankl* mRNA expression (Fig. 2) in tibia of UUO mice as well as the microarchitectural changes in the proximal tibia, likely to be precursors of the early stage during CKD-MBD [62]. The pathological alterations of proximal tibia in UUO group were characterized by a marked expansion of hypertrophic zone of chondrocytes and a dramatic decrease in osteoid content of the primary spongiosa zone, where the immature, poorly mineralized woven bones were present, indicating impaired mineralization of the newly formed bones (Fig. 3B). Above all, in addition to established genetic pathways, we suggest that the local skeletal renin-angiotensin system may be involved in the bone deteriorations associated with CKD as demonstrated by the marked up-regulation of protein expression of angiotensin II and its type 2 receptor in tibia of UUO mice (Fig. 4) [62].

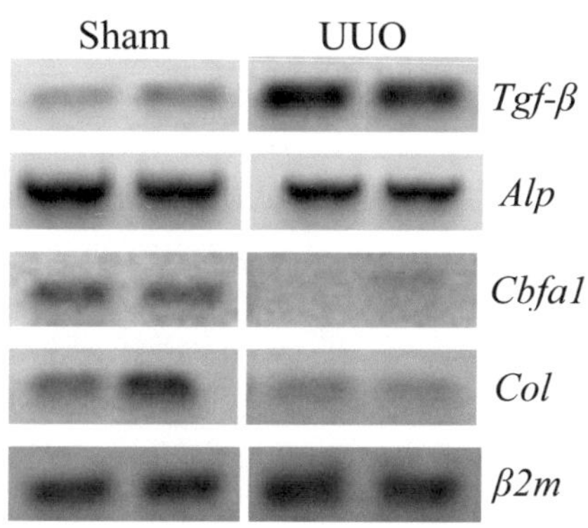

Figure 1. mRNA expression of osteoblast-specific genes in tibia of sham-operated and UUO mice

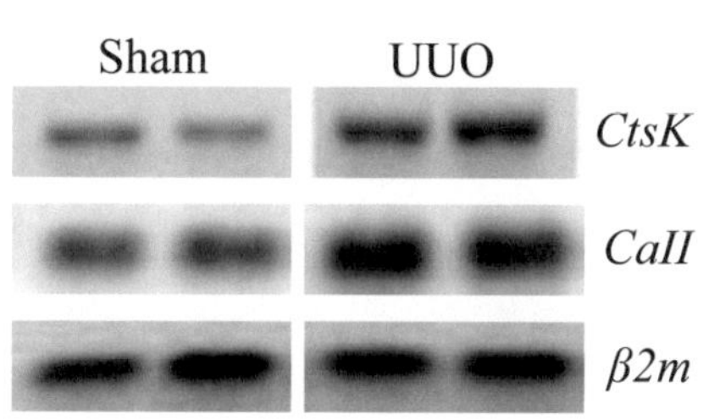

Figure 2. mRNA expression of osteoclast-specific genes in tibia of sham-operated and UUO mice

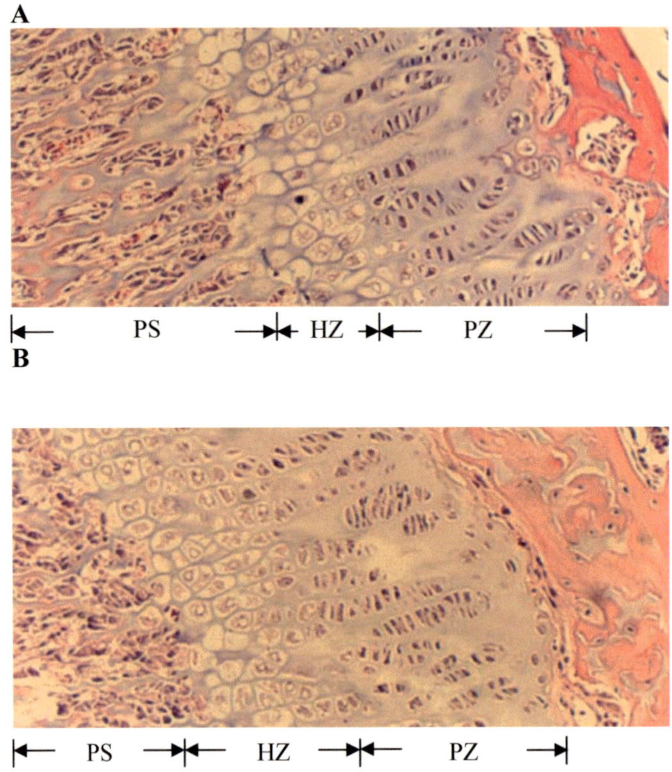

Figure 3. Hematoxylin and Eosin staining of the proximal tibia. The chondrocyte zone at growth plate was shown in A (Sham) and B (UUO) and it was visually separated into two areas, proliferative zone (PZ) and hypertrophic zone (HZ). Calcified cartilage with overlying newly bone underneath growth plate is known as the primary spongiosa (PS). Magnification, ×100.

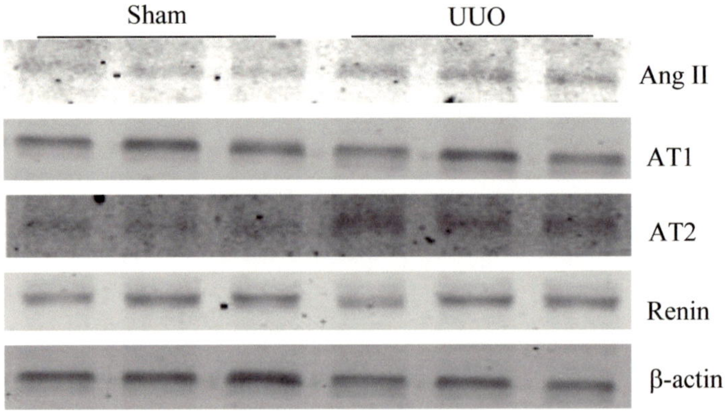

Figure 4. Protein expression of RAS components in mice tibia

http://dx.doi.org/10.5772/54238

6. Conclusion

In summary, the present review demonstrates that the main pathological mechanisms involved in CKD-MBD are secondary hyperparathyroidism and vascular calcification. Therefore the main focus of the therapeutic research and the further molecular investigations should be on these main abnormalities associated with CKD. This can be achieved by employing the proper animal models for each of these complications including genetically modified mouse models. The animal models can play a great role in understanding the underlying mechanisms for CKD-MBD. The clinical treatment approaches should depend on the specific levels of the biomarkers of CKD patients. Further studies are needed to discover other pathological mechanisms for CKD-MBD other than those explained here. More advanced basic medical sciences should also be performed on the research and development of novel drugs with less adverse effects.

This work was sponsored by Shanghai Pujiang Program (10PJ1407700) and Innovation Program of Shanghai Municipal Education Commission (11ZZ137) for Yan Zhang.

Author details

Yan Zhang[1,2*] and Yoseph Asmelash Gebru[1]

*Address all correspondence to: medicineyan@yahoo.com.cn

1 Center for Systems Biomedical Sciences, University of Shanghai for Science and Technology, Shanghai, P.R.China

2 Department of Applied Biology and Chemical Technology, The Hong Kong Polytechnic University, Hung Hom, Kowloon, Hong Kong, P.R.China

References

[1] Mejía N, Roman-García P, Miar AB, Tavira B, Cannata-Andía JB. Chronic Kidney Disease – Mineral and Bone Disorder: A Complex Scenario. Nefrologia 2011;31(5) 514-519.

[2] Anca G, Stuart MS. Role of Vitamin D Deficiency in Chronic Kidney Disease. J Bone Miner Res 2007;22(S2) S91–94.

[3] Nickolas TL, Stein E, Cohen A, Thomas V, Staron RB, McMahon DJ, Leonard MB, Shane E. Bone Mass and Microarchitecture in CKD Patients with Fracture. J Am Soc Nephrol 2010;21(8) 1371-1380.

[4] Chauhan V, Kelepouris E, Chauhan N, Vaid M. Current Concepts and Management Strategies in Chronic Kidney Disease-Mineral and Bone Disorder. South Med J 2012;105(9) 479-485.

[5] Tomasello S. Secondary Hyperparathyroidism and Chronic Kidney Disease. Diabetes Spectrum 2008;21(1) 19-25.

[6] Schumock GT, Andress DL, Marx SE, Sterz R, Joyce AT, Kalantar-Zadeh K. Association of Secondary Hyperparathyroidism with CKD Progression, Health Care Costs and Survival in Diabetic Predialysis CKD Patients. Nephron Clin Pract 2009;113(1) 54–61.

[7] Goodman WG. Medical Management of Secondary Hyperparathyroidism in Chronic Renal Failure. Nephrol Dial Transplant 2003;18(S3) 2-8.

[8] Kiattisunthorn K, Moe SM. Chronic Kidney Disease-Mineral Bone Disorder (CKD-MBD). IBMS BoneKEy 2010;7(12) 447-457.

[9] Riggs MM, Peterson MC, Gastonguay MR. Multiscale Physiology-Based Modeling of Mineral Bone Disorder in Patients with Impaired Kidney Function. J Clin Pharmacol 2012;52(1) 45-53.

[10] Lips P. Vitamin D Deficiency and Secondary Hyperparathyroidism in the Elderly: Consequences for Bone Loss and Fractures and Therapeutic Implications. Endocr Rev 2001;22(4) 477-501.

[11] Kuro-O M. Phosphate and Klotho. Kidney Int Suppl 2011;(121) S20-23.

[12] Komaba H. CKD-MBD (Chronic Kidney Disease-Mineral and Bone Disorder). Role of FGF23 Klotho Axis in CKD-MBD. Clin Calcium 2010;20(7) 1028-1036.

[13] Rodríguez M, López I, Muñoz J, Aguilera-Tejero E, Almaden Y. FGF23 and Mineral Metabolism, Implications in CKD-MBD. Nefrologia 2012;32(3) 275-278.

[14] Moe SM, Chen NX, Seifert MF, Sinders RM, Duan D, Chen X, Liang Y, Radcliff JS, White KE, Gattone VH 2nd. A Rat Model of Chronic Kidney Disease-Mineral Bone Disorder (CKD-MBD) and the Effect of Dietary Protein Source. Kidney Int 2009;75(2) 176-184.

[15] Vattikuti R, Towler DA. Osteogenic Regulation of Vascular Calcification: An Early Perspective. Am J Physiol Endocrinol Metab 2004;286(5) 686-696.

[16] Covic A, Kanbay M, Voroneanu L, Turgut F, Serban DN, Serban IL, Goldsmith DJ. Vascular Calcification in Chronic Kidney Disease. Clin Sci 2010;119(3) 111-121.

[17] Shao JS, Cai J, Towler DA. Molecular Mechanisms of Vascular Calcification: Lessons Learned From the Aorta. Arterioscler Thromb Vasc Biol 2006;26(7) 1423-1430.

[18] Proudfoot D, Shanahan CM. Molecular Mechanisms Mediating Vascular Calcification: Role of Matrix Gla Protein. Nephrology 2006;11(5) 455-461.

[19] Speer MY, McKee MD, Guldberg RE, Liaw L, Yang HY, Tung E, Karsenty G, Giachelli CM. Inactivation of the Osteopontin Gene Enhances Vascular Calcification of Matrix Gla Protein–Deficient Mice: Evidence for Osteopontin as an Inducible Inhibitor of Vascular Calcification In Vivo. J Exp Med 2002;196(8) 1047-1055.

[20] Shanahan CM, Proudfoot D, Farzaneh-Far A, Weissberg PL. The Role of Gla Proteins in Vascular Calcification. Crit Rev Eukaryot Gene Expr 1998;8(3-4) 357-75.

[21] Kidney Disease: Improving Global Outcomes (KDIGO) CKD-MBD Work Group. KDIGO Clinical Practice Guideline for the Diagnosis, Evaluation, Prevention and Treatment of Chronic Disease -Mineral and Bone Disorder (CKD-MBD). Kidney Int 2009;(113) S1-130.

[22] Morrone LF, Russo D, Di Iorio B. Diagnostic Workup for Disorders of Bone and Mineral Metabolism in Patients with Chronic Kidney Disease in the Era of KDIGO Guidelines. Int J Nephrol DOI: 10.4061/2011/958798

[23] Gao P, D'Amour P. Evolution of the Parathyroid Hormone (PTH) Assay--Importance of Circulating PTH Immunoheterogeneity and of its Regulation. Clin Lab 2005;51(1-2) 21-29.

[24] Kidney Disease: Improving Global Outcomes (KDIGO) CKD-MBD Work Group. KDIGO Clinical Practice Guideline for the Diagnosis, Evaluation, Prevention, and Treatment of Chronic Kidney Disease-Mineral and Bone Disorder (CKD-MBD). Kideny Int Suppl 2009;76(113) S1-130.

[25] Hu MC, Shi M, Zhang J, Quiñones H, Griffith C, Kuro-o M, Moe OW. Klotho Deficiency Causes Vascular Calcification in Chronic Kidney Disease. J Am Soc Nephrol 2011;22(1) 124-136.

[26] Jiang JQ, Lin S, Xu PC, Zheng ZF, Jia JY. Serum Osteoprotegerin Measurement for Early Diagnosis of Chronic Kidney Disease-Mineral and Bone Disorder. Nephrology 2011;16(6) 588-594.

[27] Ford ML, Smith ER, Tomlinson LA, Chatterjee PK, Rajkumar C, Holt SG. FGF-23 and Osteoprotegerin Are Independently Associated With Myocardial Damage in Chronic Kidney Disease Stages 3 and 4. Another Link between Chronic Kidney Disease-Mineral Bone Disorder and the Heart. Nephrol Dial Transplant 2012;27(2) 727-733.

[28] Bacchetta J, Boutroy S, Juillard L, Vilayphiou N, Guebre-Egziabher F, Pelletier S, Delmas PD, Fouque D. Bone Imaging and Chronic Kidney Disease: Will High-Resolution Peripheral Tomography Improve Bone Evaluation and Therapeutic Management? J Ren Nutr 2009;19(1) 44-49.

[29] Bacchetta J, Boutroy S, Vilayphiou N, Juillard L, Guebre-Egziabher F, Rognant N, Sornay-Rendu E, Szulc P, Laville M, Delmas PD, Fouque D, Chapurlat R. Early Impairment of Trabecular Microarchitecture Assessed with HR-pQCT in Patients with Stage II-IV Chronic Kidney Disease. J Bone Miner Res 2010;25(4) 849-857.

[30] Raggi P, Bellasi A. Clinical Assessment of Vascular Calcification. Adv Chronic Kidney Dis 2007;14(1) 37-43.

[31] Martin KJ, González EA. Long-term Management of CKD-Mineral and Bone Disorder. Am J Kidney Dis 2012;60(2) 308-315.

[32] Martin KJ, González EA. Prevention and Control of Phosphate Retention/Hyperphosphatemia in CKD-MBD: What is Normal, When to Start, and How to Treat? Clin J Am Soc Nephrol 2011;6(2) 440-446.

[33] Negi S, Shigematsu T. CKD-MBD (Chronic Kidney Disease-Mineral and Bone Disorder). Lanthanum Carbonate and New Phosphate Binders in Patients with Chronic Kidney Disease. Clin Calcium 2010;20(7) 1096-1102.

[34] Cozzolino M, Mazzaferro S, Brandenburg V. The Treatment of Hyperphosphataemia in CKD: Calcium-Based or Calcium-Free Phosphate Binders? Nephrol Dial Transplant 2011;26(2) 402-407.

[35] Kazama JJ. Oral Phosphatebinders: History and Prospects. Bone 2009;45(S1) S8–12.

[36] Spaia S. Phosphate Binders: Sevelamer in the Prevention and Treatment of Hyperphosphataemia in Chronic Renal Failure. Hippokratia 2011;15(1) 22-26.

[37] Frazão JM., Adragão T. Non-Calcium-Containing Phosphate Binders: Comparing Efficacy, Safety, and other Clinical Effects. Nephron Clin Pract 2012;120(2) 108-119.

[38] Ogata H, Koiwa F, Kinugasa E, Akizawa T. CKD-MBD: Impact on Management of Kidney Disease. Clin Exp Nephrol 2007;11(4) 261-268.

[39] Barreto FC, de Oliveira RA, Oliveira RB, Jorgetti V. Pharmacotherapy of Chronic Kidney Disease and Mineral Bone Disorder. Expert Opin Pharmacother 2011;12(17) 2627-2640.

[40] Wüthrich RP, Martin D, Bilezikian JP. The Role of Calcimimetics in the Treatment of Hyperparathyroidism. Eur J Clin Invest 2007;37(12) 915-922.

[41] Bover J, Aguilar A, Baas J, Reyes J, Lloret MJ, Farré N, Olaya M, Canal C, Marco H, Andrés E, Trinidad P, Ballarin J. Calcimimetics in the Chronic Kidney Disease-Mineral and Bone Disorder. Int J Artif Organs 2009;32(2) 108-121.

[42] Bacchetta J, Harambat J, Cochat P, Salusky IB, Wesseling-Perry K. The Consequences of Chronic Kidney Disease on Bone Metabolism and Growth in Children. Nephrol Dial Transplant 2012;27(8) 3063-3071.

[43] Mitu G, Hirschberg R. Bone Morphogenetic Protein-7 (BMP7) in Chronic Kidney Disease. Front Biosci 2008;13 4726-39.

[44] González EA, Lund RJ, Martin KJ, McCartney JE, Tondravi MM, Sampath TK, Hruska KA. Treatment of a Murine Model of High-Turnover Renal Osteodystrophy by Exogenous BMP-7. Kidney Int 2002;61(4) 1322-1331.

http://dx.doi.org/10.5772/54238

[45] White AP, Vaccaro AR, Hall JA, Whang PG, Friel BC, McKee MD. Clinical Applications of BMP-7/OP-1 in Fractures, Nonunions and Spinal Fusion. Int Orthop 2007;31(6) 735-741.

[46] Jha V, Kher V, Pisharody R, Sharma RK, Abraham G, Gokulnath, Almeida A, Gupta A. Indian Commentary on the 2009 KDIGO Clinical Practice Guideline for the Diagnosis, Evaluation, and Treatment of Chronic Kidney Disease-Mineral and Bone Disorders. Indian J Nephrol 2011;21(3) 143-151.

[47] Tominaga Y, Matsuoka S, Sato T. Surgical Indications and Procedures of Parathyroidectomy in Patients with Chronic Kidney Disease. Ther Apher Dial 2005;9(1) 44-47.

[48] Onoda N, Kashiwagi T, Nakamura T, Niitsu Y, Omata M, Kurihara S. Parathyroid Interventions for Secondary Hyperparathyroidism in Hemodialyzed Patients. Ther Apher Dial 2005;(S1) S11-15.

[49] Jofré R, López Gómez JM, Menárguez J, Polo JR, Guinsburg M, Villaverde T, Pérez Flores I, Carretero D, Rodríguez Benitez P, Pérez García R. Parathyroidectomy: Whom and When? Kidney Int Suppl 2003;(85) S97–100.

[50] Naranda J, Ekart R, Pečovnik-Balon B. Total Parathyroidectomy with Forearm Autotransplantation as the Treatment of Choice for Secondary Hyperparathyroidism. J Int Med Res 2011;39(3) 978-987.

[51] Cunningham J, Locatelli F, Rodriguez M. Secondary Hyperparathyroidism: Pathogenesis, Disease Progression, and Therapeutic Options. Clin J Am Soc Nephrol 2011;6(4) 913-921.

[52] Sinanoglu O, Sezgin G, Ozturk G, Tuncdemir M, Guney S, Aksungar FB, Yener N. Melatonin with 1,25-Dihydroxyvitamin D3 Protects against Apoptotic Ischemia-Reperfusion Injury in the Rat Kidney. Ren Fail 2012;34(8) 1021-1026.

[53] Shobeiri N, Adams MA, Holden RM. Vascular Calcification in Animal Models of CKD: A Review. Am J Nephrol 2010;31(6) 471-481.

[54] Padagas J, Colloton M, Shalhoub V, Kostenuik P, Morony S, Munyakazi L, Guo M, Gianneschi D, Shatzen E, Geng Z, Tan HL, Dunstan C, Lacey D, Martin D. The Receptor Activator of Nuclear Factor-Kappab Ligand Inhibitor Osteoprotegerin is a Bone-Protective Agent in a Rat Model Of Chronic Renal Insufficiency and Hyperparathyroidism. Calcif Tissue Int 2006;78(1) 35-44.

[55] Iwasaki Y, Kazama JJ, Yamato H, Fukagawa M. Changes in Chemical Composition of Cortical Bone Associated with Bone Fragility in Rat Model with Chronic Kidney Disease. Bone 2011;48(6) 1260-1267.

[56] Neven E, D'Haese PC. Vascular Calcification in Chronic Renal Failure: What Have We Learned from Animal Studies? Circ Res 2011;108(2) 249-264.

[57] Wahner HW. Measurements of Bone Mass and Bone Density. Endocrinol Metab Clin North Am 1989;18(4) 995-1012.

[58] Price PA, Roublick AM, Williamson MK. Artery Calcification in Uremic Rats is Increased by a Low Protein Diet and Prevented by Treatment with Ibandronate. Kidney Int 2006;70(9) 1577-1583.

[59] Sabbagh Y, Graciolli FG, O'Brien S, Tang W, Dos Reis LM, Ryan S, Phillips L, Boulanger J, Song W, Bracken C, Liu S, Ledbetter S, Dechow P, Canziani ME, Carvalho AB, Jorgetti V, Moyses RM, Schiavi SC. Repression of Osteocyte Wnt/B-Catenin Signaling is an Early Event in the Progression of Renal Osteodystrophy. J Bone Miner Res 2012;27(8) 1757-1772.

[60] Zhang Y, Wu SY, Gu SS, Lv FK. Changes of Renal Vitamin D Metabolic Enzyme Expression and Calcium Transporter Abundance in Obstructive Nephropathy. Nephrology 2011;16(8) 710-714.

[61] Zhang Y, Kong J, Chang A, Deb DK, Li YC. Vitamin D Receptor Attenuates Renal Fibrosis in Obstructive Nephropathy by Suppressing the Renin-Angiotensin System. J Am Soc Nephrol 2010;21(6) 966-973.

[62] Gu SS, Zhang Y, Wu SY, Diao TY, Gebru YA, Deng H. Early Molecular Responses of Bone to Obstructive Nephropathy Induced by Unilateral Ureteral Obstruction in Mice. Nephrology 2012;17(8) 767-773

Chapter 7

Osteoporosis and Nutrition — Nutrition, Anthropometry and Bone Mineral Density in Women

Olga Cvijanović, Sandra Pavičić Žeželj,
Silvija Lukanović, Nenad Bićanić, Robert Domitrović,
Dragica Bobinac and Željka Crnčević Orlić

Additional information is available at the end of the chapter

http://dx.doi.org/10.5772/54433

1. Introduction

Osteoporosis affects millions of people all around the world and it is the most common metabolic bone disease, characterized by low bone mass, disrupted bone micro architecture and increased bone brittleness [1].

Interaction of numerous factors, such as: genetic, medical, anthropometric, pharmacological, lifestyle and nutrition, lead to loss of bone mass and to increased risk for the osteoporotic fractures in female [2].

The most of the studies which have explored the effect of calcium on bone mass in females, demonstrated that high calcium intake is related to greater bone mass, compared to smaller bone mass in respondents who had less dietary calcium intake [3]. Besides calcium, sufficient dietary intake of other micronutrients, such as: zinc, magnesium, potassium, dietary fibers as well as vitamin C are believed to have favorable effect on the bone metabolism too [4].

The study of osteoporotic fractures reports that higher intake of animal proteins compared to vegetable proteins is associated to increased risk of loss of the bone mass and occurrence of the osteoporotic fractures [5]. High protein and sodium intake increases calcium excretion in urine, which increases the need for dietary calcium. It has been also found that a high dietary total protein intake, increases production of endogenous acid, which results in accelerated bone resorption and reduced bone formation. This is especially expressed in diets high in animal proteins [6]. It is believed that unfavorable effect of the animal proteins on the bone metabolism can be repaired by higher fruit and vegetable intake [7].

Recent researches indicate a risk of excessive fat intake, which leads to metabolic bone disorders. High fat intake is considered to be a risk factor for osteoporosis, because it reduces the calcium absorption, since calcium forms insoluble compounds with fatty acids [7].

The aim of this study was to quantify the intake of trace elements in fruit and vegetable: zinc, magnesium, potassium and dietary fats as well as fat derivatives intake in examinees and to explore their relation to the bone mass. The aim was to examine the extent to which these nutritional parameters are predictors of values of bone mineral density.

2. Patients and methods

2.1. Subjects

The study population consisted of women with sedentary occupations in age ranged from 40 to 67 years. Women are inhabitants of the down town Rijeka, Croatia. Exclusion criteria for further participation in the survey were: smoking and any medical therapy which can alter bone metabolism, including food supplements with added calcium. Dietary habits, anthropometric characteristics, serum concentration of the biochemical markers and values of the bone densitometry parameters were comprised by this study. 200 women were included in this investigation, of which 120 menopausal women constituted experimental group, and 80 fertile women represents the control group.

2.2. Dietary intakes

Participants completed an anonymous, encrypted questionnaire, conducted in accordance with ethical and bioethical principles and their privacy and protection of confidential information was ensured.

For the assessment of dietary habits and the average daily energy and nutrients intake, we used data obtained from semi- quantitative Food Frequency Questionnaire- sq-FFQ, the main method for collecting data about a foodstuff choice, as well as the type and quantity of food intake in the study population. This method of identifying the dietary habits is a questionnaire validated by the Department of Nutrition, Harvard School of Public Health [8], from which are obtained informations about daily intake of energy and nutrients. Women were asked to note the frequency and the quantity of offered food items. The amount of each food item was offered as one portion and declared as small, medium and large. This method quantified the values of nutritional parameters that are essential for bone health, such as: calcium, phosphorus, vitamin D, proteins, zinc, magnesium, potassium, dietary fibers and vitamin C. We also determined a total fat intake and the emphasis was placed on the intake of total fat, saturated fatty acids, monounsaturated fatty acids and polyunsaturated fatty acids. The nutritive and energy values of each food noted were calculated using the composition tables of raw and cooked food [9].

http://dx.doi.org/10.5772/54433

2.3. Anthropometric, biochemical and bone mineral status measurements

Bodyweight was measured on a portable electronic scale (SECA, Hamburg, Germany), with accuracy of ± 0,1 kg. Body height was measured on a portable stadiometer, which is a part of a specified scale (SECA, Hamburg, Germany), to the nearest ± 0,5 cm. Body mass index was calculated as bodyweight divided by body height squared, BMI (kg/m^2) [10].

Biochemical indicator of bone resorption, deoxypyridinolin (DPD) and biochemical indicator of bone formation, bone alkaline phosphatase (ALP) and vitamin D were determined from urine and blood of the respondents by immune-enzymatic method (Enzyme Linked Immunosorbent Assay, ELISA), according to manufacturer's protocol [11,12,13].

Bone density in the anterior-posterior images of the spine and hip was measured using the device for bone densitometry (Hologic, Bedford, MA, USA). The obtained values were quantified according to the following parameters: bone mineral content (BMC, mg), bone mineral density (BMD, mg/cm^2) and T-score (represents a deviation from the BMD measured values of peak bone mass of young people expressed in standard deviations) and Z-score (deviation of the measured values BMD of the average bone mass of persons of the same age, expressed in standard deviations) [14].

2.4. Statistical analysis

Statistical analysis of data was performing by using Statistica for Windows, release 9.1 (Stasoft, INC, Tulsa, USA). Normality of distribution for the data interval scale (quantitative data), was tested using the Kolmogorov- Smirinov test. The results were shown as arithmetic mean and standard deviation. Results were distributed normally and in the analytical statistics, one-way analysis of variance (one-way ANOVA) was used. To determine the significance of the contribution of the percentage of nutrients on the metabolic bone status, multiple regression analysis was used. All statistical values were considered significant at the level $P<0,05$ [15].

2.5. Results

Age, anthropometric characteristics, values of the bone densitometry parameters and concentrations of the bone remodeling markers are presented in Table 1. Women of generative age are significantly taller than women in menopause ($P=0,01$) and have significantly higher body weight than women in menopause ($P<0,001$). The average value of Body Mass Index (BMI) was 27 kg/m^2.

Subjects of generative age have significantly higher values of BMD and BMC of the spine ($P<0,001$, $P<0,001$), as well as the values of T-score and Z-score ($P<0,001$, $P<0,001$), than menopausal women, respectively. Values of BMD and BMC of the hip ($P<0,001$, $P<0,001$) and the value of T-score ($P<0,001$) were also significantly higher in women of generative age.

Regarding the bone remodeling markers, significantly lower values of DPD ($P<0,001$) and bone ALP ($P=0,004$) were found in fertile women compared to menopausal women.

Parameters	Fertile women (n =80)	Menopausal women (n = 120)	Total (n = 200)	P-value
Age	47,6 ±4,1	59,9 ± 5,1	54,9 ± 7,7	<0,001*
Body height (cm)	74,0 ± 6,4	71,7 ± 13,3	72,6 ± 11,1	0,001*
Body weight (kg)	166,8 ± 0,05	161,9 ± 0,06	163,8 ± 0,06	<0,001*
BMI (kg/m^2)	26,6 ± 2,3	27,3 ± 4,7	27,0 ±3,9	0,210
BMD LS (g/cm^2)	1,074 ± 0,1	0,897 ± 0,1	0,968 ± 0,2	<0,001*
BMC LS (g)	67,49 ± 9,4	52,84 ± 9,7	58,70 ± 11,9	<0,001*
T-score	0,400 ± 1,3	-1,325 ± 1,3	-0,635 ± 1,9	<0,001*
Z-score	0,835 ± 1,3	0,033 ± 1,4	0,354 ± 1,4	<0,001*
BMD LH (g/cm^2)	0,944 ± 0,1	0,860 ± 0,1	0,893 ± 0,1	<0,001*
BMC LH (g)	37,29 ± 5,9	30,83 ± 5,5	33,41 ± 6,5	<0,001*
T-score	0,122 ± 0,8	-0,647 ± 1,1	-0,339 ± 1,1	<0,001*
Z-score	0,453 ± 0,9	0,298 ± 1,0	0,360 ± 1,0	0,269
DPD (nmol/l)	5,26 ± 1,4	6,85 ± 2,5	6,22 ± 2,2	<0,001*
ALP (ng/ml)	22,77 ± 8,1	26,0 ± 7,4	24,71 ± 7,8	0,004*
Vitamin D (nmol/l)	62,03 ± 25,8	68,90 ± 29,1	66,16 ± 27,9	0,09

* statistical significance on level P < 0,05

LS – lumbar spine

LH – left hip

Table 1. Age, anthropometry, bone densitometry parameters, bone remodeling markers and vitamin D ($\bar{X}$ ± SD)

Dietary habits of the study participants are presented in the Table 2. One-way analysis of variance (ANOVA) showed that women of generative age have significantly higher average daily intake of vitamin D, vitamin C, potassium, magnesium and zinc, while menopausal women have significantly higher average daily phosphorus intake (P<0,001).

Parameters		**Fertile women (n =80)**	**Menopausal women (n = 120)**	**Total (n = 200)**	**P- values**
Energetic food equivalent	kcal	2851,91 ± 1034,4	2448,65 ± 716,37	2609,95 ± 877,9	<0,001*
	kJ	11932,38 ± 4327,8	10,245 ± 2997,3	10920,04 ± 3673,5	<0,001*
Proteins (total) (g)		90,76 ± 65,4	60,52 ± 28,9	75,64 ± 50,7	<0,001*
Proteins (vegetable) (g)		21,95 ± 22,5	19,70 ± 9,2	20,71 ±16,7	<0,001*
Proteins (animal) (g)		67,88 ± 45,5	40,20 ± 24,7	54,04 ± 37,0	<0,001*
Total fat (g)		101,74 ± 63,9	74,76 ± 45,37	87,30 ± 56,3	<0,001*
Saturated fatty acids (g)		45,35 ± 28,3	31,41 ± 22,6	38,38 ± 25,8	<0,001*
Monounsaturated fatty acids (g)		34,40 ± 25,32	26,37 ± 18,2	30,39 ± 22,1	<0,001*
Polyunsaturated fatty acids (g)		20,89 ± 13,05	16,98 ± 8,2	18,94 ± 11,5	<0,001*
Carbohydrates (g)		180,16 ± 215,9	152,05 ± 90,2	166,10 ± 163,8	<0,001*
Vegetable fibers (g)		26,72 ± 24,1	14,27 ± 11,5	20,50 ± 18,7	<0,001*
Vitamin D (µg)		9,91 ± 5,1	6,32 ± 7,6	7,76 ± 6,9	<0,001*
Vitamin C (mg)		131,62 ± 111,1	118,36 ± 112,0	123,66 ± 166,8	<0,001*
Calcium (mg)		953,91 ± 316,32	918,79 ± 232,0	932,74 ± 268,7	0,366
Phosphorus (mg)		1012,23 ± 315,23	1132,21 ± 235,25	1072,22 ± 235,2	<0,001*
Potassium (mg)		6441,99 ± 3231,4	4453,70 ± 1362,0	5294,02 ± 2482,4	<0,001*
Magnesium (mg)		546,16 ± 245,9	404,70 ± 136,1	461,28 ± 199,8	<0,001*
Zinc (mg)		17,38 ± 8,0	13,02 ± 4,2	14,77 ± 6,4	<0,001*

* statistical significance on the level P < 0,05

Table 2. The average daily nutrient intake in fertile and in menopausal women ($\bar{X} \pm SD$)

DXA parameters which were extracted by ROC analyses as excellent predictors of bone metabolism were included in multiple regression analyses. Those include: LS BMC, LS BMD, LS T-score, LS Z-score, LH BMC, LH T-score.

The results of multiple regression analysis by which are defined total shares and significance of contributions of menstrual status, age, anthropometry and nutrition on the bone densitometry parameters. The largest total share of contributions to all the bone densitometry parameters was observed for menstrual status and diet (Table 3).

Parameters	Menstrual status	Age	Anthropometry	Nutrition
	Share of contributions (%)	Share of contributions (%)	Share of contributions (%)	Share of contributions (%)
LS BMC	40,1	8,4	8,5	44,8
LS BMD	29,6	3,3	16,6	12,7
LS T-score	29,6	6,1	19,3	27,4
LS Z-score	20,8	7,2	13,0	12,7
LH BMC	27,8	12,0	24,2	23,2
LH T-score	24,5	0,5	27,0	18,6

LS – lumbar spine

LH – left hip

Table 3. Total shares of contributions of menstrual status, age, anthropometry and nutrition on DXA (%)

Parameters	LS BMC		LS BMD		LS T-score		LS Z-score		LH BMC		LH T-score	
	ß	P	ß	P	ß	P	ß	P	ß	P	ß	P
Menstrual status	-0,632	<0,001*	-0,560	<0,001*	-0,632	<0,001*	-0,529	<0,001*	-0,568	<0,001*	-0,389	<0,001*
Age	-0,156	0,057	-0,097	0,251	-0,156	0,057	-0,365	0,001*	-0,210	0,010*	-0,017	0,831
Nutrition												
Energy	0,346	0,014*	0,238	0,150	0,667	0,016*	0,627	0,002*	0,400	0,048*	0,063	0,529
Proteins (g)	0,008	0,580	0,010	0,445	0,081	0,481	0,004	0,978	0,349	<0,001*	0,786	0,082
Total fat (g)	-0,273	0,036*	-0,103	0,386	-0,098	0,016*	-0,191	0,127	-0,427	0,016*	-0,500	0,054
Saturated fatty acids (g)	-0,234	0,810	-0,141	0,166	0,148	0,005*	-0,016	0,332	-0,414	0,053	-0,259	0,244
Monounsaturated fatty acids (g)	0,079	0,551	0,029	0,875	0,144	0,019*	0,031	0,145	0,328	0,182	0,258	0,312
Polyunsaturated fatty acids (g)	0,086	0,546	0,044	0,782	0,209	0,049*	0,013	0,104	0,310	0,069	0,329	0,063
Calcium (mg)	2,045	0,256	0,538	0,168	0,007	0,145	-0,219	0,032*	0,034	0,626	0,023	0,748
Potassium (mg)	0,211	0,004*	0,536	0,006*	0,213	0,005*	0,103	0,004*	0,089	0,001*	0,750	0,414
Phosphorus (mg)	-0,623	0,277	-0,078	0,053	0,139	0,031*	0,071	0,033*	-0,078	0,851	-0,234	0,588
Magnesium (mg)	0,073	0,002*	0,054	0,053	0,133	0,036*	0,031	0,010*	0,157	0,002*	0,422	0,187

*statistical significance on level $P < 0,05$

β – regression coefficient

LS – lumbar spine

LH – left hip

Table 4. Statistically significant interactions of predictors (menstrual status, age, and nutrients) to categorical variables (LS BMC, LS BMD, LS T-score, LS Z-score, LH BMC, LH T-score) are shown

Menstrual status, age, total fat, saturated fatty acids, are inversely proportional to the values of the bone densitometry parameters, while energy, proteins, monounsaturated fatty acids, polyunsaturated fatty acids, calcium, potassium and magnesium are exactly proportional to the values of the bone densitometry parameters.

http://dx.doi.org/10.5772/54433

Parameters	Milkand milk products		Fish		Vegetables		Fruit	
LS BMD	β	P	β	P	β	P	β	P
	0,008	0,169	0,031	0,677	0,034	0,742	0,027	0,733
LS BMC	0,109	0,128	0,171	0,014*	0,006	0,346	0,016	0,645
LS T-score	0,077	0,301	0,043	0,577	0,089	0,150	0,047	0,556
LS Z-score	0,105	0,163	0,008	0,024*	0,127	0,135	0,092	0,256
LH BMC	0,039	0,598	0,086	0,005*	0,214	0,002*	0,156	0,050
LH T-score	0,178	0,015*	0,135	<0,001*	0,178	0,004*	0,107	0,178

*statistical significance on level P < 0,05

β – regression coefficient

LS – lumbar spine

LH – left hip

Table 5. Interactions of predictors (milk and milk products, fish, vegetables and fruit) to categorical variables (LS BMD, LS BMC, LS T-score, LS Z-score, LH BMC, LH T-score) are shown

Milk and milk products, fish, vegetables and fruit are exactly proportional to the bone densitometry parameters.

Parameters	LS BMC	LS BMD	LS T-score	LS Z-score	LH BMC	LH T-score
	share of contribution (%)	share of contribution (%)	share of contribution (%)	share of contribution (%)	share of contribution (%)	share of contribution (%)
Menstrual status	40,1	29,6	29,6	20,8	27,8	24,5
Age	8,4	3,3	6,1	7,2	12,0	0,5
Energy	2,7	0,5	2,8	3,2	1,4	0,2
Proteins (g)	0,2	0,1	0,2	0	5,8	4,8
Total fat (g)	5,8	0,9	2,4	1,8	1,5	2,4
Saturated fatty acids (g)	0,5	1,6	3,3	0,2	1,7	0,7
Monounsaturated fatty acids (g)	1,4	0,2	2,2	0,3	1,5	0,7
Polyunsaturated fatty acids (g)	1,6	0,5	1,6	0,1	0,2	0,6
Calcium (mg)	0,9	0,7	1,0	1,8	0,2	0
Potassium (mg)	8,8	5,9	3,4	4,1	7,3	5,1
Phosphorus (mg)	5,3	0,6	3,5	4,5	0	0,9
Magnesium (mg)	10,1	0,2	3,1	2,4	2,8	0,8

Table 6. Total shares of contributions of menstrual status, age and nutrition on DXA (%)

3. Discussion

It is considered that menopausal women have the highest risk of osteoporotic fractures and the incidence of osteoporosis in this group is increased by 25% compared to fertile women [3]. Furthermore, the frequency of osteoporotic vertebral and hip fractures in both genders increases exponentially with age [1]. Results obtained by this study coincide with the majority of results of similar studies, showing that menopausal women have significantly lower values of the bone densitometry parameters [17,18,19]. The latter is additionally confirmed by our finding of inversely proportional relationship between menopause and bone mineral density parameters. Our result of inversely proportional relationship between age and bone mineral density parameters, corresponds to a study conducted on 450 000 participants from Sweden [20].

Bone remodeling markers provide information about the dynamic state of bone metabolism, and those are very useful tools to predict early changes in the bone metabolism. Along with the bone densitometry, bone remodeling markers are needy in diagnosis and follow up of diseases of the bone mass deficit [21]. We have demonstrated that women of generative age have significantly lower values of DPD ($P<0,001$) than women in menopause. This is consistent to increased excretion of DPD in postmenopausal women [22]. Menopausal women had significantly higher levels of bone ALP ($P=0,004$) compared to women in generative age. The latter could be explained by the fact that high serum concentration of bone formation markers is associated with greater bone loss [23]. Average concentration of vitamin D in all study participants amounted 66,16 nmol/l, out of which average value in fertile women amounted 62,03 nmol/l, and 68,9 nmol/l in menopausal women (Table 2). Similar values of vitamin D concentrations were observed in a study of postmenopausal women of nine European countries [24]. By adding our results of low vitamin D concentrations to similar results published by Kraljević et al. [25] and by Žerjavić et al. [26], we can summarize that some action should be done by Croatian Health Care system, such as food-based strategies, to prevent vitamin D deficiency in Croatia.

Nutrition has a unique role in processes of growth and modeling of the human skeleton, as well as in maintaining the peak bone mass in adulthood [2]. The most of the studies are focused on dietary calcium intake [19], some of the researchers have analyzed the impact of some other nutrients such as proteins, carbohydrates, fat and energy intake [27], and only a few studies have explored the influence of vitamins and minerals on bone mass [7]. Calcium in a form of the calcium phosphate or calcium carbonate is the major mineral constituent of the bone tissue. High calcium intake, within the normal diet, does not protect against fractures, but low calcium intake represents a risk factor for the osteoporosis [19].

By means of the multiple regression analysis we have determined that the greatest contribution of the anthropometry is to values of the BMC and the T-score of the left hip

(Table 3). A positive relationship between increased body weight or body mass index (BMI) to bone mass has been already reported [28,29]. Some authors have considered that increased body weight can improve bone mass, by stimulation of the osteoblast differentiation. Body weight increase in postmenopausal period is correlated to increased number of adipocytes. Adipocytes are an important source of estrogen, a hormone which stimulates bone formation [30]. The opposite theories to afore mentioned have been reported too [31] and amongst those is a research of Kroke et al. [32], who did not find strong influence of anthropometric parameters on bone mineral density neither in women of generative age, nor in postmenopausal women.

It has been proposed that high energy intake, leads to body weight increase and finally to increased values of the bone mineral density [33,34]. Similarly to results obtained by Kumar et al. [35], our results indicate that daily energy intake is exactly proportional to the values of the bone densitometry parameters (Table 4).

Total daily protein intake is directly proportional to the values of the bone densitometry parameters, which was significant for the LH BMC ($P<0,001$) (Table 4). Such result is in agreement to results obtained by Misra et al. [36]. These researchers have documented a positive correlation between total protein intake and increased bone mineral density. Further protein analysis revealed a positive influence of proteins of vegetable origin and negative influence of proteins of animal origin on the bone mass. SOF study (Study of osteoporotic fractures) found that women with increased animal proteins intake have low values of the bone mineral density and increased risk of osteoporotic fractures [5].

Total fat and saturated fatty acids are inversely proportional to DXA parameters, while monounsaturated and polyunsaturated fatty acids are exactly proportional to DXA parameters (Table 4). Greater shares of contribution of all four types of fat were found for DXA parameters of the lumbar spine than of the left hip (Table 6). Significance was observed for the T-score of the lumbar spine (Table 4). Corwin et al., conducted the survey on menopausal women, and found a negative correlation between total fat intake and bone mineral density [37]. Another research of Hogstroma et al. corresponds to our results since they have also found positive correlation between monounsaturated fatty acids intake and bone mineral density [38].

Regarding daily calcium intake, total shares of calcium contribution are greater in lumbar spine than in the left hip. Interestingly calcium does not contribute at all to the values of the LH T-score (Table 6). Calcium is directly proportional to the values of DXA parameters, but the only statistical significance relates to LS Z-score (Table 4). Similarly was found in the study of H. F. Saadi et al., where dietary calcium intake of fertile women and postmenopausal women is positively, but not significantly correlated to bone mineral density [39]. Average daily calcium intake amounted 932,74 g, which are adequate amounts of dietary calcium according to existing recommendations in Croatia (Table 2).

Daily intake of the minerals magnesium and potassium has the greatest contribution of all the given minerals to DXA parameters (Table 6). Both of the minerals are directly proportional to DXA parameters (Table 4). Studies published so far argue that sufficient magnesium and potassium intake is related to increased bone mineral density [40,41], or as contrast opinions state, to reduced bone mass and increased risk of wrist fracture [43]. Magnesium is important in processes of bone mineralization, and potassium has important role in systemic acid-base (pH) homeostasis. Potassium salts neutralize bone-depleting metabolic acids, and therefore conditions that require drain of alkalizing compounds from bone lead to loss of bone tissue. Positive influence of potassium on bone health has been reported [3,4,40,45].

Zinc is a cofactor for alkaline phosphatase, an enzyme, necessary for bone mineralization. Low concentration of the zinc in serum and its increased secretion in urine is associated with osteoporosis [44]. Considering that calcification of the bone is reduced with insufficient zinc intake, we analyzed influence of the dietary zinc on bone health. Results revealed that daily zinc intake is directly proportional to DXA parameters, but the influence was not significant (data not shown).

Analyzing the impact of fruit and vegetables on DXA parameters in women, we have found that vegetables are directly proportional to the parameters of the left hip, which is statistically significant (table 5). Similar results were obtained by New et al. [3] who have that bone mineral density in premenopausal women was positively related to fruit and vegetable intake, as well as to magnesium, calcium, zinc and plant fibers. Similarly, Tucker et al. have found better bone mass in women who consumed more fruits, vegetables, potassium and magnesium [41]. However, other study which has included postmenopausal women, showed no relationship between bone mass to fruit or vegetable intake [7,46].

Regarding the mechanisms fruit and vegetables influence bone metabolism, it is important to mention that these nutrients create an alkaline environment and therefore reduce urinary calcium excretion. Besides, fruits and vegetables are rich in vitamins with antioxidant properties such as vitamin C and beta-carotene. Vegetables are an important source of vitamin K, which also has a role in the mineralization of bone since it induces carboxylation of osteocalcin [40].

4. Conclusion

Analyses of the impact of age, anthropometric parameters, menstrual status and nutrition on the bone status, represents the age and menstrual status as predictors with the highest influence on the bone mineral density in women.

Fruits and vegetables have pleiotropic effects on bone metabolism, which include: alkalinity, antioxidant properties of vitamins and as it was determined by this study, beneficial influence of minerals magnesium, potassium and zinc.

http://dx.doi.org/10.5772/54433

Author details

Olga Cvijanović[1*], Sandra Pavičić Žeželj[2], Silvija Lukanović[1], Nenad Bićanić[3], Robert Domitrović[4], Dragica Bobinac[1] and Željka Crnčević Orlić[3]

*Address all correspondence to: olgac@medri.hr

1 Department of Anatomy, Rijeka Faculty of Medicine, Rijeka, Croatia

2 Department of Ecology Health, Teaching Institute of Public Health Mountain-Littoral County, Rijeka Faculty of Medicine, Rijeka, Croatia

3 Department of Endocrinology, Clinics for Internal Medicine Rijeka Clinical Centre, Rijeka Faculty of Medicine, Rijeka, Croatia

4 Department of Chemistry and Biochemistry, Rijeka Faculty of Medicine, Rijeka, Croatia

References

[1] Prentice, A. Diet, nutrition and prevention of osteoporosis. Pub Health Nutr (2004)., 7, 227-243.

[2] Bainbridge, K. E, Sowers, M, Lin, X, & Harlow, S. D. Risk factors for low bone mineral density and the 6-year rate of bone loss among premenopausal and perimenopausal women. Osteoporos Int (2004)., 15, 439-446.

[3] New, S. A, Robins, S. P, Campbell, M. K, Martin, J. C, Gorton, M. J, Bolton-smith, C, Grubb, D. A, Lee, S. J, & Reid, D. M. Dietary influences on bone mass and bone metabolism: further evidence of a positive link between fruit and vegetable consumption and bone health. Am J Clin Nutr (2000)., 71, 142-51.

[4] Nieves, J. W. Osteoporosis: the role of micronutrients. Am J Clin Nutr (2005). S-9S.

[5] Sellmeyer, D. E, Stone, K. L, Sebastian, A, & Cummings, S. R. For the Study of Osteoporotic Fractures Research Group. A high ratio of dietary animal to vegetable protein increases the rate of bone loss and the risk of fracture in postmenopausal women. Am J Clin Nutr (2001)., 73, 118-22.

[6] Weikert, C, Dietmar, W, Hoffman, K, Kroke, A, Bergmann, M. M, & Boeing, H. The Relation between Dietary Protein, Calcium and Bone Health in Women: Results from the EPIC-Postdam Cohort. Ann Nutr Metab (2005)., 49, 312-318.

[7] Mecdonald, H. M, New, S. A, Golden, M. H, Cambel, M. K, & Reid, D. M. Nutritional associations with bone loss during the menopausal transition: evidence of a benefi-

cial effect of calcium, alcohol, and fruit and vegetable nutrients and of a detrimental effect of fatty acids. Am J Clin Nutr (2004). , 79, 155-65.

[8] Willet, W. C, Sampson, L, Stampfer, M. J, Rosner, B, Bain, C, Witschi, J, Hennekens, C. H, & Speizer, F. E. Reproducibility and validity of a semi quantitative food frequency questionnaire. Am J Epidemiol (1985). , 122, 51-65.

[9] Kaic-rak, A, & Antonic, K. Tablice o sastavu namirnica i pića. Zagreb: Zavod za zaštitu zdravlja Hrvatske; (1990).

[10] WHO: Technical Report Series 53Geneva ((1976).

[11] QuidelAn enzyme immunoassay for the quantitation of pyridinum crosslinks (PYD and DPD) in human urine. Metra PYD EIA kit.

[12] QuidelAssays for Bone-specific Alkaline Phosphatase. Metra BAP EIA kit.

[13] IDSHydroxy Vitamin D EIA. Enzymeimmunoassay for the quantitative determination of 25-hydroxyvitamin D and other hydroxylated metabolites in serum or plasma., 25.

[14] Favus, M. J. Primer on the Metabolic Bone Diseases and Disorders of Mineral Metabolism, 4th ed. An Official Publication of The American Society for Bone and Mineral Research. USA: Lippincott Williams & Wilkins (1999). , 113-174.

[15] Petz, B. Osnove statističke metode za nematematičare. Jastrebarsko: Naklada Slap; (2001).

[16] Wallace, L, Boxall, M, & Riddick, N. Influencing exercise and diet to prevent osteoporosis: lessons from three studies. Br J Community Nurs (2004). , 9, 544-552.

[17] Okano, H, Mizunuma, H, Soda, M, Kagami, I, Miyamoto, S, Ohsawa, M, Ibuki, Y, Shiraki, M, Suzuki, T, & Shibata, H. The long-term effect of menopause on postmenopausal bone loss in Japanese women: results from a prospective study. J Bone Miner Res (1998). , 13, 303-309.

[18] Poullies, J. M, Tremolliers, F, & Ribot, C. The effects of menopause on longitudinal bone loss from spine. Caitiff Tissue Int (1993). , 52, 340-343.

[19] Filip, R. S, & Zagorski, J. Osteoporosis risk factors in rural and urban women from the Lublin Region of Poland. Ann Agric Environ Med (2005). , 12, 21-6.

[20] Landin-wilhelmsen, K, Johansson, S, Rosengren, A, Dotevall, A, Lapass, G, Bengntsson, B. A, & Wilhelmsen, L. Calceneal ultrasound measurements are determined by age and physical activity. Studies in two Swedish random population samples. J Inter Med (2000). , 247, 269-278.

[21] Garnero, P. Biomarkers for osteoporosis management: utility in diagnosis, fracture risk prediction and therapy monitoring. Mol Diagn Ther (2008). , 1283, 157-70.

[22] Cepelak, I, & Cvorišcec, D. Biokemijski biljezi pregradnje kostiju-pregled. Biochemia Medica (2009). , 19(1), 17-35.

[23] Garnero, P, & Delmas, P. D. Contribution of bone mineral density and bone turnover markers to the estimation of risk of osteoporotic fracture in postmenopausal women. J Musculoskel Neuron Interact (2004). , 4(1), 50-63.

[24] Bruyere, O, & Malaise, O. Neuprez, Collette J, Reginster JY. Prevalence of vitamin Dinadequancy in European postmenopausal women. Curr Med Res Opin (2007). , 23, 1212-1221.

[25] Kraljevic, I, Kastelan, D, Gorsic, I, Solak, M, Giljevic, Z, Kasovic, M, Sertic, J, & Korsic, M. Vitamin D deficiency in postmenopausal women receiving osteoporosis therapy. Liječnički Vjesnik (2007).

[26] Laktasic-zerjavic, N, Korsic, M, Crncevic-orlic, Z, Kovac, Z, Polasek, O, & Soldo-juresa, D. Vitamin D status, depedence on age, and seasonal variations in the concentracion of vitamin D in Croatian postmenopausal women initially screened for osteoporosis. Clin Rheumatol (2010). , 29, 861-867.

[27] Babaroutsi, E, Magkos, F, Manios, Y, & Sidossis, L. S. Lifestyle factors affecting heel ultrasound in Greek females across different life stages. Osteoporos Int (2005). , 16, 552-561.

[28] Guney, E, Kisakol, G, Ozgen, G, Yulmaz, C, Yilmal, Z, & Kabalak, T. Effect of weight loss on bone metabolism: comparison of vertical banded gastroplasty and medical intervention. Obes Surg (2003). , 13, 383-8.

[29] Radak, T. L. Caloric restriction and calciums effect on bone metabolism and body composition in overweight and obese premenopausal women. Nutr Rev (2004). , 62, 468-81.

[30] Kyong-chol, K, Dong-hyuk, S, Sei-young, L, Jee-aee, I, & Duk-chul, L. Relation berween Obesity and Bone Mineral Density and Vertebral Fractures in Korean Postmenopusal Women. Yonsei Med J (2010). , 51(6), 857-863.

[31] Zhao, L. J, Liu, Y. J, Liu, P. Y, Hamilton, J, Recker, R. R, & Deng, H. W. Relationship of obesity with osteoporosis. J Clin Endocrinol Metab (2007). , 92, 1640-6.

[32] Kroke, A, Klipstein-grobusch, K, Bergmann, M. M, Weber, K, & Boeing, H. Influence of body composition on quantitative ultrasound parameters of the os calcis in a population-based sample of pre-and postmenopausal women. Calcified Tissue Int (2000). , 66, 5-10.

[33] Felson, D. T, Zhang, Y, Hannan, M. T, & Anderson, J. J. Effects of weight and body mass index in bone mineral density in men and women: the Framingham study. J Bone Mineral Res (1993). , 8, 567-573.

[34] Harris, S. S, & Dawson-huges, B. Weight, body composition and bone density in postmenopausal women. Calcif Tissue Int (1996). , 59, 428-432.

[35] Kumar, A, Mittal, S, Orito, S, Ishitani, K, & Ohta, H. Impact of dietary intake, education nad physical activity on bone mineral density among North Indian women. J Bone Miner Metab (2010). , 28(2), 192-201.

[36] Misra, D, Berry, S. D, Broe, K. E, Mclean, R. R, Cupples, L. A, Tucker, K. L, Kiel, D. P, & Hannan, M. T. Does Dietary Protein Reduce Hip Fracture Risk in Elders? The Framingham Osteoporosis Study. Osteoporos Int (2011). , 22(1), 345-349.

[37] Corwin, R. L, Hartman, T. J, Maczuga, S. A, & Graubard, B. I. Dietary saturated fat intake is inversely associated with bone density in humans: analysis of NANES III. J Nutr (2006). , 136, 159-65.

[38] Hogstrom, M, Nordstrom, P, & Nordstrom, A. n. fatty acids positively associated with bone mineral density and bone accrual in healthy men: the Study. Am J Clin Nutr (2007). , 85(2), 803-7.

[39] Saadi, H. F, Reed, R. L, Carter, A. O, Duun, E. V, Qazaq, H. S, & Al-suhaili, A. R. Quantitative ultrasound of the calcaneus in Arabian women: relation to anthropometric and lifestyle factors. Maturitas (2003). , 44, 215-223.

[40] Prynne, C. J, Mishra, G. D, Connell, O, Muniz, M. A, Laskey, G, Yan, M. A, Prentice, L, Ginty, A, & Fruit, F. and vegetable intakes and bone mineral status: a cross-sectional study in 5 age and sex cohorts. Am J Clin Nutr (2006). , 83, 1420-1428.

[41] Tucker, K. L, Hannan, M. T, Chen, H, Cupples, L. A, Wilson, P. W, & Kiel, D. P. Potassium, magnesium and fruit and vegetable intakes are associated with grater bone mineral density in elderly men and women. Am J Clin Nutr (1999). , 69, 727-36.

[42] Schaafsma, A. Vries PJF, Saris WHM. Delay of natural bone loss by higher intakes of specific minerals and vitamins. Crit Rev Food Sci Nutr (2001). , 41(3), 225-249.

[43] Jackson, R. D. LaCroix AZ, Cauley JA, McGowan J. The impact of magnesium intake on fractures: results from the women's health initiative observational study (WHI-OS). ASBMR (2003). abstr.

[44] Ilich, Z. J, & Kerstetter, J. E. Nutrition in bone health revisited: A story beyond calcium. J Am Coll Nutr (2000). , 19, 715-37.

[45] Kaptoge, S, Welch, A, Mctaggart, A, Mulligan, A, Dalzell, N, Day, N. E, Birgham, S, Knaw, K. T, & Reeve, J. Effects of dietary nutrients and food groups on bone loss from the proximal femur in men and women in 7th and 8th decades of age. Osteoporos Int (2003). , 14, 418-28.

[46] Macdonald, H. M, New, S. A, Fraser, W. D, Cambell, M. K, & Reid, D. V. Low dietary potassium intakes and high dietary estimates of net endogenous acid production are associated with low bone mineral density in premenopausal women and increased markers of bone resorption in postmenopausal women. Am J Clin Nutr (2005). , 81, 923-33.

Chapter 8

Bone Mineral Density and High-Performance Aerobic Activity in Older Adults Experience in Brazil

Luiz Eugênio Garcez Leme and
Maria do Carmo Sitta

Additional information is available at the end of the chapter

http://dx.doi.org/10.5772/55661

1. Introduction

Population aging has exhibited a significant increase in the last decades. For instance, in Brazil, recent projections by the IBGE 1 (Instituto Brasileiro de Geografia e Estatística/Brazilian Institute of Geography and Statistics) forecast a threefold increase of the elderly population by 2050 from the current 10.8% to 29.7% of the country's total population, corresponding to almost 65 million people. The life expectancy at birth of the overall population increased to 73 years in the last decade (1999-2009), ranging from 73.9 to 77 years among females and 66.3 to 69 years among males. Such aging of the Brazilian population will pose increasing challenges to the national public health system, SUS (Sistema Único de Saúde/Unified Health System), as older adults exhibit a larger number of chronic diseases, which contribute to loss of functionality and decline of the quality of life.

The expected and, indeed, already occurring consequences include the progressive increase of the demand for public healthcare services, higher numbers of hospital admissions, and the use of long-term care facilities [2, 3]. The growth of the elderly population may cause a significant increase of the prevalence of chronic diseases, frailty syndrome, and femoral head fractures, which are frequent occurrences in developed countries.

In a Brazilian population-based study involving more than 2,400 individuals older than 40 years, Pinheiro et al. 4 reported incidences of frailty fractures of 15.1% among females and 12.8% among males. A study conducted by the National Institute of Traumatology and Orthopedics (Instituto Nacional de Traumato-Ortopedia - INTO) in Rio de Janeiro reported that the incidence of osteoporosis was 36.4% among men older than 80 years 5. Cost studies indicate that the average cost of in-hospital intervention and surgery per patient is approximately BRL 24,000.00 (USD 11,700.00) 6.

As the number of hospital admissions due to bone fractures among the Brazilian population older than 40 years is higher than 250,000 per year [7], a total cost of approximately 3 billion dollars (BRL 6.5 billion) might be estimated. This estimate comprises only hospital expenses; the cost of home and outpatient care and the loss of patient and caregiver productivity must be added to this estimate together with the incalculable costs associated with loss of quality of life and health. Consequently population aging is an emerging and serious problem.

2. Frailty

Aging is associated with progressive manifestations of frailty, poorer capacity of adaptation, and less resilience, which is defined as the ability of individuals to address problems, overcome obstacles, or resist the pressure imposed by adverse conditions.

The conference on frailty in older adults sponsored by the American Geriatrics Society (AGS) and the National Institute on Aging (NIA) defined frailty as a "state of greater vulnerability to stressors due to age and declines related with the neuromuscular, metabolic and immune physiological reserve [8].

The correlation between frailty and orthopedic risks is patent among older adults.

Fried et al. [9] created a definition of the phenotype of frailty that is widely used in research protocols and was validated in the Cardiovascular Health Study (CHS), which was conducted with more than 5,000 men and women aged 65 years or older. According to this study, frailty corresponds to the presence of three or more of the following criteria (pre-frailty corresponds to the presence of less than three):

1. Weight loss (≥ 5% of the body weight in the past year)
2. Exhaustion (positive answers to questions on the effort needed for physical activity)
3. Weakness (reduced grip strength)
4. Slow walking speed (> 6 to 7 minutes to walk 15 m)
5. Low physical activity (Kcal per week: men < 383 Kcal, women < 270 Kcal)

In a study on the index of osteoporotic fractures, Ensrud et al. [10] applied a simpler index to define frailty, whereby it corresponds to the presence of at least two out of the three following criteria:

1. Loss of 5% of the body weight in the past year
2. Inability to rise from a chair five times without using the arms
3. Answering "no" to the question, "Do you feel full of energy?"

Several studies [11, 12] found that the two abovementioned indices were comparable in the prediction of the risk of fall, deficiency, fracture, hospital admission, and death.

http://dx.doi.org/10.5772/55661

There is a clear correlation between the criteria used in the definition of frailty and the factors related with fall risk and osteoporosis. From the syndromic perspective, a strong correlation exists indicating that frailty as such might be considered as a predisposing factor for falls, fractures, and their complications among the elderly population.

3. Falls

Falls are most likely the main health problem among the elderly population, frail people in particular. The risks of fractures and their complications increase together with osteoporosis.

A cohort study conducted in the city of São Paulo and involving more than 1,500 participants [13] found that 35% to 40% of the elderly individuals aged 60 years or older fall at least once per year, and this rate grows to 50% among individuals older than 80 years.

In the abovementioned study, the variables that independently and significantly correlated with increased probability of falls were female gender, previous history of fractures, difficulty to perform physical activity, and reported poor or very poor vision.

Upon investigating falls, another cohort study in São Paulo involving more than 2,000 older adults [14] reported that 33.5% of the studied population reported falls in the past year, whereby 20.2% of the participants reported one single episode, 5.9% reported two episodes, and 7.4% reported three or more episodes.

That same study clearly established a direct correlation between frailty and number and severity of falls.

4. Osteoporosis and aging

Osteoporosis and falls represent the main risk factors for the occurrence of fractures, which possibly are the main health problem of older adults.

4.1. Physiopathology

The skeleton performs a double function related with metabolism and body support.

A reduction of bone mass associated with deterioration of its microarchitecture predisposes an individual to fractures. The bone is a metabolically active tissue, undergoing constant remodeling through the action of the cells responsible for bone resorption (osteoclasts – derived from the monocyte lineage) and formation (osteoblasts – derived from the fibroblast lineage).

The control of bone resorption and formation is coordinated and synchronized by a system known as RANK-RANKL-OPG, which allows for a better understanding of bone physiology and paves the way for the development of novel treatments[1].

The cytokine RankL, a member of the TNF (tumor necrosis factor) superfamily, is expressed and secreted by osteoblasts. Interaction between RankL (expressed on the osteoblast surface) and RanK (expressed on the surface of the osteoclast precursors) mediates differentiation and activation of osteoclasts in the presence of M-CSF (macrophage colony-stimulating factor). Mature osteoclasts initiate the process of bone resorption. The interaction between RankL and its receptor on osteoclasts is controlled by osteoprotegerin (OPG). OPG is a soluble receptor belonging to the TNF family that inhibits the binding of RankL to RanK, thus preventing the recruitment, proliferation, and activation of osteoclasts, and this receptor also exerts inhibitory effects on the osteoclast precursor cells. The balance between OPG and RankL controls bone remodeling.

The balance of the RANK/RANKL/OPG system is regulated by cytokines and hormones.

Parathormone (PTH), glucocorticoids, and E2 prostaglandins increase the activity of RANKL and reduce the activity of OPG. However, transforming growth factor beta (TGF-β), 17 β-estradiol, interleukin 1 (IL-1), and TNF-α exhibit the opposite actions, i.e., they reduce the activity of RANKL and activate OPG. [3]

During growth and aging, the predominance of formation and resorption alternate in the development of bone. Formation is greater until the age of 25 years, stabilizes until the age of 35 years, then decreases progressively, exhibiting a greater decline starting at the age of 70 years. Resorption predominates starting at the age of 35 years and accelerates during the postmenopausal period and until the age of 70 years.

Osteoporosis can be classified as primary or secondary. In turn, primary osteoporosis is subdivided into

- Type I or postmenopausal, which is characterized by increased bone resorption.
- Type II or senile, which is characterized by decreased bone formation.

Secondary osteoporosis, resulting from other pathologies, may be triggered by

- Endocrine disorders: Hyperthyroidism, Diabetes, Hyperparathyroidism, Hypercortisolism, Hypogonadism
- Rheumatic disorders: Rheumatoid arthritis, Spondylitis
- Malabsorption syndromes, Inflammatory Bowel Disease, Coeliac Disease, Post-Gastrectomy
- Kidney Failure
- Neoplasias: Myeloma, Lymphoma
- Drugs: corticosteroids, anticonvulsants, alcohol, thyroid hormone.

Osteoporosis is universal among the elderly population, exhibits progressive incidence, and is directly correlated with age and lifestyle, including the practice of sports.

---

1 RANK – is the abbreviation of receptor activator of nuclear factor kappa B; RANKL – receptor activator of nuclear factor kappa-B ligand; and OPG –osteoprotegerin.

http://dx.doi.org/10.5772/55661

5. Physical activity

Given the growth of the elderly population, the establishment of health promotion measures to reduce the prevalence of chronic diseases, improve functionality, and control multimorbidity is notably important. The goal in this regard is to improve the quality of life of older adults and to reduce healthcare expenses. Among such health-promoting measures, physical activity is one of the main factors associated with control of comorbidities and the reduction of the risk of morbimortality by cardiovascular diseases [15], diabetes [16], obesity [17], and osteoporosis [18]. Physical activity has also been correlated with improved cognition [19, 20, 21, 22] and reduced risk of the incidence of Alzheimer's disease [23].

Regular exercise is important for healthy aging because it has an influence on chronic diseases and functionality. Exercise seems to be a protective factor against genetic and molecular aging and is associated with longevity [24]. Exercise protects [25] the organism against oxidative stress [26] and inflammation [27], which cause damage to the deoxyribonucleic acid (DNA) and other cell structures, resulting in progressive loss of metabolic and physiological functions and greater propensities for cardiovascular, neurodegenerative, and oncological diseases.

The beneficial effects of physical exercise have been demonstrated in the prevention and control of cardiovascular and osteomuscular diseases and diabetes and in the prevention of neoplasias. [28] In recent years, research has focused on the beneficial effects of physical activity on cognitive functions and prevention of dementias [29].

Together with nutritional measures, hormone and calcium replacement, and use of bisphosphonates, programmed physical exercise has been reported as a protective factor against osteoporosis in older adults. Programmed physical exercise is an acknowledged source of countless benefits in all population sectors, including the elderly. Several authors have correlated the absence or reduction of such physical activity with a higher prevalence of osteoporosis.

Nevertheless, the prescription of physical activity involves a heterogeneous range of interventions, with each one possessing particular risks and benefits. Therefore, in addition to stimulating the practice of physical activities by their patients, healthcare professionals must carefully and thoroughly analyze the types of activity that are most appropriate for their intended purposes.

6. The rule of aerobic exercises

Aerobic exercises and, more particularly, walking and running, are the activities most often recommended by healthcare professionals and most widely practiced by the elderly population.

However, overly intense exercise (ultramarathon, running > 64 km per week) is associated with a larger number of osteoarticular lesions and immunosuppression. In addition, the ideal level of physical activity promoting cognitive benefits and modulating neuroprotectors and the inflammatory activity is still unknown.

Data in the literature regarding the benefits of long-distance running in the prevention of osteoporosis among older adults are controversial. Novotny et al. [30] assessed an Olympic and world champion long-distance runner 35 years after the end of his racing career and found that his joints were free of signs of arthrosis but that he presented with exceptionally advanced osteoporosis. Conversely, Maud et al. [31] studied a similar case of a long-distance runner older than 70 years who had more than 50 years of training and did not find any alterations in any system (including musculoskeletal). Additionally, regarding resistance exercise, the consensus seems to point to reduction of falls [32] and thus of fractures [33], although not necessarily of osteoporosis [34].

Several authors reported increases in bone density among high-performance runners, mainly in the femoral neck [35], whereas according to other authors, similarly to what appears to be the case of women [36], such runners exhibited reductions in bone mass 37 with debatable physiopathology but with a possible association with the metabolism of PTH. Finally, a third group of investigators did not identify any significant differences in bone density among the various groups. [38, 39]

When aerobic activity is combined with resistance training, the increase in bone mass becomes more evident, at least at the experimental level. [40]

6.1. Metanalyses

As the literature data concerning the benefits of aerobic activity in the elderly are conflicting, conducting metanalysis can be a real benefit in his assessment.

Metanalyses of studies on anaerobic exercise and osteoporosis in women produced notably modest results [41]. Several meta-analyses studies published by the Cochrane Collaboration [42] report that both resistance and aerobic exercises might improve bone density among women, and even walking might increase bone density at the hip. It is worth noting that the authors of the abovementioned study stated that the quality of the articles included in the review was modest, whereby the reliability of the results is limited. Still, in this regard, Yamasaki et al. reported that walking improved bone density at the lumbar spine and hip in postmenopausal women. [43]

7. Our experience

To analyze the effects of high-performance physical activity among older Brazilian adults, a cohort of senior athletes from IOTFMUSP (Instituto de Ortopedia e Traumatologia do Hospital das Clínicas da USP/Institute of Orthopedics and Traumatology of the Clinical Hospital of USP) was established in 2001. During the last 11 years, athletes older than 60 years and a control group consisting of healthy non-athlete individuals older than 60 years have been followed periodically by the assessment of several parameters, including bone density and body composition.

http://dx.doi.org/10.5772/55661

To analyze those parameters, 44 male athletes older than 60 years (mean 64 years) who regularly run more than 15,000 meters were compared; this group included several marathon runners and a number of super-marathon runners. The control group included 18 non-athlete individuals older than 60 years (mean 66.72 years) who had positive self-perceptions of their health and were independent in their everyday life activities. The groups were comparable with p=0,419.

Data were collected by means of double-absorption densitometry and were subjected to descriptive statistical analysis and Student's t-test for paired samples; the chi-square test was used in calculating sport activity as an intervention factor in controls and study subjects in a 2 x 2 table.

Comparisons of bone density, measured at the femoral neck and lumbar spine, between athletes and controls did not reveal any statistical significance (tables 1 and 2).

As a complementary measure, comparative analysis of the bone density in a subgroup of athletes over a 6-year period was performed. Although that group maintained its physical activity, no significant differences were identified among the measurements (table 3).

	Athletes –Femoral Neck Density	
	BMD	T - VALUE
Mean	0.958	-0.898
SD	0.152	1.175
Median	0.933	-1.100
	Controls –Femoral Neck Density	
	BMD	T - VALUE
Mean	0.90	-1.22
SD	0.10	0.77
Median	0.88	-1.45
	p=0.169	

BMD – Bone Mass Density in g/cm^2 /T-Score or Young Adults compared in standard deviations

Table 1. Density of the femoral neck in athletes and controls

	Athletes –Lumbar Spine Density	
	BMD	T Score Value
Mean	1.01	-0.21
SD	0.57	1.54
Median	1.23	-0.02
	Controls –Lumbar Spine Density	
	BMD	T Score Value
Mean	1.15	-0.89
SD	0.17	1.69
Median	1.12	-0.95
	p=0.501	

BMD – Bone Mass Density in g/cm² /T-Score or Young Adults compared in standard deviations

Table 2. Density of the lumbar spine in athletes and controls

Athlete	**Year**	
	T – VALUE	T Score Value
Year	*2001*	*2007*
Mean	1.02	1.02
SD	0.20	0.20
Median	1.03	1.03
	p=0.464	

T-Score or Young Adults compared in standard deviations

Table 3. Progression of bone density in athletes, 2001-2007

8. Discussion and conclusions

The first noteworthy aspect of our study is that only men were included, whereas most studies on osteoporosis, including those addressing physical activity, focus on women. This condition, resulting from the overall design of our cohort, was employed because although osteoporosis is less frequent among men, the consequences of its major complication, i.e., fractures, are more severe, resulting in higher indices of morbimortality among men compared to women [44].

In addition, several studies demonstrated that the incidence of osteoporosis among men increases quickly and progressively with age; in the studied area, osteoporosis may affect up to 40% of the male population older than 80 years [5].

Our data showed that predominantly aerobic activity, such as high-performance running, did not exhibit a statistically significant correlation with increased bone density; however, the density also did not decrease over a 6-year period. Therefore, our data agree with the findings by Kemmler [37] and Wisswell [38].

However, this finding places us at the center of the debates on aerobic exercise and osteoporosis.

The participants of this study belonged to a group of senior athletes with good athletic performance. An average running distance of 15 km and the fact that those athletes exhibited statistically significant improvement over the years denote effective training and follow-up.

As a measurement of bone mineral density (BMD), the femoral neck was preferentially used because it is location one most commonly tested. However, our data show that there is a statistically significant difference between the femoral neck and total body bone density that prevents their undifferentiated use.

In regard to the incidence of osteoporosis among older adults, analysis of the participants' bone densities in 2001 and 2007 (table 3) did not reveal any statistically significant differences.

Despite the small number of controls in this group, which may compromise its reliability, the data couldn't show us any perceptible difference between athletes and controls in respect to incidence of osteoporosis in concordance with international refereed data.

In the other hand we could not find alterations in bone density between comparisons with seven years of interval in the athletes group. This find may indicate that, if there were no gain in bone mass, on the other hand there were no losses, which might lead us to imagine a protective effect of bone loss in this group, confirming literature data.

These data lead us to conclude that regarding the prevention or treatment of osteoporosis in older adults, the practice of aerobic physical activity alone is controversial. In the best of cases, physical activity leads to reduced bone loss, although this finding is also poorly supported by evidence.

We are currently studying a subgroup of our cohort consisting of senior athletes practicing high-performance aerobic activity and simultaneously being subjected to parallel resistance training. We believe that the results obtained from this group might shed new light on this currently unclear aspect of the prevention and treatment of osteoporosis in older adults.

Acknowledgements

This chapter was partially funded by FAPESP - Fundação de Amparo à Pesquisa do Estado de São Paulo, Brasil (Foundation for Research Support of the State of São Paulo, Brazil), by process number 2013/00480-2.

Author details

Luiz Eugênio Garcez Leme and Maria do Carmo Sitta

Faculty of Medicine of University of São Paulo, Universidade de São Paulo – USP, Brazil

References

[1] IBGE, Diretoria de Pesquisas. Coordenação de População e Indicadores Sociais. Gerência de Estuidos e Análises de Dinâmicas Demográficas [Board of Research. Coordination of Population and Social Indicators. Management of Dynamic Demographic Studies and Analyses]. Projeção da População do Brasil por sexo e idade: 1980-2050 - Revisão 2010 [Projection of the Brazilian Population per gender and age: 1980-2050. 2010 Revision].

[2] Hazzard W, Blass J, Halter J, Ouslander J, Tinetti M. Principles of Geriatric Medicine & Gerontology. McGraw-Hill Companies, 2003.

[3] Freitas EV, Py L, Cançado FAX, Doll J, Gorzoni Ml. Tratado de Geriatria e Gerontologia [Treatise on Geriatrics and Gerontology]. 2ª edição , Rio de Janeiro: Guanabara Koogan, 2006.

[4] Pinheiro Marcelo M, Ciconelli Rozana M, Jacques Natielen de O, Genaro Patrícia S, Martini Lígia A, Ferraz Marcos B. O impacto da osteoporose no Brasil: dados regionais das fraturas em homens e mulheres adultos [Impact of osteoporosis in Brazil: regional data on fractures in adult men and women] - The Brazilian Osteoporosis Study (BRAZOS). Rev. Bras. Reumatol. [serial on the Internet]. 2010 Apr [cited 2012 Nov 11]; 50(2): 113-120. Available at: http://www.scielo.br/scielo.php?script=sci_arttext&pid=S0482-50042010000200002&lng=en. http://dx.doi.org/10.1590/S0482-50042010000200002.

[5] Ministério da Saúde: Pesquisa revela realidade da Osteoporose Masculina [Health Ministry: Study discloses the reality of male osteoporosis]. In: http://portal.saude.gov.br/portal/arquivos/pdf/saude_brasil_junho_2005.pdf - Accessed on November 11 2012.

[6] Araújo Denizar Vianna, Oliveira Juliana H. A. de, Bracco Oswaldo Luís. Cost of osteoporotic hip fracture in the Brazilian private health care system. Arq Bras Endocrinol Metab [serial on the Internet]. 2005 Dec [cited 2008 Feb 18]; 49(6): 897-901.

[7] Data obtained at SUS database (Datasus) at URL: http://tabnet.datasus.gov.br/cgi/tabcgi.exe?sih/cnv/niuf.def. Accessed on November 11 2012.

[8] Walston J, Hadley EC, Ferrucci L, Guralnik JM, Newman AB, Studenski SA, Ershler WB, Harris T, Fried LP. SOJ Research agenda for frailty in older adults: toward a better understanding of physiology and etiology: summary from the American Geriat-

http://dx.doi.org/10.5772/55661

rics Society/National Institute on Aging Research Conference on Frailty in Older Adults. J. Am Geriatr Soc. 2006; 54(6):991.

[9] Fried LP, Tangen CM, Walston J, Newman AB, Hirsch C, Gottdiener J, Seeman T, Tracy R, Kop WJ, Burke G, McBurnie MA: Frailty in older adults: evidence for a phenotype Cardiovascular Health Study Collaborative Research Group. J Gerontol A Biol Sci Med Sci. 2001; 56(3):M146.

[10] Ensrud KE, Ewing SK, Taylor BC, Fink HA, Cawthon PM, Stone KL, Hillier TA, Cauley JA, Hochberg MC, Rodondi N, Tracy JK, Cummings Comparison of 2 frailty indexes for prediction of falls, disability, fractures, and death in older women. SR. Arch Intern Med. 2008; 168(4): 382.

[11] Ensrud KE, Ewing SK, Cawthon PM, Fink HA, Taylor BC, Cauley JA, Dam TT, Marshall LM, Orwoll ES, Cummings SR. A comparison of frailty indexes for the prediction of falls, disability, fractures, and mortality in older men. Osteoporotic Fractures in Men Research Group. J Am Geriatr Soc. 2009; 57(3):492.

[12] Kiely DK, Cupples LA, Lipsitz LA: Validation and comparison of two frailty indexes: The MOBILIZE Boston Study. J Am Geriatr Soc. 2009; 57(9):1532.

[13] PERRACINI, Monica Rodrigues; RAMOS, Luiz Roberto. Fatores associados a quedas em uma coorte de idosos residentes na comunidade [Factors associated with falls in a cohort of community-residing older adults]. Rev. Saúde Pública, São Paulo, v. 36, n. 6, Dec. 2002. Available at <http://www.scielo.br/scielo.php?script=sci_arttext&pid=S0034-89102002000700008&lng=en&nrm=iso>. Accessed on 12 Nov. 2012.

[14] Lebrão, M.L. et al. Saúde, bem-estar e envelhecimento: o estudo SABE no Município de Sã Paulo [Health, wellbeing and aging: SABE study at the São Paulo Municipality]. Rev Bras Epidemiol 2005; 8(2): 127-41.

[15] Berlin JA, Colditz GA. A meta-analysis of physical activity in the prevention of coronary heart disease. Am J Epidemiol. 1990; 132(4):612-628.

[16] Albright A, Franz M, Hornsby G. American College of Sports Medicine position stand: exercise and type 2 diabetes. Med Sci Sports Exerc. 2000; 32(7): 1345-1360.

[17] Warburton DE, Nicol CW, Bredin SS. Health benefits of physical activity: the evidence. CMAJ. 2006; 174(6):801-809.

[18] Layne JE, Nelson ME. The effects of progressive resistance training on bone density: a review. Med Sci Sports Exerc 1999; 31:25-30.

[19] Yaffe K, Barnes D, Nevitt M, Lui LY, Covinsky K. A prospective study of physical activity and cognitive decline in elderly women: women who walk. Arch Intern Med 2001; 161:1703-1708.

[20] Barnes DE, Yaffe K, Satariano WA, Tager IB. A longitudinal study of cardiorespiratory fitness and cognitive function in healthy older adults. J Am Geriatr Soc 2003; 51:459-465.

[21] Abbot RD, White LR, Ross GW. Walking and dementia in physically capable elderly men. JAMA 2004; 292:1447-1453.

[22] Weuve J, Kang JH, Manson JE, et al. Physical activity, including walking, and cognitive function in older women. JAMA 2004; 292:1454-1461.

[23] Larson EB, Wang L, Bowen JD, et al. Exercise is associated with reduced risk for incident dementia among persons 65 years of age and older. Ann Intern Med 2006; 144:73.

[24] Yates L B, Djoussé L, Kurth T, Buring JE, Gaziano JM. Exceptional Longevity in Men. Arch Intern Med. 2008; 168(3):284-290.

[25] Radak Z, Chung HY, Goto S. Exercise and hormesis: oxidative stress-related adaptation for successful aging. Biogerontology. 2005; 6(1):71-75.

[26] Finkel T, Holbrook NJ. Oxidants, oxidative stress and the biology of ageing. Nature. 2000; 408(6809):239-247.

[27] Finch CE, Crimmins EM. Inflammatory exposure and historical changes in human life-spans. Science. 2004; 305(5691):1736-1739.

[28] Bean JF, Vora A, Frontera WR. Benefits of exercise for community-dwelling older adults. Arch Phys Med Rehabil. 2004; 85(3 Supl):S31-42.

[29] Qiang MA. Beneficial effects of moderate voluntary physical exercise and its biological mechanisms on brain health. Neurosci Bull. 2008; 24(4): 265-270.

[30] Novotny V, Brandejsky P, BarackovaM, Boudova L, Vilikus Z, Streda A, Novotny Medical and anthropological study of a world and Olympic champion, long-distance runner, 35 years after the end his racing career. Sb Lek. 1994; 95(2):139-55.

[31] Maud PJ, Pollock ML, Foster C, Anholm JD, Guten G, Al-Nouri M, Hellman C, Schmidt DH Fifty years of training and competition in the marathon: Wally Hayward, age 70--a physiological profile S Afr Med J. 1981 Jan 31; 59(5):153-7.

[32] Consuelo H. Wilkins MD and Stanley J. Birge MD. Prevention of osteoporotic fractures in the elderly. The American Journal of Medicine 118, 11, 1190-1195.

[33] M.E. Tinetti, Preventing falls in elderly persons, N Engl J Med 348 (2003), pp. 40–49.

[34] C. Becker, M. Kron and U. Lindermann et al., Effectiveness of a multifaceted intervention on falls in nursing home residents, J Am Geriatr Soc 51 (2003) 316-313.

[35] MacKelvie K J, Taunton J E, McKay H A, Khan K M. Bone mineral density and serum testosterone in chronically trained, high mileage 40–55 year old male runners. Br J Sports Med 2000; 34:273–278.

[36] Hind K, Truscott J.G. Evans, J.A. Low lumbar spine bone mineral density in both male and female endurance runners. Bone 39 (2006) 880–885.

[37] Lund M, Jens H H & Christiansen C. Low Bone Mass and High Bone Turnover in Male Long Distance Runners. J. Clin. Endocrinol Metab 77: 770-7751993.

[38] . Kemmler W; Engelke K; Baumann H; Beeskow C; von Stengel S; Weineck J et al. Bone status in elite male runners. Eur J Appl Physiol (2006) 96: 78–85.

[39] .Wiswell R.A., Hawkins S.A., Dreyer H.C. & Jaque S.V. Maintenance of BMD in older male runners is independent of changes in training volume or VO2 peak. J. Gerontol. Ser. A Biol. Sci. Med. Sci. 2002 57:4 (M203-M208).

[40] Ishihara A., Roy R.R., Ohira Y., Kawano F., Nonaka K., Yamamoto K. and Edgerton V.R. Effects of aging and exercise on density and cross-sectional area of femur in senescence-accelerated mouse prone 6. J. Musculoskelet. Neuronal Interact. 2003 3:2 (162-169).

[41] George A. Kelley. Aerobic Exercise and Bone Density at the Hip in Postmenopausal Women: A Meta-Analysis. PREVENTIVE MEDICINE 27, 798–807 (1998)

[42] Bonaiuti D, Shea B, Iovine R, Negrini S,Welch V, KemperHHCG,WellsGA, Tugwell P, Cranney A. Exercise for preventing and treating osteoporosis in postmenopausal women. Cochrane Database of Systematic Reviews 2002.

[43] Satoshi Yamazaki, Shoichi Ichimura, Jun Iwamoto, Tsuyoshi Takeda, and Yoshiaki Toyama. Effect of walking exercise on bone metabolism in postmenopausal women with osteopenia/osteoporosis. J Bone Miner Metab (2004) 22:500–508.

[44] Garcia R, Leme MD, Garcez-Leme LE.. Evolution of Brazilian elderly with hip fracture secondary to a fall. Clinics (Sao Paulo). 2006 Dec; 61(6):539-44.

Chapter 9

Influence of the Nutrition on Bone Health of Children and Adolescents

Emilio González-Jiménez

Additional information is available at the end of the chapter

http://dx.doi.org/10.5772/54773

1. Introduction

Maintaining adequate nutritional status, is an essential factor for bone growth and mineralization. Both processes, both the increase in size and development through the deposit of minerals pass alongside and under the regulation by different factors [1]. In this sense, acquired during childhood and adolescence adequate bone mass will be a prime target for complications, not only in childhood and adolescence but during adulthood [2].

Currently, in developed countries, osteoporosis is a serious public health problem that affects mainly children and adolescents as a consequence of sedentary lifestyle and unhealthy eating habits [3].

Recent studies suggest that osteoporosis prevention should begin in childhood. Children and adolescents should achieve an adequate peak bone mass (PMO) before the end of its growth. Otherwise, they may develop osteopenia or osteoporosis early, with a high risk of fractures and consequently a lower quality of life [4].

Given that the risk of developing osteoporosis depends in 60-80% of genetic factors on which we can not intervene, we must act on those other environmental factors involved which if capable of being corrected, mainly food [5]. It is known that bone mineral density (BMD) is modifiable by diet and exercise as much as 20%. Nutrients ingested daily through food involved in the development and maintenance of adequate bone mineralization by means of different processes, favoring the differentiation of bone tissue functional cells (osteoblasts and osteoclasts) and acting as plastics elements. In addition, provide adequate nutrition essential vitamins involved in bone matrix synthesis and calcium absorption at intestinal level, also allowing the synthesis of certain hormones and growth factors involved [6].

Therefore, based on the above premises, childhood and adolescence are important periods in which an adequate nutrition will firmly prevent the development of osteopenia or osteoporosis at an early age [7].

2. Nature of bone tissue and skeletal development

Bone consists of cells (2-5%) and in a largely inert matter (95-98%), ie basically protein and minerals [8]. From a structural standpoint, the protein component is composed of fibers of collagen type I and gla protein (osteocalcin, osteonectin, fibronectin, osteopontin and bone sialoprotein). Its component consists mainly of hydroxyapatite mineral-rich carbonates (37-40% calcium and phosphate 50-58%) and to a lesser extent sodium, potassium, magnesium and citrate [8].

At birth, the newborn already has 70 to 95 grams of bone mass approximately equivalent to 4% by weight. During adolescence, girls have 2,400 grams of bone [9]. The boys, meanwhile, are at increased volume estimated at approximately 3,300 grams. Both quantities correspond to a 85% to development of the cortical bone and 15% of the cancellous bone development [9].

In this sense, it is considered that the girls get their peak bone mass at age 18 as opposed to boys who reach it some years later, at the age of 23 years or so [9]. The gain of this peak is mediated by the action of sex hormones on growth factor 1 (IGF-1), which is stimulated in parallel mode by proteins [10].

Once acquired peak bone mass, it will tend to stabilize. After bone mass will be reduced only to certain pathological processes involving a state of prostration of the patient or following the administration of certain drugs such as glucocorticoids [11]. Although the bone loss does not occur evenly across the skeleton. Normally, women aged between 20 and 30 begin to develop a reduced bone loss (<1%) level of the vertebrae [12]. It will be during the first 5 years post-menopause when the loss increases between 2 and 6% annually. Among men, the loss occurs at older ages, ie from 50 years of age [12].

3. Nutritional factors involved in the process of bone mineralization

Energy intake

Maintain adequate caloric intake permitted during childhood and adolescence to ensure growth, maturation and bone mineralization process [13].

Protein intake

Protein intake, is another important factor for the formation of bone matrix. However, protein intake appears to be important risk factor among our child population as they often exceed recommendations [14]. This mainly because the food in Western countries usually contain plenty of eggs, meat, fish and dairy products which guarantees a significant amount of protein [14]. Moreover, low consumption of protein (less than 45-55 g/day in men or 45 g/day in women) are usually accompanied by a lower muscle mass and bone, this mainly due to a reduction in bone structure protein. Meanwhile, a high protein intake (greater than 2 grams/kilogram/day) may also cause a loss of bone mass, since for each gram of protein intake in excess through the diet, results in a loss of 1 mg of calcium [14].

Calcium and phosphorus

Both nutrients are the substances most studied for their influence on the prevention and treatment of osteoporosis. Calcium is the most abundant mineral in the human skeleton. 99% is deposited in the bone and passing about 30 grams at birth [10 grams per kilogram of body weight) to about 1,300 grams in adult (19 grams per kilogram of body weight) [15]. Now, by weight, calcium accounts for 40% of bone mineral and 60% phosphorus. From a metabolic point of view, the absorption of calcium from food depends on several factors. First of its bioavailability in the diet, the deposits of vitamin D, the calcium / phosphorus (Ca/P) and the presence in food of substances that facilitate or interfere with its absorption [16]. In the case of phosphorus (P), this also deposits in the bone by 85%. The high presence among foods in our diet (60-70%), guaranteed to meet the needs of our food without difficulty, especially among the young. While its excessive intake may alter the Ca/P thus hindering the absorption of calcium [17].

Calcium-phosphorus balance

The study of calcium-phosphorus balance is complex when you consider its high fecal excretion. In the case of calcium, their daily loss (through excretion in the urine, fecal and dermal) are estimated at 420 mg/day. Calcium is absorbed in the intestine not ever exceeding 30% of the total amount ingested [18]. For absorption, calcium must compete with other substances such as phytates and oxalates act by inhibiting its absorption. The solubilized calcium in foods like milk or juice is absorbed supplemented with ease. In the case of phosphates, these are found in a wide variety of foods thereby showing a higher bioavailability than calcium. His diet recommendations are estimated at 700-800 mg / day in adults compared to 1200 mg/day estimated as necessary during adolescence. For its part, has a phosphorus antiosificante effect by increasing the secretion of PTH and reduced intestinal calcium absorption [18].

Recommendations for calcium intake

In the case of calcium, recommendations vary depending on the stage of life where we are. For children under 1 year and for both sexes, the recommended intake of between 400-600 mg/day of calcium. During adolescence, the recommendations are found up to 1200 mg/day for both sexes [19]. For adult males, the recommendations provide a daily intake of between 800 to 1000 mg/day. For adult women the recommendations are higher, between 1200 and 1500 mg/day for those postmenopausal women in gestation and during lactation [20]. According to recent studies, 60% of the calcium in our diet comes from foods such as dairy products, followed by 13% from foods such as cereals, 15% from fruits, vegetables, legumes, while not as only 6% comes from foods like meat, fish or eggs. This entails risks if it is very sedentary children and adolescents and women with menopause. In some cases this will be indicated calcium supplementation, especially through the diet is not achieved optimal calcium intake. In the study by Johsnton et al (1992) [21], from a population of prepubertal twins who are supplemented with a dose of 700 mg/day of calcium, managed to increase its process of mineralization and bone mass in a 5%.

Sodium intake

Excessive sodium intake in the diet may be accompanied by a reduction in bone mineral density. This decrease in bone mass is mediated by a renal calcium excretion [22]. In this regard, given an approximate intake of 450 mg of sodium in the diet, the kidney is capable of removing in parallel up to 10 mg of calcium. Accordingly, the recommendations established for calcium intake in adolescents, they must not exceed a daily sodium intake greater than 2000 mg or what is just 5 grams of salt [22].

Intake of vitamin D and K and its importance in the process of bone mineralization

Vitamin D belongs to the group of so-called fat-soluble vitamins. Their presence in food is by way of cholecalciferol (D3) and ergocalciferol. Usually has its origin in cholesterol or ergosterol derivative which is converted to ergocalciferol (D2) the effect of ultraviolet radiation. However, the active form of this vitamin is called calcitriol [23]. Its synthesis is closely associated with sun exposure, that is, with a daily sun exposure is insufficient to meet the physiological needs of the vitamin in our body [24]. Their presence facilitates the absorption of calcitriol in the intestine. In this regard, serum levels of this vitamin have been correlated with bone density in certain locations such as the lumbar spine and femoral neck. Another vitamin involved in the process of bone mineralization during childhood and adolescence is vitamin K. Participates in the process of carboxylation of osteocalcin and thereby cause a deficit decreased and carboxylation of osteocalcin synthesis [25]. *Fluorine* Within the elementary ions, fluoride in nature and chemical behavior is the most active of all elementary ions. Its concentration is high in mineral water, fish, tea and certain meals [26]. Fluoride ingested through the diet, is rapidly absorbed from the gastrointestinal tract to blood from which will be distributed to tissues and organs by simple diffusion. Among its benefits to bone level highlights its ability to stimulate osteoblast activity, increasing the mainly trabecular bone. In this regard, it has been demonstrated that administration of 25 mg/day slow-release fluoride supplied for 4 years reduces the incidence of vertebral fractures [26]. *Consumption of carbonated drinks*

The increased consumption of carbonated beverages is associated with a progressive decrease in milk intake, has led to high consumption of phosphoric acid associated with calcium deficiency [27]. This eating pattern will have consequences for bone health, because when a diet is high in phosphorus and low in calcium, bone resorption increases to recover the serum levels of this mineral. There are epidemiological studies that linked the consumption of carbonated beverages to an increased risk of fracture in children and young girls. However, there is some controversy about this relationship [28]. Many authors, conclude that the major effect of carbonated beverages is mainly due to displacement of milk in the diet, especially among young people.

Alcohol consumption, snuff and caffeine

Excessive alcohol consumption, is an important risk factor for osteoporosis, especially among young males. Ingestion, causes a decrease in bone mass through an alteration of the formation and bone remodeling [29]. During adolescence, a high intake of alcohol reduces bone mass peak. This circumstance enables the development of osteopenia or osteoporosis at an early age [30]. In addition, alcohol intake is associated with dietary disorders, which adversely affect the bone metabolism. Thus, their intake is related to a deficiency of vitamin D and parathyroid hormone (PTH), hypoproteinemia, liver, hypomagnesemia, deficit B vitamins and folic acid, iron overload and decreased testosterone [31].

Regarding the consumption of snuff in adolescents, it has been associated with a significant reduction in bone mineral density (BMD). It has been shown that adolescent smokers, especially girls, have a lower bone mineral density and increased rate of bone loss that girls do not smoke. This has been demonstrated also among male adolescents [32].

Regarding caffeine intake, it increases urinary calcium excretion during the first 3 hours after ingestion. It has been found that a daily intake of two or more cups of coffee, is correlated with lower bone mineral density in these subjects.

4. In conclusion

Among all the factors involved in the mineralization of bone mass, maintaining a balanced diet is a key factor. A balanced and varied diet will be the best procedure to ensure proper bone development among young people. Therefore, an adequate energy and protein intake, coupled with a contribution provided essential nutrients such as calcium, phosphorus or fluorine and certain vitamins such as D and K Assume the basic nutritional elements to ensure adequate bone mass during the later stages early in life. Given that bone development achieved during childhood and adolescence will influence the health status and bone mass in adulthood and that this depends largely on food, care for the food of the young should be a prime target order.

Author details

Emilio González-Jiménez*

Address all correspondence to: emigoji@ugr.es

Department of Nursing. Faculty of Nursing (Campus of Melilla), University of Granada, Melilla, Spain

References

[1] Jones, G. Early life nutrition and bone development in children. Nestle Nutr Workshop Ser Pediatr Program (2011). , 68, 227-33.

[2] Tristán Fernández JMRuiz Santiago F, Pérez de la Cruz A, Lobo Tañer G, Aguilar Cordero MJ, Collado Torreblanca F. Influencia de la nutrición y del entorno social en la maduración ósea del niño. Nutr Hosp (2007). , 22, 417-24.

[3] Quesada Gómez JMSosa Henríquez M. Nutrición y osteoporosis. Calcio y vitamina D. Rev Osteoporos Metab Miner (2011). , 4, 165-82.

[4] Adami, S, Isaia, G, Luisetto, G, Minisola, S, Sinigaglia, L, Silvestri, S, et al. ICARO Study Group. Osteoporosis treatment and fracture incidence: the ICARO longitudinal study. Osteoporos Int (2008). , 19, 1219-23.

[5] Bechtold-Dalla Pozza SBone density measurements on growing skeletons and the clinical consequences. Z Rheumatol (2011). , 70(10), 844-52.

[6] Cashman, K. D. Diet, Nutrition, and Bone Health. J Nutr (2007). S, 2507-12.

[7] Hirota, T, & Hirota, K. Nutrition in bone growth and development. Clin Calcium (2011). , 21(9), 1329-33.

[8] Qiu, Z. Y, Li, G, Zhang, Y. Q, Liu, J, Hu, W, Ma, J, & Zhang, S. M. Fine structure analysis and sintering properties of Si-doped hydroxyapatite. Biomed Mater (2012).

[9] Mora, S, & Gilsanz, V. Establishment of peak bone mass. Endocrinol Metab Clin N Am (2003). , 32, 39-63.

[10] Zofková, I. Soft tissues, hormones and the skeleton. Vnitr Lek (2012). , 58(2), 135-39.

[11] Krall, E. A, & Dawson-hughes, B. Osteoporosis: En: Shils ME, Olson JA, Ross AC, editores. Nutrición en Salud y Enfermedad. México, Interamericana, (2002).

[12] Zatonski, T, Temporale, H, & Krecicki, T. Hearing and balance in metabolic bone diseases. Pol Merkur Lekarski (2012). , 32(189), 198-201.

[13] Zagarins, S. E, Ronnenberg, A. G, Gehlbach, S. H, Lin, R, & Bertone-johnson, E. R. Are existing measures of overall diet quality associated with peak bone mass in young premenopausal women? J Hum Nutr Diet (2012). , 25(2), 172-79.

[14] Bonjour, J. P. Protein intake and bone health. Int J Vitam Nutr Res (2011).

[15] Caroli, A, Poli, A, Ricotta, D, Banfi, G, & Cocchi, D. Invited review: Dairy intake and bone health: a viewpoint from the state of the art. J Dairy Sci (2011). , 94(11), 5249-62.

[16] Food and Nutritional BoardDietary Reference Intakes (DRI) for calcium, phosphorus, magnesium, vitamin D and fluoride. Washington: National Academy of Sciences. National Academy Press; (1997).

[17] Bonjour, J. P. Bone mineral adquisition in adolescente. En: Markus R, Felman D, Kesley J, editores. Osteoporosis. San Diego: Academic Press; (1996). , 465-476.

[18] Loui, A, Raab, A, Obladen, M, & Brätter, P. Calcium, phosphorus and magnesium balance: FM 85 fortification of human milk does not meet mineral needs of extremely low birthweight infants. Eur J Clin Nutr (2002). , 56(3), 228-35.

[19] Basabe, B, Mena, M. C, Faci, M, Aparicio, A, López-sobaler, A. M, & Ortega, R. M. Influencia de la ingesta de calcio y fósforo sobre la densidad mineral ósea en mujeres jóvenes. Arch Latinoam Nutr (2004). , 54, 203-8.

[20] Jackson, R. D. LaCroix AZ, Gass M, Wallace RB, Robbins J, Lewis CE, et al. Calcium plus vitamin D supplementation and the risk of fractures. N Engl J Med (2006). , 354, 669-83.

[21] Johsnton, C. C, Miller, J. Z, Siemenda, C. W, Reister, T. K, Hui, S, & Christian, J. C. Calcium supplementation and increases in bone mineral in children. N Engl J Med (1992). , 82-87.

[22] Chan, R, Woo, J, Lau, W, Leung, J, Xu, L, Zhao, X, Yu, W, Lau, E, & Pocock, N. Effects of lifestyle and diet on bone health in young adult Chinese women living in Hong Kong and Beijing. Food Nutr Bull (2009). , 30(4), 370-78.

[23] Holick, M. F, & Chen, T. C. Vitamin D deficiency: A world wide problem with health consequences. Am J Clin Nutr (2008). , 87, 1080-86.

[24] Holick, M. F. Vitamin D deficiency. N Engl J Med (2007). , 357, 266-81.

[25] Ahmadieh, H, & Arabi, A. Vitamins and bone health: beyond calcium and vitamin D. Nutr Rev (2011). , 69(10), 584-98.

[26] Grajeta, H. Nutrition in prevention and treatment of osteoporosis. Przegl Lek (2003). , 60(10), 649-53.

[27] Ma, D, & Jones, G. Soft drink and milk consumption, physical activity, bone mass, and upper limb fractures in children: a population-based case-control study. Calcif Tissue Int (2004). , 75(4), 286-91.

[28] Wyshak, G. Teenaged girls, carbonated beverage consumption, and bone fractures. Arch Pediatr Adolesc Med (2000). , 154(6), 610-13.

[29] Chakkalakal, D. A. Alcohol-induced bone loss and deficiente bone repair. Alcohol Clin Exp Res (2005). , 29, 2077-90.

[30] Turner, R. T. Skeletal response to alcohol. Alcohol Clin Exp Res (2000). , 24, 1693-701.

[31] Kim, M. J, Shim, M. S, Kim, M. K, Lee, Y, Shing, Y. G, Churg, C. H, et al. Effect of chronic alcohol ingestión on bone mineral density in males without liver cirrosis. Korean J Intern Med (2003). , 18, 174-80.

[32] Vogt, M. T, Hanscom, B, Lauerman, W. C, & Kang, I. D. Influence of smoking on the health patients. The National Spine network data base. Spine (2002). , 27, 313-19.

Chapter 10

The Effectiveness of Progressive Load Training Associated to the Proprioceptive Training for Prevention of Falls in Women with Osteoporosis

Lucas Teixeira, Stella Peccin, Kelson Silva,
Tiago Teixeira, Aline Mizusaki Imoto,
Joelma Magalhães and Virgínia Trevisani

Additional information is available at the end of the chapter

http://dx.doi.org/10.5772/54554

1. Introduction

In most of the cases, osteoporosis is a related condition to aging. It can be seen in both genders, but it especially manifests in women after menopause due to estrogen production rate fall.

For understanding what happens, it is necessary to bear in mind that the bones are compounded of a matrix in which mineral complexes such as calcium are laid up. Another important feature is that they are in constant renewal process, since they are formed by cells called osteoclasts which are responsible for reabsorbing the aged areas and others, the osteoblasts, which is responsible for producing new bones. This permanent and constant process makes possible the bone reconstitution when fractures happen and it explains why around every ten years the human skeleton is entirely renewed. Along the time, however, the old cells absorption increases and the bone new cells formation decreases. The outcome is that the bones become more porous, losing resistance. Bone mass lighter loss features osteopenia. Greater losses are in the osteoporosis area.

If it is not early prevented, or if it is not treated, the bone mass loss is progressively increasing, in an asymptomatic fashion, without any manifestation, until a fracture occurrence. What features the osteoporotic fractures, is when they take place with a minimum trauma, what would not cause fractures in a normal bone. Therefore, they are also called fragility fractures.

The incidence of osteoporotic fractures is strictly related to the individual bone mass that depends on the speed of loss throughout life as well as the amount of bone tissue in the end of puberty and beginning of adulthood. The great variation in bone mass peak is explained not only by hereditary factors but also by gender, race, eating habits, several hormone influence, body composition of lean mass and body fat, intercurrent diseases, chronic use of medications and physical activity (Brandão & Vieira, 1999).

Like any other chronic disease, the ethiology of osteoporosis is multifactorial. Genetic factors contribute approximately with 46% to 62% of bone mineral density (BMD) whereas other causes include lifestyle, diet and physical exercise (Neto et al., 2002).

Osteoporosis clinical symptoms do not usually occur before a fracture occurrence. Osteoporosis is considered an asymptomatic disease. Indeed, during the disease progression, the bones become progressively more fragile without affecting the individuals. This characteristic of being a silent disease exposes the population to even a greater risk of suffering a fracture.

Osteoporosis is considered a "silent disease" until a fracture occurs. Approximately 1.5 million fractures per year are attributable to this disease. Only in the USA, these fractures result in 500.000 hospitalizations, 800.000 emergency room visits, 2.6 million physician visits. The treatment cost is high. In 2002, 12 billion dollars to 18 billion dollars were spent (Gass & Huges, 2006). In 1998, cost management of osteoporosis fractures in the UK recorded 942 million pounds per year (Szejnfeld et al., 2007). Osteoporosis has become one of the major public health problems. Nowadays, the impact of osteoporosis is compared to the impact caused by most important health problems, such as cardiovascular diseases and cancer (Froes et al., 2002).

It exposes the fallers to a high risk of fractures (Johnell et al., 2005; Siris et al., 2006). The first hip fracture is associated to 2.5-fold increased risk of subsequent fracture (Cólon-Emeric et al., 2003) with a high level of morbidity and mortality (Cathleen et al., 2006).

It is believed that about 25% of menopausal women in the USA will exhibit some kind of fracture as a consequence of osteoporosis. The most severe fractures are the fractures of femur and they are associated with higher medical expenses than all other osteoporotic fractures together (Moreira & Xaxier, 2001). The incidence of these fractures has doubled in the last 25 years and it is estimated that six million people in the world will suffer fracture of the proximal femur in 2050. Fractures resulted from the decrease of bone mineral loss are considered an orthopedic epidemic leading to an increase in costs for several countries and consequently representing a big social and economic problem (Ramalho et al., 2001).

There have been a significant number of evidences showing that the decrease in bone quality, from generation to generation, is caused by a change in life style, having as a main determinant the lack of physical activity. This evidence varies with the biology of the basic bone. However, epidemiological studies indicate that physical activity is the most important factor to maintain bone mass and prevent fractures (Mosekilde, 1995).

Almost all hip fractures (more than 90%) occur as a result of a fall and these fractures are related not only to the decreased bone mass, but also to other factors such as reduction of balance, muscle strength and power in the lower extremities (American College of Sports Medicine [ACSM], 1995; Parkkari et al. 1999). Therefore, aging and alterations in balance and muscle strength, as well as sensorial changes, predispose patients with osteoporosis to a higher risk of having fractures due to falls.

http://dx.doi.org/10.5772/54554

Falls are multifactorial (Cathleen et al., 2006), (Tinetti et al., 1989) and their intrinsic causes include altered balance, gait, muscle strength, visual acuity, cognition and the presence of chronic diseases (van Schoor et al., 2002).

The participation of environmental risk factors might reach up to 50% of the falls in elderly that live in the community. These factors include poor lighting, slippery surfaces, loose or folded rugs, high or narrow stairs, obstacles in the way (low furniture, small objects, wires), lack of rails in halls and bathrooms, extremely low or high shelves, inadequate shoes and clothes, poorly maintained streets with holes or irregularities and inappropriate orthosis.

A reduction of approximately 30% in the strength is found in individual ages ranging from 50 to 70. These changes are more common in women than in men, more prevalent in lower limbs than in upper limbs and a great amount of this reduction in strength is caused by a selective atrophy of Type IIB fibers (American College of Sports Medicine Position, 1998).

Evidences have shown that specific exercises might reduce the risk factors for falls and the number of falls in the elderly.

The purpose of our study was to evaluate the efficacy of the resistance training associated to a proprioceptive training in the prevention of falls and reduction of the respective risk factors in postmenopausal women with osteoporosis.

2. Physical exercise to prevent falls

Prevention in individuals older than 60 years has an important role in avoiding adverse consequences resulting from falls (Weatherall, 2004).

The work to prevent fractures related to osteoporosis should focus the prevention or increase of material and structural properties of the bone, the prevention of falls and improvement of total mass of lean tissue (American College of Sports Medicine, 1995).

The American College of Sports Medicine recommends that:

1. physical activity of transporting weight is essential to the normal development and maintenance of a health skeleton. Activities that focus the increase of muscle strength might also be beneficial, particularly for bones that do not support weight;
2. a sedentary woman might progressively increase her bone mass by becoming active, but the primary benefit of increasing the activity is to prevent a future bone reduction that resulting from the lack of activity;
3. exercise should not be recommended as a replacement to medications treatment;
4. the optimal program for an older woman might include activities that improve the strength, flexibility and coordination which might indirectly, but effectively decrease the incidence of osteoporotic fractures by reducing the probability of falls. Therefore, the treatment of osteoporosis should aim the prevention of falls and fractures and preservation or improvement of bone mineral density.

2.1. Exercises for postural control

Postural control is a result of the combination of several types of sensorial information, such as visual, vestibular and somatosensorial information, and passive and active properties of the nervous system and skeletomuscle system that composes the human postural control system (Figure 2), (Shumway-Cook et al., 2000).

The postural control system use three functions that are required to maintain balance: support, stabilization and balance. The body should contract the adequate muscles to sustain the body against gravity; the articular segments should be stabilized and the body should be stabilized in the body's support base (Rothwell, 1994). This way the treatment program which aims at falls prevention should contain strength and resistance increasing components for promoting the articular coaptation and to face the gravity, it also should prevent the posture reorganization aligning the body gravity center.

Currently, proprioception is defined as a set of afferent information provided by joints, muscles, tendons and other tissues that reaches the Central Nervous System (CNS) where it is processed, having an influence on reflex responses and voluntary motor control. Proprioception contributes to postural control, joint stability and several conscious sensations (Lephart & Fu, 2000).

Therefore the sensorial-motor training becomes indispensable for an appropriate falls prevention program, since it potentializes the propriocetive information captation and transmission providing to SNC information regarding the contraction speed, movement speed, articular position and angle, which are fundamental for a good motor control.

It is extremely important to understand that proprioception is only limited to the acquisition of the mechanical stimulus and its transduction in neural stimuli, not having any influence on the CNS processing and its motor response (Lephart & Fu, 2000).

Proprioception is part of a system denominated somatosensorial system. This includes all mechanical information provided by the mechanoreceptors. The feeling of pain is provided by the nociceptors and the thermal information provided by thermoreceptors (Guyton & Hall, 2006).

All propriocetive information are originated at the muscular and tendon receptors called muscular fusion and Golgi tendon organ and receptors located in ligaments, articular capsule, meniscus and cutaneous tissues (Guyton & Hall, 2006).

Four elements should be focused to reestablish the sensorimotor deficits: proprioception, stabilization, reactive neuromuscular control and functional motor patterns (Lephart & Henry, 1995).

The proprioceptive mechanism comprises both conscious and unconscious pathways. Therefore, the prescribed exercises need to include conscious exercises to stimulate the cognition as well as sudden and unexpected alterations of joint position that initiate reflex muscle contraction. These exercises should involve balance in an unstable surface while the individual perform functional activities. The purpose of the dynamic stabilization training is to improve the co-activation between the antagonist muscles (Hurd et al., 2006)

Exercises to stimulate proprioception and dynamic stabilization should be performed in closed-chain activities and with small movements, since the compression stimulates the articular receptors and the changes in the curve length-tension stimulate the muscle receptors. Limbs repositioning exercises should also be performed to stimulate the sense of joint position and neuromuscular control (Lephart & Henry, 1995).

The improvement of dynamic stiffness is another important aspect. It is suggested that muscle receptors increase its sensitivity through the increase of dynamic stiffness (Adler et al., 2008).

Exercises that involve eccentric training, like going down the stairs and landing after jumps, are the most efficient to increase anticipatory and reactive muscular stiffness (Bastian et al., 2006).

The reactive neuromuscular control is reached through exercises that create unexpected situations, such as perturbations in unstable surfaces in unipodal support and during gait. Apparently, this kind of training improves the preparatory and reactive muscle activation (Swanik et al., 2002).

The training protocol might include:

1. 5 – 10 minutes of warm-up, with stretching movements for upper and lower limbs, 03 repetitions for each movement being kept for 30 seconds, with 30-second intervals among the series. After stretching, movements of fast gait as previous warm-up were performed and in the end of the session, slow gait movements and stretching.

2. Proprioceptive exercises followed an evolution sequence based on the use of stable surfaces to unstable, walking straight forward progressing to changes in direction, from gait with no obstacles to gait with obstacles, alteration in the support base (from open to closed), exercises with eyes open to closed eyes, always respecting the functional capacity of each patient and progressively increasing the difficulty of each exercise. To aid the training, cones, balance boards, sticks, mats and trampolines were used. According to the patient's evolution, the exercises were combined creating the circuits.

2.2. Stretching

Stretching should be performed during the warm up and in the last phase. A great joint range of motion (ROM) increases the muscle, reduces the risk of lesion and increases the cartilage nutrition. Painful joints should not be stretched excessively to a point that will result in more pain; all movements should be made in order to get the maximum pain-free ROM. The use of heat before stretching reduces pain and increases the range. At least three sessions of stretching might be performed a week. In the beginning, three to five repetitions and a gradual increase up to 10 repetitions is the ideal. The muscle should be stretched during 10 to 30 seconds.

2.3. Muscle strengthening

Muscle strengthening should be acquired with weights or elastic bands which will give endurance to the movement. The training protocols should include the following principles:

- muscle contraction exercises should be made in a moderate speed;
- exercises should be chosen according to joint stability and degree of pain and edema;
- muscles should not be exercised to fatigue;
- exercise endurance should be submaximal;
- inflamed articular joints should be strengthen with isometric exercises and at first it should include few repetitions;
- pain or edema in a joint after an hour of exercise indicates excessive activity.

Isometric exercises are indicated for unstable or swollen joints. On the other hand, isometric contractions result in a low articular pressure and are well tolerated by older patients. It should start with contractions with an intensity of approximately 30% of maximal strength, slowly increasing to 80%. The contraction should not be kept for more than 6-10 seconds and the repetitions should be increased from 8 to 10, if tolerated by the patient. It should be performed twice a day during the inflammatory period and after the inflammation is over, it should be increased from 5 to 10 times a day.

Isotonic exercises should include from 8 to 10 exercises involving the major muscle groups (four exercises for the upper limbs and from four to six for the lower limbs). At first, patients should use weights with 40% of the individual's maximal load, increasing up to 80%. Generally, a series of four to six repetitions should be made, avoiding the muscle fatigue. At first, the frequency should be at most twice a week but in case of individuals with advanced age or significant fragility the exercises should be made only once a week. Between the sessions, there might be at least one full day of rest.

Changes in strength after resistance exercise training RET are assessed using a variety of methods, including isometric, isokinetic, one-repetition maximum (1-RM), and multiplerepetition (e.g., 3-RM) maximum-effort protocols. In general, strength increases after RET in older adults seem to be greater with measures of 1-RM or 3-RM performance compared with isometric or isokinetic measures. Older adults can substantially increase their strength after RET—with reported increases ranging from less than 25% to greater than 100% (American College of Sports Medicine, 2009).

3. Material and methods

The present research was approved by the Research Ethics Committee of the Federal University of São Paulo. The clinical trial was registered in the Australian New Zealand Clinical Trials Registry (ANZCTR).

Among the 758 bone densitometries tests made in the Image Diagnosis Service at the Ambulatório de Especialidades de Interlagos, São Paulo - Brazil, 284 were found positive for Osteoporosis, where 162 of these densitometries tests were from patients which ages were within the age group proposed by the present research and 80 of them were included in the study, since they met the required inclusion criteria (Fig. 1).

Patients were from 65 to 75 years old and only individuals with a postmenopausal osteoporosis, according to the OMS, with a bone mineral density (BMD) T-score of −2.5 standard deviation (SD), in the lumbar spine, femoral neck or total femur region (Lewiecki et al., 2004) were included.

The following women were excluded: those with secondary osteoporosis, visual deficiency with no possibilities of previous corrections; severe auditive deficiency; with vestibular alteration of important clinical status; as well as women who used assisted walking devices (orthesis or prosthesis); those who planned to be out of town for two consecutive weeks during the 18-week study and also women who presented absolute contraindications for physical exercise, according to the American College of Sports Medicine.

All patients selected according to the inclusion and exclusion criteria signed an informed consent (IC). The randomization was performed by a technical assistant not involved in the research using a computer program and the sequential numbers were kept in opaque, not translucent and sealed envelope being given to one of the two groups based on the Consort recommendations.

The volunteers were included in two groups: the first group (G1) comprised 40 patients who underwent 18-week proprioceptive and progressive muscular strength training associated to a drug treatment of Osteoporosis; and the second called G2 also included 40 patients that only underwent a conventional drug treatment.

3.1. Evaluation

The registration of patients was made during the medical evaluation in order to include or exclude the individuals in the research and their personal and clinical data were also registered.

All patients were evaluated by a physical therapist who was blinded to the group to which the patient belonged. The quality of life, functional skills and the risk and number of falls were evaluated.

The quality of life was evaluated using the Short Form Health Survey (SF-36), a questionnaire displayed in a scale from 0 to 100, where 0 means the worst quality of life and 100 points corresponds to the best quality of life, according to what is proposed by the survey (Ciconelli et al., 1999).

The Berg Balance Scale, a test where the maximum score that can be achieved is 56 and where each item has an ordinal scale of five alternatives which varied from 0 to 4 points, was used to evaluate the balance (Berg et al., 1996), Miyamoto et al., 2004).

The functional mobility was evaluated by the Timed "Up & Go" Test which measures the time an individual takes to get up of a chair, walks to a line on the floor 3 meters away as fast and safe as possible, turn around, walk back to the chair and sits down again allowing the buttocks and lumbar region to touch the seat surface (Podsiadlo et al., 1991, Shumway-Cook et al.,

1997). The TUG was performed along with other balance and functional mobility tests (Bohannon et al., 2006) since it is a sensitive and specific measurement of the fall probability among elderly adults (Large et al., 2006, Kristensen et al., 2007).

The dynamic strength of the quadriceps muscle was evaluated by the One Repetition Maximum (1 RM) Test that measures the maximum weight a subject can lift with one repetition when making a standard weight lifting exercise. Three attempts were made to reach the plateau in the 1-RM score with 3-minute intervals between each attempt (Weier 1997, Hortobagyi et al., 1998).

The number of falls was evaluated by monitoring the immediate report of falls from patients of both groups during 24 weeks. The patients were also questioned if they experienced falls six months preceding the study.

3.2. Treatment protocol of Teixeira & Silva et al., 2010

The protocol consisted of a routine where: 1) the patients participated in a 5-10 minutes warm-up in a treadmill, static stretching exercises (global and segmentary) for the upper and lower limbs, lumbar, cervical and thoracic region with 3 repetitions for each muscle or muscular group, maintaining the stretching for 30 seconds between the 2 series of exercises. 2) The functional exercises (proprioception and balance) were performed in a routine that follows a progressive order beginning with stable surface and changing to unstable surfaces, gait training without obstacles and then performance of gait training with obstacles, exercises first with eyes opened and then eyes closed, first low speed exercises and according to the patient performance high speed exercises, bipedal training and then unipedal, also using resources such as balance, trampoline and proprioceptive boards always using the same progressive order (table 1). 3) Strengthening exercises included leg extensions with a load up to 80% of 1-RM, following a protocol of two weeks of adjustment wearing 1 to 2 kilos ankle weight, progressing for 50%, 60%, 70% up to 80% of 1-RM (American College of Sports Medicine, 2002).

Examples of exercises: ten repetitions with one-minute intervals for antero-posterior and latero-lateral gait; gait with obstacles (20 cm high); gait over mattress; going up and down the stairs; change in direction according to the sound stimulus; balance exercises lasting 30 seconds and with one-minute interval for unipodal and bipodal support on the floor with eyes open and/or closed; change in floor for a more unstable surface such as a trampoline and balance board; exercises with dissociation of waist and use of a stick (Table 1).

3.3. Data analysis

After evaluating 758 patients, 80 were randomized and only 65 concluded the study, being 33 patients from G1 and 32 from G2. Three patients included in the G1 group did not complete the study because they did not have appropriate means of transportation, two others due to financial conditions, another one moved to a different city and the last one abandoned the study due to personal reasons. Two patients from G2 group did not complete the study for personal reasons, three started exercising regularly in another place, one quit due to illness of a family member and two others because we could not contact them by phone in order to

http://dx.doi.org/10.5772/54554

schedule their re-evaluations, as illustrated in the chart based on the Consort recommendations (Moher et al., 2001) (Fig. 1).

Options of Exercises	Evolution of Exercises	Time or # of repetitions
Balance exercises (balance board, mini-trampoline. Dyna disc)	Eyes open or closed / stable or unstable	10 rep / 30s
Stability exercises	Unipodal or bipodal support / open or close base	10 rep / 30s
Anteroposterior and latero-lateral gait	With or without obstacle and Variation in speed	10 rep (3 m)
Mat exercises	Go up/down: 1 to 3 mats	10 rep / 3 series
Exercises on the stairs	Variation in speed	10 rep / 3 series
Exercises with sticks	With or without arm movements	10 rep / 3 series

Table 1. Examples of exercises

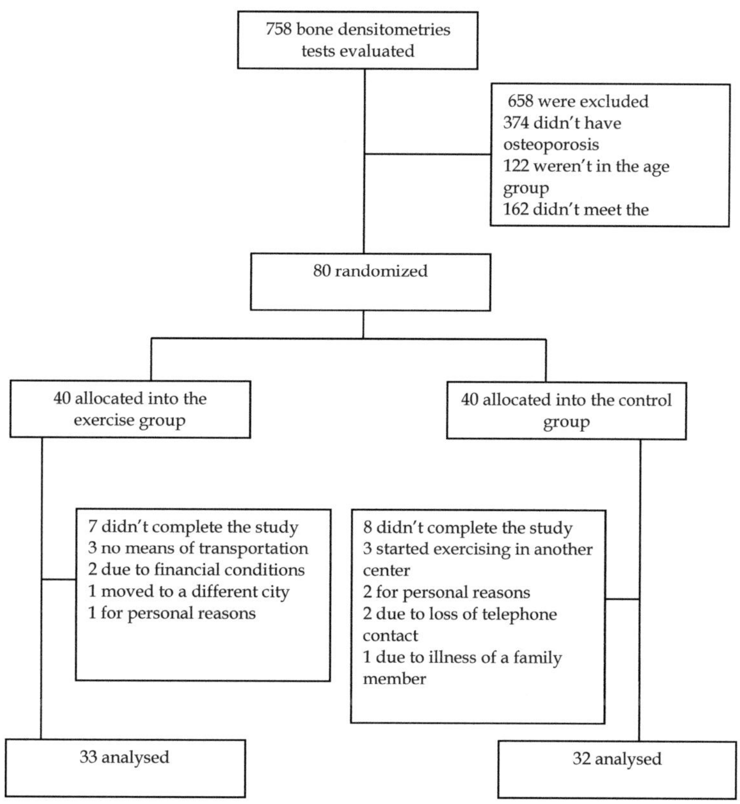

Figure 1. Organizational chart (based on Consort recommendations) including the inclusion and exclusion analysis, randomization, group allocation, losses and patients who concluded the study.

3.4. Statistical analysis

In order to verify the presumed normality in the data distribution, the Shapiro-Wilk test was used, as well as the Q-Q plot. Since the studied variable distribution could not be rounded up by the normal distribution the median and quartile 1 and 3 were calculated to describe the variables in the study.

The chi-square test was employed to evaluate the epidemiological data in the baseline.

The significance of the influence of the time the treatment was performed (pre and post-intervention) and influence of the groups (control and experimental) was evaluated by using the nonparametric hypothesis test (Robertson et al., 2005).

The statistical significance was set at $P \leq 0.05$. All the statistical process was performed with the statistical language R (version, 2.6.2; R Foundation for Statistical Computing, Vienna, Austria).

3.5. Results

The basal characteristics of the patients of both groups were similar in relation to age, bone mineral density, history of fractures, osteoporosis treatment, use of diuretics, hypnotics, and antidepressants, other rheumatic diseases and number of individuals that fell 6 months prior to the study.

According to data described in Table 2, it is possible to conclude that the scores for SF-36 in the intervention group were better in all eight sub-scales after the rehabilitation period compared to the admission time, as well as the control group. These changes were statistically ($p \leq 0.007$) and clinically significant (a change of at least 13.5 points in each sub-scale of the SF-36) for all sub-scales.

According to what was described in Table 3, there was a significant difference in the results of the Timed Up & Go Test in the pre and post- training ($p < 0.001$) for the experimental group. Furthermore, the post-training values for the experimental group were significantly greater than the ones shown by the control group ($p < 0.001$). In terms of maximum dynamic load, a significant increase between pre and post-training in the experimental group ($p < 0.001$) was observed. Besides that, the post-training values in the experimental group were significantly greater than the ones of the control group ($p < 0.001$).

Variables such as physical activity, rotational component and decreased base showed a significant increase when compared to the admission data and the control group ($p \leq 0.003$). The general score of the Berg Scale (TABLE 4) showed a significant increase in the experimental group ($p < 0.001$), where the post-training values were significantly greater in the experimental group compared to the control ($p < 0.001$). No significant differences were found in the items Transference and Static Tests. Although the changes in numbers are not huge they are consistent. A lot of people in the experimental group showed increased scores; therefore the possibility of a small score may not be great. No statistical reduction in the number of falls per patient was observed.

Variables	Moment	Control (N=32)	Intervention (N=33)	Δ (intervention-control)	p-value
Functional skills	t0	54,4(26,42)	63,95(22,56)	—	—
	t18	50,6(29,45)	82,44(17,3)	25,11[17,7;32,52]	< 0.0001
Physical aspects	t0	44,05(33,95)	36,05(34,63)	—	—
	t18	43,57(37,42)	92,44(17,71)	51,62[39,97;63,28]	< 0.0001
Pain	t0	38,88(20,63)	38,21(19,94)	—	—
	t18	44,93(21,51)	65,58(23,2)	20,98[12,29;29,68]	< 0.0001
General Health Status	t0	52(22,38)	51,09(17,72)	—	—
	t18	55,88(23,81)	73,67(17,54)	18,38[11,29;25,47]	< 0.0001
Vitality	t0	50,71(22,4)	58,26(20,26)	—	—
	t18	54,05(23,51)	74,88(15,49)	16,55[9,61;23,48]	< 0.0001
Social aspects	t0	63,62(29,4)	69,4(26,69)	—	—
	t18	68,05(28,51)	93,12(13,68)	23,06[14,32;31,81]	< 0.0001
Emotional aspects	t0	52,4(44,29)	55,79(40,38)	—	—
	t18	61,12(44,15)	85,28(28,49)	22,7[8,69;36,7]	< 0.0018
Mental health	t0	48,29(21,08)	64,3(20,52)	—	—
	t18	52,86(21,05)	78,84(17,41)	15,26[9,03;21,48]	< 0.0001

The data were expressed as the mean (standard deviation) or average [95% confidence interval].

Table 2. Pre and post-training values for SF-36 scores

Variables	Moment	Control (N=32)	Intervention (N=33)	Δ(intervention-control)	p-value
Maximum load (kg)	t0	7.6(2.27)	8.02(1.81)	—	—
Maximum load (kg)	t18	8.1(2.81)	14.81(3.14)	3.65[2.74;4.57]	< 0.0001
Time up and go (s)	t0	11.35(2.88)	10.74(2.23)	—	—
Time up and go (s)	t18	11.15(2.55)	6.9(1.11)	-3.96[-4.63;-3.29]	< 0.0001

The data were expressed as the mean (standard deviation) or average [95% confidence interval].

Table 3. Pre and Post-Training Values for the Time Up and Go Test (s), maximum load (Kg) and Berg Balance Scale (scores).

Variables	Moment	Control (N=32)	Intervention (N=33)	$\Delta_{(intervention-control)}$	p-value
Decreased base	t0	9.98(2.31)	10.05(1.4)	—	—
	t18	9.67(2.2)	11.28(1.44)	1.56[1.04;2.08]	< 0.0001
Static Tests	t0	11.88(0.33)	11.95(0.21)	—	—
	t18	11.71(0.99)	12(0)	0.19[-0.07;0.45]	0.1537
Rotational component	t0	11.21(1.14)	11.37(1.75)	—	—
	t18	11.17(099)	11.91(0.37)	0.7[0.43;0.97]	< 0.0001
Transference	t0	11.24(1.16)	11.53(1.05)	—	—
	t18	11.26(1.21)	11.81(0.93)	0.35[0.01;0.69]	0.0533
General score	t0	51.71(4.1)	52.07(3.63)	—	—
	t18	51.26(4.66)	55.12(1.73)	3.58[2.75;4.42]	< 0.0001

The data were expressed as the mean (standard deviation) or average [95% confidence interval].

Table 4. Table 4. Pre and Post-Training Values for the Berg Balance Scale (scores).

Based on the positive results of the protocol used for the physical status, an expressive reduction in the number of total falls (Figure 2) was observed. We could also observe a significant reduction between the pre and post-training in the experimental group ($p < 0.001$).

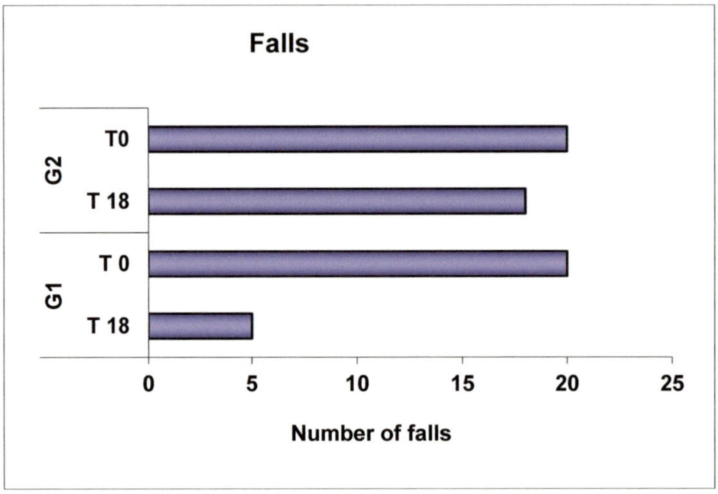

Figure 2. Number of falls 24 weeks preceding the treatment (Before) and 24 weeks after the treatment (After), in the Intervention (G1) and Control Groups (G2)

Besides that, the post-training values in the experimental group were significantly lower than the ones shown by the control group ($p < 0.001$), confirmed by the odds ratio (TABLE 5).

http://dx.doi.org/10.5772/54554

	Control (n=32)	Intervention (n=33)
T0	0,5625 ($^{18}/_{32}$)	0,6060 ($^{20}/_{33}$)
T18	0,6250 ($^{20}/_{32}$)	0,1515 ($^{5}/_{33}$)
Razão $^{T18}/_{T0}$	1,111	0,25

The data were expressed as ratio and odds ratio.

Table 5. Comparison of odds ratio falling between the control and intervention groups.

4. Discussion

Evidences have shown that specific exercises might reduce the risk factors for falls and number of falls in older people (Table 6, 7).

Muscle Strength Training and Balance Training			
Autor	**Objective**	**Desing**	**Results**
Carter, et al, 2002	Exercise programs improve balance, strength and agility in elderly people and thus may prevent falls. However, specific exercise programs that might be widely used in the community and that might be "prescribed" by physicians, especially for patients with osteoporosis, have not been evaluated. We conducted a randomized controlled trial of such a program designed specifically for women with osteoporosis.	We identified women 65 to 75 years of age in whom osteoporosis had been diagnosed by dual-energy X-ray absorptiometry in our hospital between 1996 and 2000 and who were not engaged in regular weekly programs of moderate or hard exercise. Women who agreed to participate were randomly assigned to participate in a twice-weekly exercise class or to not participate in the class. We measured baseline data and, 20 weeks later, changes in static balance (by dynamic posturography), dynamic balance (by a timed figure-eight run) and knee extension strength (by dynamometry).	Of 93 women who began the trial, 80 completed it. Before adjustment for covariates, the intervention group tended to have greater, although nonsignificant, improvements in static balance (mean difference 4.8%, 95% confidence interval [CI] –1.3% to 11.0%), dynamic balance (mean difference 3.3%, 95% CI –1.7% to 8.4%) and knee extension strength (mean difference 7.8%, 95% CI – 5.4% to 21.0%).
Madureira et al; 2007	The purpose of this study was to investigate the effect of a 12-month Balance Training	Sixty-six consecutive elderly women were selected from the Osteometabolic Disease	Sixty women completed the study and were analyzed. The BBS difference was significant

Muscle Strength Training and Balance Training			
Autor	**Objective**	**Desing**	**Results**
	Program on balance, mobility and falling frequency in women with osteoporosis	Outpatient Clinic and randomized into 2 groups: the 'Intervention', submitted for balance training; and the 'Control', without intervention. Balance, mobility and falling frequency were evaluated before and at the end of the trial, using the Berg Balance Scale (BBS), the Clinical Test Sensory Interaction Balance (CTSIB) and the Timed "Up & Go" Test (TUGT). Intervention used techniques to improve balance consisting of a 1-hour session each week and a home-based exercise program.	higher in the Intervention group compared to Control (5.5±5.67 vs differences between the TUGT were reduced in the Intervention group compared to Control (–3.65±3.61 vs 2.27±7.18 seconds, p< 0.001). Notably, this improvement was paralleled by a reduction in the number of falls/patient in the Intervention group compared to Control (–0.77 ± 1.76 vs 0.33 ± 0.96, p=0.018).
Chyu, et al, 2010	To evaluate the effects of tai chi exercise on risk factors for falls in postmenopausal women with osteopaenia through measurements of balance, gait, physical function and quality of life.	Sixty-one independently living elderly females aged 65 years and older with low bone. Subjects were recruited and randomly assigned to 24 weeks of tai chi (60 minutes/session, three sessions/week, n = 30) or a control group (n = 31). Computerized dynamic posturography, gait, 'timed up and go', five-chair sit-to-stand and quality of life assessed at baseline, 12 and 24 weeks.	After 24 weeks, subjects in the tai chi group demonstrated an increase in stride width (P = 0.05) and improvement in general health (P = 0.008), vitality (P = 0.02) and bodily pain (P = 0.03) compared with those in the control group.

Table 6. Studies that used different methods of muscle strength training and balance training

Muscle Strength Training and Balance Training			
Autor	**Objective**	**Desing**	**Results**
Smulders E et al; 2010	To evaluate the efficacy of the Nijmegen Falls Prevention Program (NFPP) for persons with osteoporosis and a fall	Persons with osteoporosis and a fall history (N=96; mean ± SD age, 71.0±4.7y; 90 women). Randomized in two groups. Primary outcome	The fall rate in the exercise group was 39% lower than for the control group (.72 vs 1.18 falls/person-year; risk ratio, .

Muscle Strength Training and Balance Training			
Autor	**Objective**	**Desing**	**Results**
	history in a randomized controlled trial.	measure was fall rate, measured by using monthly fall calendars for 1 year. Secondary outcomes were balance confidence (Activity-specific Balance Confidence Scale), quality of life (QOL), and activity level (LASA), assessed posttreatment subsequent to the program and after 1 year of follow-up.	61; 95% confidence interval, .40-.94). Balance confidence in the exercise group increased by 13.9% (P=.001). No group differences were observed in QOL and activity levels.
Burke TN et al; 2010	To assess the efficacy of an exercise program aiming to improve balance and muscular strength, for postural control and muscular strength of women with osteoporosis.	Sample consisted of 33 women with osteoporosis, randomized into one of two groups: intervention group, in which exercises for balance and improvement of muscular strength of the inferior members were performed for 8 wks (n = 17, age 72.8 +/- 3.6 yrs); control group, which was women not practicing exercises (n = 16, age 74.4 +/- 3.7 yrs).At baseline and after 8 wks of treatment, postural control was assessed using a force plate (Balance Master, Neurocom), and muscular strength during ankle dorsiflexion, knee extension, and flexion was assessed by dynamometry.	When compared with the control group, individuals in the intervention group significantly improved the center of pressure velocity (P = 0.02) in the modified clinical test of sensory interaction for balance test, center of pressure velocity (P < 0.01), and directional control (P < 0.01) in limits of stability test, isometric force during ankle dorsiflexion (P = 0.01), knee extension (P < 0.01), and knee flexion (P < 0.01).
Teixeira, et al, 2010	To evaluate the effect of a progressive muscular strength and proprioception training program on the muscle strength of the quadriceps, balance, quality of life and reduction in the risk of falls in postmenopausal women with osteoporosis.	One hundred sedentary postmenopausal women with osteoporosis, ages ranging from 55 to 75, were randomized into two groups: the intervention group comprised of 50 patients who underwent a 18-week of progressive load training for the quadriceps and proprioception training and the control group that included 50 patients of osteoporosis. The muscular strength, balance, functional	Eighty-five patients concluded the research. The program promoted a significant difference among the groups for SF-36 in the eight sub-scales (p ≤ 0.007), Timed Up & Go Test (p < 0.001), 1-RM test (p < 0.001), Berg Balance Scale (p < 0.001) and also a decrease in the total number of falls in the intervention group compared to control (p < 0.001).

Muscle Strength Training and Balance Training			
Autor	**Objective**	**Desing**	**Results**
		mobility, quality of life were evaluated in the beginning and end of the research. The number of falls was evaluated 24 weeks post treatment.	
Wayne, et al, 2012	Tai Chi (TC) is a mind-body exercise that shows potential as an effective and safe intervention for preventing fall-related fractures in the elderly.	In a pragmatic randomized trial, 86 post-menopausal osteopenic women, aged 45-70, were recruited. Primary outcomes were changes between baseline and nine months of bone mineral density (BMD) of the proximal femur and lumbar spine (dual-energy X-ray absorptiometry) and serum markers of bone resorption and formation. Secondary outcomes included quality of life.	Changes in sway parameters were significantly improved by TC vs. UC (average sway velocity, P = 0.027; anterior-posterior sway range, P = 0.014). Clinical measures of balance and function showed non-significant trends in favor of TC.

Table 7. Studies that used different methods of muscle strength training and balance training

Because of the strong interaction between osteoporosis and falls, the selection of participants in protocols for the prevention of fractures should be based on factors related to bones and falls (Pfeifer et al., 2004).

The German Society of Sport Medicine and the American College of Sport Medicine also recommend that the ideal program for women with osteoporosis should include activities that improve strength, flexibility and coordination that might indirectly and more effectively decrease the incidence of osteoporotic fractures by the reduction in the probability of falls (Lange et al., 2005).

Few studies take into consideration the importance of the proprioceptive training as a fundamental and unseparable part of a muscular strengthening program. Mechanoreceptors located in the joints, tendons, muscles and neighbor tissue provide information to the Nervous System about the position and articular movements and about the forces generated in the muscles (Huntlei, 2003) (van der Esch, 2007).

The knee proprioception is essential for the modulation and accurate activation of the muscle contraction, once the functional skill and muscular balance are strongly affected by the proprioceptive inaccuracy and muscle weakness (van der Esch, 2007). Studies including patients with knee ligament lesions show that the proprioceptive training promotes additional sensorial information that contributes to the improvement in postural control (Bonfin, 2008).

This relationship becomes even more important when the muscle strengthening program aims to improve the functional balance and prevention of falls.

Despite the knowledge on muscular strength power and the proprioception for a good motor control, and consequently a lower unbalance and fall risk, previous studies to this one ignore the association importance of sensorial-motor training to strength training.

The significant results found in the present research might be explained by the concern in following the ACSM recommendations when prescribing exercises, respecting the basic concepts of prescription exercises.

Additionally, one should take into consideration that the skill to develop muscle strength decreases with aging (Hakkinen et al, 1998) explaining the importance of the gradual progression (Adams et al, 1999). With sedentary elderly people, a period of adaptation and low working load for two weeks should be applied for further implementation of a loading progression protocol (American College of Sports Medicine, 2002).

Data combined from three studies conducted by Gillespie et al., 2006 (Cochrane Library review) with a total of 556 women aged 80 years or older, who underwent to the same progressive muscular strengthening program, balance training and gait training indicate that this intervention decreased the number of individuals that fell during a year, having also reduced the number of injurious falls. Although the studies had methodological limitations, there is a determined consistency as for the decrease of falls in multiple interventions exercises (Gillespie et al., 2009). As for the physical exercise, we only know that it improves balance without a direct association with the decrease in the number of falls (Howe Tracey et al., 2009) and that although the decline in muscle strength is a risk factor for falls, the muscle strength training could not be associated to the reduced number of falls (Sherrington et al, 2009), (Gillespie, et al., 2009).

During strength training elderly people respond positively presenting exponential gains in muscular strength, on explosion as well in muscular resistance. This is explained due to muscular mass decreases in approximately 50% between twenty and ninety years old and the number of muscular fibers in an elder person is around 20% less than in an adult person, being clear the latent capability for recovery of a strength pattern nearly to an adult.

In this study, after a 18-week training, an average increase of 89.5% in the maximum dynamic strength of the quadriceps muscle (1RM) in the intervention group was observed, being within the values described by Humphries et al., 2000 which shows increases of 20 to 200% in the dynamic muscle strength of the quadriceps depending on the initial values and duration of the training. This increase in the knee extension force is significantly important because this force is an independent risk factor for falls and fractures caused by osteoporosis (Nguyen et al., 1993). The increase in the force occurs as a result of neural changes and muscle adjustments (Resende et al, 2006).

The body balance depends on information appropriate receiving through sensorial, cognitive components from the nervous system and from the musculoskeletal system in an integrated manner by the proprioception. The association of muscle strengthening and proprioceptive training was fundamental to the increase of functional mobility and skills, which can be related to the reduction of 36% in the time spent to the performance of the TUG. In this case, the lower the time spent to make the exercise, the better the balance (Resende et al, 2006).

Although the changes in the numbers were small, the improvement in the balance evaluated by the BBS was consistent, and they are in agreement with the results found by Madureira et al, 2007.

Bemben (2000) compared the effects of high and low-intensity training in 25 postmenopausal women (41 to 60 years old) using a high repetition (40% 1-RM, 16 repetitions) and high load (80 % 1-RM, 8 repetitions) protocols for six months showing increases from 30 to 40%, respectively in the dynamic strength in quadriceps.

In a randomized controlled trial of 10 weeks of strength, balance and stretching training in 53 postmenopausal women with osteoporosis, Malmros and colleagues (1998) showed that strength and muscle mass and also the static balance improved significantly.

In another randomized clinical trial, physiotherapy-directed exercise in 30 patients with osteoporosis significantly improved static balance measured by functional reach and increased quadriceps dynamic strength (Mitchell et al, 1998).

These two studies indicate that the exercises programs improved the profile of fall risk but showed limitations because of the small number of samples and short time of the interventions.

Hartard et al. (1996) studied the effects of muscle strength training in 16 postmenopausal women with osteopenia, where fifteen belonged to the control group. Although they used a small group, a proper load protocol for 6 months, twice a week at 70% 1RM was applied demonstrating a considerable increase in muscle strength ranging from 44 to 76%, with results similar to the ones found in the present investigation.

Kemmler et. al (2002) evaluated the dynamic force (1RM tests) in 137 postmenopausal women with osteopenia divided in two groups and observed a significant increase of 43% in the leg press in the intervention group training at 70% of 1-RM for fourteen months.

Carter et al. (2002) in a program that trains instructors to work with the community selected 93 postmenopausal women with osteoporosis who were randomized and underwent physical exercises of balance and muscle strength for twenty weeks. No improvement in the quality of life was found, which might be explained by the high quality of life at baseline. Researchers observed an improvement of 6.3% in the dynamic balance and an increase of 12.8% in the muscular strength.

On the other hand, this study contradicts other researches since it shows a significant improvement in the quality of life evaluated by the SF-36, where the values for the physical aspects and mental aspects were considerably higher than the ones found in the control group and the values in the baseline. These outcomes might be related to the systemic physiologic benefits provided by the exercises, which improves the capability of performing daily activities. The results can also be explained by the psychological effects the physical exercise provides, the socialization with other patients and the low levels of quality of life the patients had in the beginning of this study.

Madureira et. al (2006) conducted a randomized clinical trial that included 66 postmenopausal women with osteoporosis assigned to two groups. One of the groups underwent a 12-month of balance training once a week combined with oriented training at home showing significant results concerning balance, mobility and decrease in the number of falls.

Swanenburg et. al (2007) studied 24 women (65 years old or older) with osteoporosis or osteopeny who underwent three months of strength, balance and coordination training. After twelve months, they observed a reduction in the risk of fall (Berg Scale) and increase in the muscle strength of lower limbs. They also found a decrease in the number of falls in the intervention group (89%), showing a significant number although it was a pilot study.

Our figures concerning the reduction of number of falls are similar to the ones found in other studies, although an average of 40% (Barnett et al., 2003) is still not well-substantiated, which can be explained by the differences in the population and mainly in the interventions used in the different researches.

The programmed answers execution by the central nervous system is performed by the musculoskeletal system and the reflex answers, voluntary motor control, postural control and articular stability influence it, fundamental components for falls risk decrease. Therefore the proposed and performed program in this study took in consideration the effector system optimization importance and the neural components, thus, by associating the strength training to sensorial-motor training we obtained effective outcomes and even more vigorous than those that only use muscular strength or balance without taking in consideration the integrated action among the central nervous system, peripheral nervous system (through proprioceptors) and the effecting organs.

As we could observe, several studies have shown to be effective to increase the strength, balance and functional skills, decreasing the risk of falls. Only the research conducted by Madureira et al. 2007 and Swanenburg et al. 2007 direct related these outcomes with the number of falls. However, it is difficult to compare the studies because the training programs and the evaluation methods are different.

The possible limitations of the present study include the tests and functional scales used, that are validated but are not so accurate as the lab tests considered the gold pattern. On the other side, we used the BBS, TUG and 1-RM Test which are highly reproducible in the daily clinic practice, where the access to lab tests is not very often.

A high adherence rate to the exercises, the thorough evaluation made by a blinded physical therapist, the size of the sample and also the strict methodology used when prescribing the exercises might have contributed to the outcomes in this present study.

The purpose of this study was to implement a muscle and proprioceptive training program that would follow the recommendations stated by ACSM, promoting a program that would be strictly followed and prescribed, but easy to use and reproduce.

5. Conclusion

The association of progressive strength training for the quadriceps and the proprioceptive training is effective for the prevention of falls, increasing the muscle power, the static and dynamic balance and increasing the speed of the motor responses, therefore improving the performance of daily activities.

Acknowledgements

The authors would like to thank Federal University of São Paulo, University of Santo Amaro and Federal University of Amazonas for all the support given when developing this project.

Author details

Lucas Teixeira[1,3], Stella Peccin[1,4], Kelson Silva[1], Tiago Teixeira[2], Aline Mizusaki Imoto[1], Joelma Magalhães[5] and Virgínia Trevisani[1,2]

1 Department of Internal and Therapeutic Medicine – Federal University of São Paulo, Brazil

2 Department of Rheumatology - University of Santo Amaro, Brazil

3 Department of Physical Therapy - Federal University of Amazonas, Brazil

4 Department of Physical Therapy - Federal University of São Paulo, Brazil

5 Department of Physical Therapy - Uninorte Laureat University, Brazil

References

[1] Adams KL, Barnard KL, Swank AM, Mann E, Kushnick MR, Denny M (1999) Combined high-intensity strength and aerobic training in diverse phase 11 cardiac rehabilitation patient. J Cardiopulm Rehabil 19:209-215.

[2] Adler, SS.; Beckers, D. & Buck M. (2008). *PNF in practice: an illustrated guide.* 3rd ed. Berlin: Springer.

[3] American College of Sports Medicine (2002) Position Stand on Progression Models in Resistance Training for Healthy Adults. Med Sci Sports Exerc 34 (2):364-380.

[4] American College of Sports Medicine. (1995). *Guidelines for Exercise Testing and Prescription.* 5th Ed. Baltimore: Williams and Wilkins, pp. 1–373.

[5] American College of Sports Medicine. (1998). Position Exercise and physical activity for older adults. *Med Sci Sports Exerc*. 30: 992-1008.

[6] American College of Sports Medicine. (2002). Position Stand on Progression Models in Resistance Training for Healthy Adults. *Med Sci Sports Exerc*. 34 (2): 364-380.

[7] Barnett A, Smith B, Lord SR, Williams M, Baumand A (2003) Community-based group exercise improves balance and reduces falls in at-risk older people: a randomized controlled trial. Age Aging 32:407-414.

[8] Bastian, AJ. (2006). Learning to predict the future: the cerebellum adapts feedforward movement control. *Curr Opin Neurobiol*. 16 (6): 645-9.

[9] Bemben DA, Fetters NI, Bemben MG, Nabavi N, Koh ET (2000) Musculoskeletal responses to high- and low-intensity resistance training in early postmenopausal women. Med Sci Sports Exerc 32:1949-1957.

[10] Berg KO, Norman KE (1996) Functional assessment of balance and gait. Clin Geriatr Med 12 (4): 705-723.

[11] Berg KO, Norman KE (1996) Functional assessment of balance and gait. Clin Geriatr Med 12 (4): 705-723.

[12] Bohannon RW (2006) Reference values for the timed up and go test: a descriptive meta-analysis. J Geriatr Phys Ther 29: 64–68.

[13] Bohannon RW (2006) Reference values for the timed up and go test: a descriptive meta-analysis. J Geriatr Phys Ther 29: 64–68.

[14] Brandão, CMA. & Vieira, JGH. (1999). Fatores envolvidos no pico de massa óssea. *Arq Bras Endocrinol Metabol*. 43(6):401-408.

[15] Brunner E, Langer F (2000) Nonparametric analysis of ordered categorical data in designs with longitudinal observations and small sample sizes. Biom J 42:663-675.

[16] Burke TN, França FJ, Ferreira de Meneses SR, Cardoso VI, Marques AP: Postural control in elderly persons with osteoporosis: Efficacy of an intervention program to improve balance and muscle strength: a randomized controlled trial. *Am J Phys Med Rehabil*;89(7):549-56, 2010.

[17] Carter ND, Kannus P, Khan KM (2001) Exercise in the prevention of falls in older people. Sports Med 31(6):427-438.

[18] Carter Nd, Kannus P, Khan Km (2002). Community-Based exercise program reduces risk factors for falls in 65- To 75-year-old women with osteoporosis: Randomized Controlled Trial. Cmaj; October 29, Vol. 167 No. 9; 997-1004.

[19] Cathleen, S.; Colón-Emeric, C. & Saag, KG. (2006). Osteoporotic fractures in older adults. *Best Pract Res Clin Rheumatol*. August; 20(4): 695–706.

[20] Cathleen, S.; Colón-Emeric, C. & Saag, KG. (2006). Osteoporotic fractures in older adults. *Best Pract Res Clin Rheumatol*. August; 20(4): 695–706.

[21] Chyu MC, James CR, Sawyer SF, Brismée JM, Xu KT, Poklikuha G, Dunn DM, Shen CL (2010). Effects of tai chi exercise on posturography, gait, physical function and quality of life in postmenopausal women with osteopaenia: a randomized clinical study. *Clin Rehabil;* 24(12):1080-90

[22] Ciconelli RM, Ferraz MB, Santos W, Meinão I, Quaresma MR (1999) Tradução para a língua portuguesa e validação do questionário genérico de avaliação de qualidade de vida SF-36 (Brasil SF-36). Rev Bras Reumatol 39: 143-150.

[23] Ciconelli RM, Ferraz MB, Santos W, Meinão I, Quaresma MR (1999) Tradução para a língua portuguesa e validação do questionário genérico de avaliação de qualidade de vida SF-36 (Brasil SF-36). Rev Bras Reumatol 39: 143-150.

[24] Cólon-Emeric, C.; Kuchibhatla, M.; Pieper, C.; Hawkes, W.; Fredman, L.; Magaziner, J.; Zimmerman, S. & Lyles, KW. (2003). The contribution of hip fracture to risk of subsequent fractures: data from two longitudinal studies. *Osteoporos Int.* 14 (11): 879–883.

[25] Froes, NDTC.; Pereira, ES. & Negrelli, WF. (2002). Fatores de risco da osteoporose: prevenção e detecção através do monitoramento clínico e genético. *Acta Ortop Bras.* 10 (1): 52-57.

[26] Gass, M. & Huges, BD. (2006). Preventing osteoporosis – related fractures: An overview. *Am J Med.* 119(4A): 3-11.

[27] Guyton, AC. & Hall, JE. (2006). *Textbook of medical physiology*. 11 ed. Philadelphia: WB Saunders.

[28] Häkkinen K, Kallinen M, Izquierdo M, Jokelainen K, Lassila H, Mälkiä E, Kraemer WJ, Newton RU, Alen M (1998) Changes in agonist-antagonist EMG. Muscle CSA. And force during strength training in middle-aged and older people. J Appl Physiol 84 (4):1341:1349.

[29] Hartard M, Haber P, Ilieva D, Preisinge E, Seidl G, Huber J (1996) Strength training as a model of therapeutic intervention: A Controlled Trial in Postmenopausal Women with Osteopenia. Am J Phys Med Rehabil 75(1):21-28.

[30] Hartard M, Haber P, Ilieva D, Preisinge E, Seidl G, Huber J (1996) Strength training as a model of therapeutic intervention: A Controlled Trial in Postmenopausal Women with Osteopenia. Am J Phys Med Rehabil 75(1):21-28.

[31] Hortobagyi,T, Katch FI, LaChance PF (1998) Interrelationships among various measures of upper body strength assessed by different contraction modes. Eur J Appl Physiol 58(7):749-755

[32] Hortobagyi,T, Katch FI, LaChance PF (1998) Interrelationships among various measures of upper body strength assessed by different contraction modes. Eur J Appl Physiol 58(7):749-755.

[33] Humphries B, Newton RU, Bronks R, Marshall S, McBride J, triplett-McBride T, Hakkinen K, Kraemer WJ,

[34] Humprhies N (2000) Effect of exercise intensity on bone density, strength, and calcium tumover in older women. Med Sci Sports Exerc 32:1043-1050.

[35] Hunter, DJ. & Sambrook, PN. (2000). Bone loss: Epidemiology of bone loss. *Arthritis Res.* 2(6): 441-445.

[36] Hurd, WJ.; Chmielewski, TL. & Snyder-Mackler L. (2006). Perturbation-enhanced neuromuscular training alters muscle activity in female athletes. *Knee Surg Sports Traumatol Arthrosc.* 14(1): 60-69.

[37] Hurley MV (2003) Muscle dysfunction and effective rehabilitation of knee osteoarthritis: what we know and what we need to find out. Arthritis & Rheum 49:444–52.

[38] Johnell, O.; Kanis, JA.; Oden, A.; Johansson, H.; De Laet, C.; Delmas, P.; Eisman, JA.; Fujiwara, S.; Kroger, H.; Mellstrom, D.; Meunier, PJ. Melton, LJ 3rd.; O'Neill, T.; Pols, H.; Reeve, J.; Silman, A. & Tenenhouse, A. (2005). Predictive value of BMD for hip and other fractures. *J Bone Miner Res.* 20 (7):1185–1194.

[39] Kemmler W, Engelke K, Lauber D, Weineck J, Hensen J, Kalendertitle WA (2002) Exercise effects on fitness and bone mineral density in early postmenopausal women: 1-year EFOPS: Med Sci Sports Exerc 34 (12):2115-23.

[40] Kristensen MT, Foss NB, Kehlet H (2007) Timed "up & go" test as a predictor of falls within 6 months after hip fracture surgery. Phys Ther 87: 24–30.

[41] Kristensen MT, Foss NB, Kehlet H (2007) Timed "up & go" test as a predictor of falls within 6 months after hip fracture surgery. Phys Ther 87: 24–30.

[42] Large J, Gan N, Basic D, Jennings N (2006) Using the timed up and go test to stratify elderly inpatients at risk of falls. Clin Rehabil 20: 421–428.

[43] Large J, Gan N, Basic D, Jennings N (2006) Using the timed up and go test to stratify elderly inpatients at risk of falls. Clin Rehabil 20: 421–428.

[44] Lephart SM, Fu FH, Borsa JP, Warner JP. (1994). *Proprioceptive of the shoulder joint in healthy, unstable, and surgically repaired shoulders.* J Shoulder Elbow Surg. 3: 371–380.

[45] Lewiecki EM, Kendler DL, Kiebzak, Schmeer P, Prince RL, Fuleihan (2004) Special report on the official positions of the International Society for Clinical Densitometry. Osteoporos Int 15: 779-784.

[46] Lewiecki EM, Kendler DL, Kiebzak, Schmeer P, Prince RL, Fuleihan (2004) Special report on the official positions of the International Society for Clinical Densitometry. Osteoporos Int 15: 779-784.

[47] Madureira MM, Takayama L, Gallinaro AL, Cparbo VF, Costa RA, Pereira RM (2007) Balance training program is highly effective in improving functional status and reducing the risk of falls in elderly women with osteoporosis: a randomized controlled trial. Osteoporos Int 18(4):419-425.

[48] Malmros B, Mortenson L, Jensen MB, Charles P (1998) Positive effects of physiotherapy on chronic pain and performance in osteoporosis. Osteoporos Int 8:215-21.

[49] Mitchell SL, Grant S, Atchison T (1988) Physiological effects of exercise on post-menopausal osteoporotic women. Physiotherapy 84:157-63.

[50] Miyamoto ST, Lombardi Junior I, Berg KO, Ramos LR, Natour J (2004) Brazilian version of the Berg balance scale. Braz J Med Biol Res 37 (9): 1411-1421.

[51] Miyamoto ST, Lombardi Junior I, Berg KO, Ramos LR, Natour J (2004) Brazilian version of the Berg balance scale. Braz J Med Biol Res 37 (9): 1411-1421.

[52] Moher D, Schulz KF, Altman D (2001) The CONSORT statement: revised recommendations for improving the quality of reports of parallel-group randomized trials. JAMA 285(15):1987-1991.

[53] Moher D, Schulz KF, Altman D (2001) The CONSORT statement: revised recommendations for improving the quality of reports of parallel-group randomized trials. JAMA 285(15):1987-1991.

[54] Moreira, C. & Xavier, JD. (2001). Doenças Ósteo-metabólicas. In: *Reumatologia, diagnóstico e tratamento*. Guanabara Koogan, 2ª ed, pp. 327-350.

[55] Mosekilde L. (1995). Osteoporosis and Exercise. *Bone.* 17(3): 193-195.

[56] Neto, AMP.; Soares, A.; Urbanetz, AA.; Souza, ACA.; Ferrari, AEM. & Amaral, B et al. (2002). Consenso Brasileiro de Osteoporose. *Rev Bras Reumatol.* 42(6):343-354.

[57] Nguyen T, Sambrook P, Kelly P, Jones G, Lord S, Freund J, Eisman J (1993) Prediction of osteoporotic fractures by postural instability and bone density. BMJ 307 (6912):1111-1115.

[58] Parkkari, J.; Kannus. P.; Palvanen, M.; Natri, A.; Vainio, J.; Aho, H.; Vuori, I. & Järvienen, M. (1999). Majority of Hip Fractures Occur as a Results of a Fall and Impact on the Greater Trochanter of the Femur: A Prospective Controlled Hip Fracture Study with 206 Consecutive Patients. *Calcif Tissue Int.* 65:1983-187.

[59] Podsiadlo D, Richardson S (1991) The timed "Up & Go": a test of basic functional mobility for frail elderly persons. J Am Geriatr Soc 39: 142–148.

[60] Podsiadlo D, Richardson S (1991) The timed "Up & Go": a test of basic functional mobility for frail elderly persons. J Am Geriatr Soc 39: 142–148.

[61] Ramalho, AC.; Castro, ML.; Hauache, O.; Vieira, JG.; Takala, E.; Calalli, F. & Tavares, F. (2001). Osteoporotic fractures of proximal femur: clinical and epidemiological features in a population of the city of São Paulo. *Sao Paulo Med J.* 119(2): 48-53.

[62] Resende SM, Rassi CM, Viana FP (2008) Effects of hydrotherapy in balance and prevention of falls among elderly. Arthritis & Rheum 12 (1):57-63.

[63] Shumway-Cook A, Baldwin M, Polissar NL, Gruber W (1997) Predicting the 21. probability for falls in community-dwelling older adults. Phys Ther 77(8) :812-819.

[64] Shumway-Cook A, Brauer S, Woollacott M (2000) Predicting the probability for falls in community-dwelling older adults using the Timed Up & Go Test. Phys Ther 80: 896 –903.

[65] Shumway-Cook, A. & Woollacott, M. (1995). *Motor Control Theory and Applications*. Williams and Wilkins: Baltimore.

[66] Shumway-Cook, A.; Brauer, S. & Woollacott, M. (2000). Predicting the probability for falls in community-dwelling older adults using the Timed Up & Go Test. *Phys Ther.* 80: 896 –903.

[67] Siris, ES.; Brenneman, SK.; Barrett-Connor, E.; Miller, PD.; Sajjan, S.; Berger, ML. & Chen, YT. (2006). The effect of age and bone mineral density on the absolute, excess, and relative risk of fracture in postmenopausal women aged 50–99: results from the National Osteoporosis Risk Assessment (NORA). *Osteoporos Int* . 17 (4): 565–574.

[68] Smulders E, Weerdesteyn V, Groen BE, Duysens J, Eijsbouts A, Laan R, van Lankveld W (2010). Efficacy of a short multidisciplinary falls prevention program for elderly persons with osteoporosis and a fall history: a randomized controlled trial. *Arch Phys Med Rehabil;* Nov; 91(11):1705-11

[69] Swanenburg J, de Bruin ED, Stauffacher M, Mulder T, Uebelhart D (2007) Effects of exercise and nutrition on postural balance and risk of falling in elderly people with decreased bone mineral density: randomized controlled trial pilot study. Clin Rehabil 21(6):523-34.

[70] Swanik, KA.; Lephart, SM.; Swanik, CB.; Lephart, SP.; Stone, DA. & Fu FH. (2002). The effects of shoulder plyometric training on proprioception and selected muscle performance characteristics. *J Shoulder Elbow Surg*. 11(6):579-86.

[71] Szejnfeld, VL.; Jennings, F.; Castro, CHM.; Pinheiro, MM. & Lopes, AC. (2007). Conhecimento dos Médicos Clínicos do Brasil sobre as Estratégias de Prevenção e Tratamento da Osteoporose. *Rev Bras Reumatol.* 47(4):251-257.

[72] Teixeira, LE.; Silva, KN.; Imoto, AM.; Teixeira, TJ.; Kayo, AH.; Montenegro-Rodrigues, R. & Trevisani, VFM. (2010). Progressive load training for the quadriceps muscle associated with proprioception exercises for the prevention of falls in

postmenopausal women with osteoporosis: a randomized controlled trial. *Osteoporosis International*; 21: 589-96.

[73] Tinetti, ME. & Speechley, M. (1989). Prevention of falls among the elderly. *N Engl J Med.* 320:1055–1059.

[74] van der Esch M, Steultjens M, Harlaar J, Knol D, Lems W, Dekker J (2007) Joint Proprioception, Muscle Strength, and Functional Ability in Patients With Osteoarthritis of the Knee. Arthritis & Rheum 57(5):787-793.

[75] Van der Esch, M.; Steultjens, M.; Harlaar, J.; Knol, D.; Lems, W. & Dekker, J. (2007). Joint Proprioception, Muscle Strength, and Functional Ability in Patients With Osteoarthritis of the Knee. *Arthritis & Rheum.* 57(5):787-793.

[76] Wayne PM, Kiel DP, Buring JE, Connors EM, Bonato P, Yeh GY, Cohen CJ, Mancinelli C, Davis RB (2012). Impact of Tai Chi exercise on multiple fracture-related risk factors in post-menopausal osteopenic women: a pilot pragmatic, randomized trial. *BMC Complement Altern Med*; 12:7

[77] Weatherall, M. (2004). Prevention of falls and falls-related fractures in community-dwelling older adults: a meta-analysis of estimates of effectivenessbased on recent guidelines. *Intern Med J.* 34:102-108.

[78] Weier, JP (1994) The effect of rest interval length on repeated maximal bench press. J Strength Cond Res 8: 58.

Chapter 11

Anabolic Agents as New Treatment Strategy in Osteoporosis

Tulay Okman-Kilic and Cengiz Sagiroglu

Additional information is available at the end of the chapter

http://dx.doi.org/10.5772/54452

1. Introduction

Osteoporosis is a systemic skeletal disease characterized by low bone mineral density (BMD), microarchitectural deterioration of bone tissue, and an increase in fracture risk [1]. Several drugs have been developed to treat osteoporosis: most of these are inhibitors of bone resorption. Effective treatment of osteoporosis requires not only resorption inhibitors, but also stimulators of bone formation especially in patients who already have lost a significant degree of bone. Although therapeutic alternatives are available for inhibiting bone resorption, options of bone anabolic agents are much more limited with regard to the bone resorption inhibitors.

Although patients included in randomised controlled trials have osteoporosis defined according to the WHO criteria, i.e. a T score below -2.5 SD and/or prevalent fragility fractures, a large proportion of fractures occurs at T-scores above -2.5 SD and in patients without prior fractures [1]. Therefore, therapies with proven fracture risk reduction efficacy in patients with osteopenia and/or clinical risk factors may contribute to earlier and more effective intervention against fractures.

The past decade has witnessed major advances in the diagnosis and treatment of osteoporosis. It would appear that anabolic drugs challenge prevailing paradigm by stimulating bone formation, therefore enhancing bone turnover. There is a great need to anabolic agents for reverse of osteoporosis. In this review, we summarize current informations about the anabolic agents.

2. Parathormon

Parathyroid hormon (PTH) is released from the parathyroid glands and is an important regulator in the bloodstream's levels of calcium phosphorus. It stimulates both bone formation and resorption [2,3]. Its intermittent low-dose using increases bone formation more than bone resorption, leading to increased bone mass. Intermittent PTH administration increases the number and activity of osteoblasts, enhances the mean wall thickness and trabecular bone volume, and improves bone microarchitecture by establishing trabecular connectivity and increasing cortical thickness [2,4].

Continuous infusions, which result in a persistent elevation of the serum parathyroid hormone concentration, lead to greater bone resorption than do daily injections, which cause only transient increases in the serum parathyroid hormone concentration [5,6]. The anabolic effects of PTH on bone formation are through the medium of PTH receptor-dependent mechanisms. Teriparatide (PTH_{1-34}) is the biological active, a recombinant form of PTH [7]. Patients with fractures of postmenopausal osteoporosis administered teriparatide 20 and 40 μg/d in FPT (Fracture Prevention Trial) [8]. After 18 months teriparatide 20 μg/d reduces the risk of spine fracture by %65 and non-spine fracture risk by %53. Over a median of 18 months spine fracture risk reduced by %69 and non-spine fracture risk reduced by %54 with the 40 μg/d regimen [8].

Subbiah et al. reported the second patient to develop osteosarcoma [9]. Although teriparatide reduces osteoporosis related fractures in select patient populations, important contraindications, such as prior radiation exposure, Paget's disease of bone, unexplained elevations of serum alkaline phosphate, open epiphysis should be considered before use.

It has been suggested teriparatide could be useful for treatment of severe and resistant forms of osteoporosis to other medications [10].

In summary, we think that the clinical benefits of parathyroid hormone reflect its ability to stimulate bone formation and thereby increase bone mass and strength. This hormone appears to be effective in preventing fractures in postmenopausal women. Hovewer, it should be used attention because of its important contraindications.

3. Stontium ranelate

Strontium ranelate is composed of an organic molecule (ranelic acid) and of two atoms of stable non-radioactive strontium [11]. Strontium naturally present in trace amounts in human body and has close similarities with calcium; act as calcium agonist in most of physiologic process [12].

Strontium is similar to calcium in its absorption in the gastrointestinal track takes place in two ways: passive diffusion and carrier mediated absorption. Both calcium and strontium share the same carrier system, which tents to be greater affinity to calcium. High dietary intake of calcium has been shown to reduce concurrent absorption of strontium [11].

Ingested strontium is distributed in the body in three compartments: plasma extracellular fluid; soft tissue and superficial zone of bone tissue; and bone itself, the greatest portion is the calcified tissues [13]. In bones, total amount of strontium relatively lower than amount of calcium. After its absorption, both strontium and calcium exhibit the same characteristics [12].

The strontium levels in bone vary according to the anatomical site. However, strontium levels at different skeletal sites are strongly correlated [14]. The strontium levels in bone also vary according to the bone structure and higher amounts of strontium are found in cancellous bone than in cortical bone. Strontium is mainly incorporated by exchange onto the crystal surface. In new bone, only a few strontium atoms may be incorporated into the crystal by ionic substitution of calcium [12, 14]. Bone strontium content is highly correlated with plasma strontium levels. Mechanism of action of strontium ranelate is shown in figure 1.

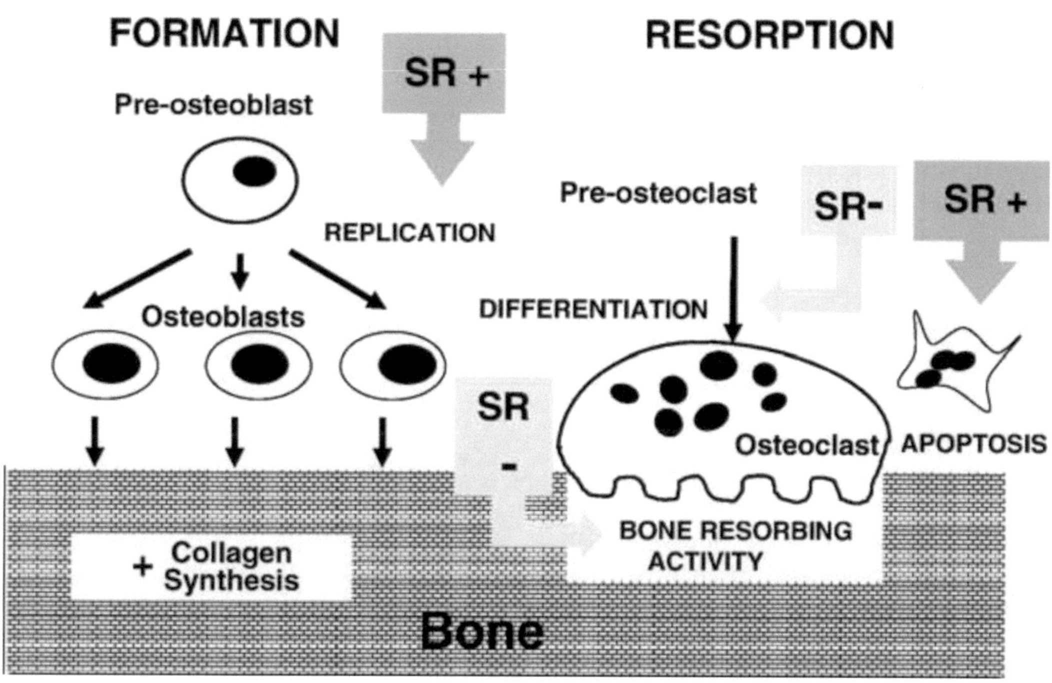

Figure 1. Mechanism of action of strontium ranelate in bone [13]

Strontium ranelate decreases osteoclast differentiation and activity [15]. Also able to increase pre-osteoblast replication, collagen type I synthesis [16]. Therefore strontium ranelate has a dual affect on bone remodeling, being able to stimulate bone formation by osteoblasts, a property shared with bone-forming agents, and to inhibit bone resorption by osteoclasts, as do anti-resorptive agents [17,18].

Strontiun ranelate shows affect by binding calcium receptor in bone. Strontium has lower affinity for calcium sensing receptor than calcium[19].

There are higher calcium ion concentrations within the bone microenvironment in case of osteoclastic resorption. Affect of calcium receptor increases in higher extracellular calcium concentrations. Strontium ranelate intake prevents bone loss with non-osteoporotic patients in early post-menopausal period [19].

In the PREVOS study (PREVention Of early postmenopausal bone loss by Strontium ranelate) usage of strontium ranelate 1g/d for period of 2 years resulted in significantly higher increase of femur BMD (bone mineral density). There was a significant increase in the bone formation markers and concurrent increase of bone resorption markers has not been recorded [20].

In the Treatment of Peripheral Osteoporosis (TROPOS) study strontium ranelate increased bone mineral density throughout the study, reaching at 3-yr 8.2% (femoral neck) and 9.8% (total hip). Same study shows %36 decrease in hip fracture risk even in high-risk subgroup over 3-yr period [21].

The Spinal Osteoporosis Therapeutic Intervention (SOTI) study investigated the safety of strontium ranelate and its efficacy against vertebral fractures. In patients used strontium ranelate 2 g/d the risk of vertebral fractures was decreased by 41% over 3-yr [22].

In both studies strontium ranelate was well tolerated. The most common adverse events consisted of nausea and diarrhea was disappeared after third month of treatment [21,22].

Therefore, we suggest that strontium ranelate has been proving antifracture efficacy in patients with osteopenia and/or clinical risk factors and very old elderly. Also, it may contribute to earlier and more effective intervention against fractures because of well- tolerated.

4. Prostaglandins

Prostaglandins act as locally acting hormones, developed as new therapeutic approach. They show the effect and are metabolized in the tissue where they are synthesized. Prostaglandins are synthesized from arachidonic acid, a polyunsaturated fatty acid with 20-carbon chain [23].

Prostaglandins are produced from bone cells by mediated cyclooxygenase. Prostaglandin production is regulated by mechanical stress, cytokines, growth factor and systemic hormones. Furthermore, prostaglandins are able to regulate their own production [24]. Prostaglandins have both inhibitory and stimulatory effects on bone structuring. The most prominent effect of prostaglandin E2 (PGE2) is to stimulate bone resorption and formation [24]. PGE2 exerts its action through the cell surface receptors. Four subtypes of prostaglandin E receptors (EP1, EP2, EP3 and EP4) [25,26] have been identified. PGE2 stimulates bone formation by EP4 receptor mediation [26]. The importance and impact of prostaglandins in bone metabolism is summarized in figure 2

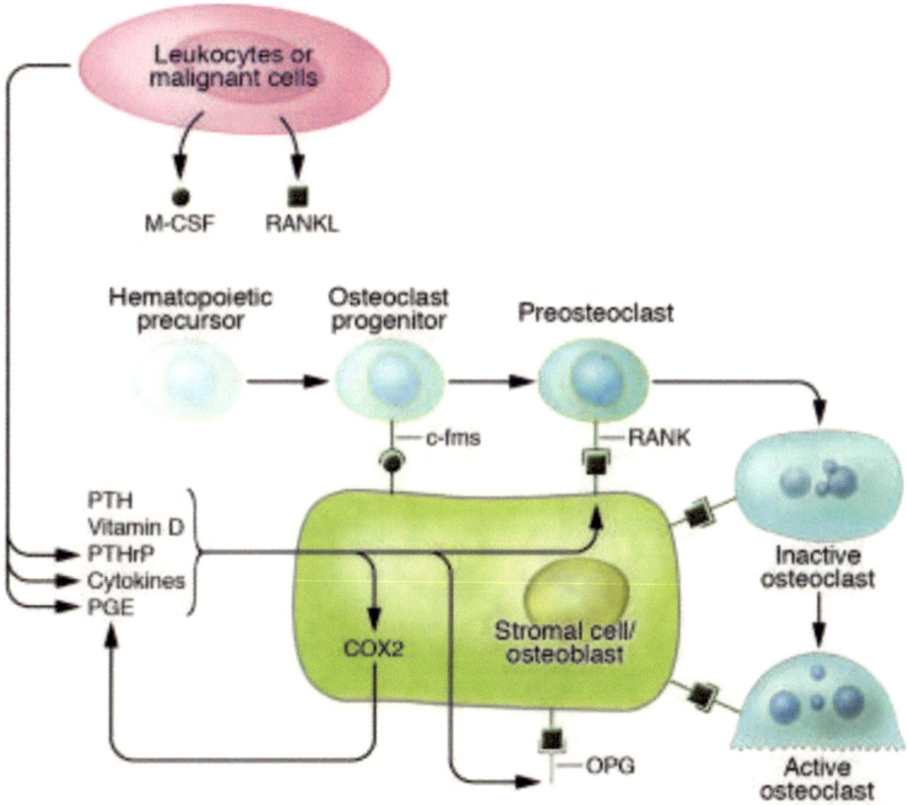

Figure 2. The mechanism of action and place of prostaglandins in bone metabolism [24]

It has been reported in certain studies that prostaglandins have anabolic effect on the bone formation, therefore can be used in osteoporosis treatment [27].

It has been demonstrated that systemic PGE2 administration stimulates proliferation of osteoblast precursors or differentiation of osteoprogenitor cells in bone marrow and 4.7% increase in bone mass eventually was found in the same study [27]. Increase of total bone surface by means of osteoblast stimulation with PGE2 administration to rats has been reported [28].

Misoprostol is a methylene analogue of prostaglandin E1 (PGE1) has been administered to oophorectomized rats. Misoprostol is being used for treatment of gastric ulcer due to its cytoprotective effect by inhibiting gastric acid and pepcin secretion [23]. Rats receiving misoprostol had significantly reduced oophorectomy related bone loss at site of lumber spine. Thus, it has been proposed that misoprostol is choice for treatment of post-menopausal osteoporosis prophylaxis [29,30].

Misoprostol 800 µg/d had been administered for 6 moths to post-menopausal osteoporotic patients. At the end of the treatment increase by 8.1% in femur bone mineral density, by 5% increase in lumber spine bone mineral density and by 3.6% increase in Ward's triangle bone mineral density have been found. It has been reported that misoprostol can be an alternative on treatment of osteoporosis [31].

We think that misoprostol may be an alternative therapy for patients with osteopenia and osteoporosis who are not suitable for hormone replacement therapy.

5. Sesamin

Sesamin is a major lignan compound in sesame seeds. Its activity on bone cell function is unclear. Recently, it has been reported that sesamin has direct effects on osteoblasts by stimulating the expression of essential genes and key enzymes of the bone mineralization process [32,33].

Wanachewin et al suggested that sesamin had the ability to trigger osteoblast differantiation by activation of the p38 and ERK/MAPK (mitogen-activated protein kinase) signaling pathway and possibility indirectly regulate osteoclast development via the expression of OPG and RANKL in osteoblasts [32].

The **MAPK/ERK pathway** is a chain of proteins in the cell that transmits a signal from a receptor on the surface of the cell to the DNA in the nucleus of the cell. MAPKs play important roles in cellular response to growth factors, cytokines, or environmental stress.

They are classified into four classes: extracellular signal-regulated kinases (ERKs), c-Jun N-terminal kinase or stress-activated protein kinase, p38 MAPKs, and ERK5 [34]. ERKs are involved in cell proliferation/transformation and survival. p38 MAPKs are involved in many cellular processes, such as inflammatory responses, osteoblast differentiation, apoptosis [35,36].

We think that sesamin which is a phytochemical agent, may be effective addition to osteoporotic therapy. Future studies are needed.

6. Statins

Statins are inhibitors of 3-hydroxy-3-methylglutaryl coenzyme A (HMG-COA) reductase. Usually, it has been known that they have efficacy and credibility on coronary artery diseases and hyperlipidemia [37,38]. First, Mundy et al showed that statins lead to increase 90 % in the trabecular bone volume by stimulating bone formation invitro and therefore it was started to studies investigating the place of statins for osteoporosis treatment [39]. Hamelin et al suggested that statins decrease the bone destruction by supressing the formation of the mevalonate that it is an important precursor on the control of osteoclastic activity as bisphosphonates [40].

It was reported that statins have efficacy on the bone metabolism, by increasing bone morphogenetic protein 2 (BMP2) activation stimulated osteoblastic cell proliferation and maturation [41]. Maeda et al showed that hydrophobic statins such as simvastatin, atorvastatin, and cerivastatin stimulated VEGF expression by osteoblasts via reduced protein prenylation and the phosphatidylinositide-3 kinase pathway, promoting osteoblastic differentiation [42].

In 2009 Pault et al revealed a dose-dependent effect and improved fracture healing under local application of simvastatin [43].

Fukui et al reported that the effect of the systemic administration of statins was limited due to its metabolism in the liver and high-dose administration may cause adverse side effects. They locally applied with gelatin hydrogel to fracture sites at a dose similar to that used in clinical settings and shown to induced fracture union in a rat unhealing bone fracture model via its effect on both angiogenesis and osteogenesis [44].

We suggest that the results of studies also point to the need for more information in order to particularly gelatin hydrogel form.

7. Growth hormone and IGF-I

It is known that growth hormone (GH) is important in the regulation of longitudinal bone growth [45]. Several *in vivo* and *in vitro* studies have demonstrated that GH is important in the regulation of both bone formation and bone resorption. In Figure 3 a model for the cellular effects of GH in the regulation of bone remodeling is showed [45].

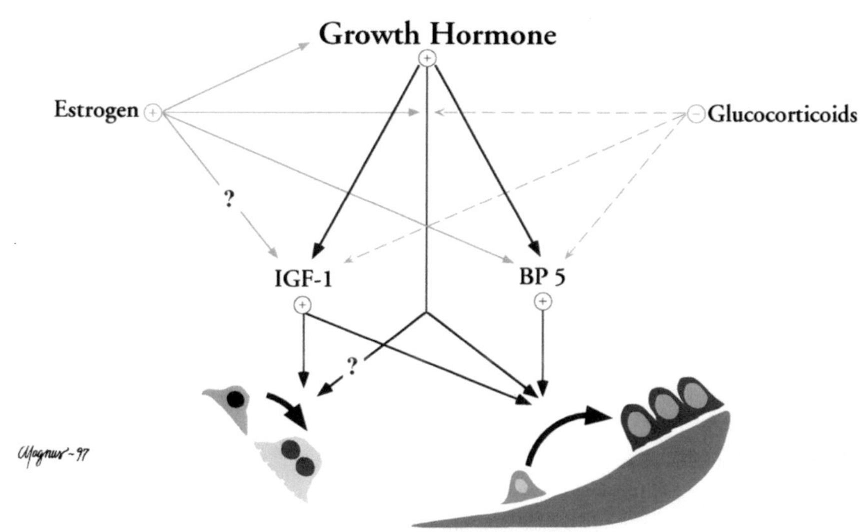

Figure 3. The mechanism of action at the cellular level for GH in regulation of bone remodeling. The left part of the figure represents osteoclast-mediated bone resorption. The right part represents osteoblast-mediated bone formation. ? indicates that both stimulatory and inhibitory effects have been shown [45]

GH increases bone formation in two ways [46]:

1. via a direct interaction with GHRs on osteoblasts
2. via an induction of endocrine and autocrine/paracrine IGF-I (Insulin like Growth Factor-1).

rhGH (recombinant human Growth Hormone) increases bone turnover in normal subjects and improves bone mineral metabolism in postmenopausal females [45]. GH treatment also results in increased bone resorption. It is still unknown whether osteoclasts express functional GHRs, but recent in vitro studies indicate that GH regulates osteoclast formation in bone marrow cultures [45, 46]. Possible modulations of the GH/IGF (Insulin like Growth Factor) axis by glucocorticoids and estrogens are also included in Fig. 3 [45].

Bone is the second richest source of IGF-I in the body. Locally this peptide promotes osteoblast differentiation and growth [48]. Recently, studies show that low levels of IGF-I are associated with a greater risk of hip and spine fractures [49–51]. Hence, there is a strong opinion for considering human GH or IGF-I as potential anabolic agents for the treatment of osteoporosis. There are potential advantages for using rhIGF-I (recombinant human Insulin like Growth Factor-1) compared with rhGH in the treatment of osteoporosis. These include

1. more direct stimulation of bone formation,
2. bypass of skeletal GH resistance that can be present, and
3. a reduction in GH-induced side-effects such as carpal tunnel and diabetes mellitus. [47]

It was reported that low doses of rhIGF-I may directly increase osteoblastic function with only a minimal increase in bone resorption [52]. In 2008, it was suggested a potential role for IGF-1 in the early identification of women at risk for low bone mass and osteoporosis. They suggested measuring the serum level of IGF-1 in women around 40 years old. When its value is 1.5 SD below the peak, BMD measurement by DXA could be considered [53]

There are limited number studies using rhIGF-I than rhGH. Therefore, these advantages have not been validated yet.

8. Sodium fluoride

Sodium fluoride is the first anabolic agentsto be used in the treatment of postmenopausal osteoporosis. Side-effects, consisting of upper gastrointestinal symptoms and a lower extremity pain syndrome, are common.

Using slow release formulation of sodium fluoride, it was showed a 50% reduction in vertebral fracture incidence with impressive increases in bone mass [54-56]. More recently, it has been suggested that a different formulation of fluoride, monofluorophosphate when is used in lower dosages and more favorable formulations, gastrointestinal side-effects are reduced [57-59]. However, consensus about its clinical utility has still not been reached.

http://dx.doi.org/10.5772/54452

9. Other potential agents for anabolic treatment of osteoporosis

Bortezomib: There are multiple potential alternative agents for increasing bone formation. A potential treatment is to target the osteoblast proteasome. It was reported that the proteasome inhibitor bortezomib (Bzb) had bone forming effects in patients with multiple myelome [60]. The mechanism for Bzb's effects on osteoblastic differentiation has not been clearly defined.

It was showed that Bzb with lenalidomide or thalidomide may increase bone formation by stimulating osteoblast activity and inhibiting osteoclastic bone destruction, respectively Figure 4.

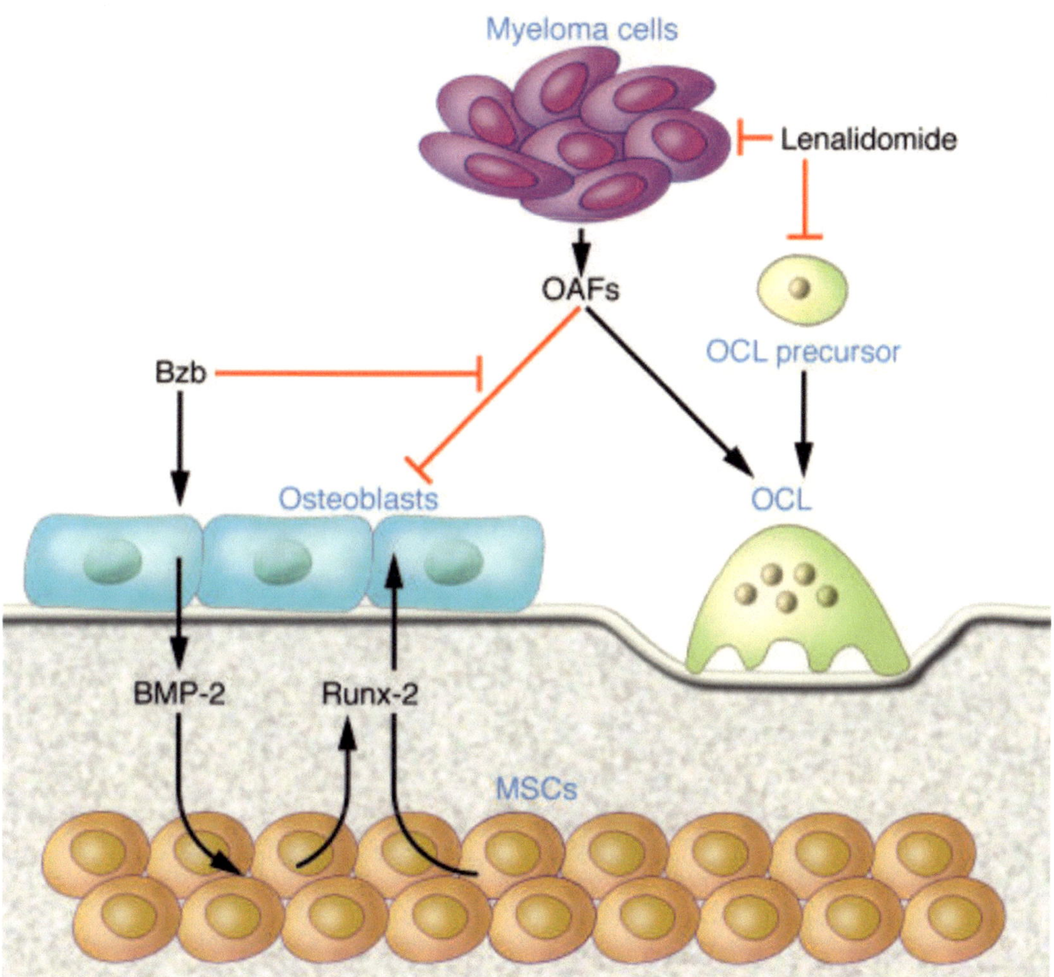

Figure 4. Bzb's action on bone formation in the patients with multiple myeloma [60]

Oxytocin: An other approach is oxytocin (OT) that increases osteoblastic bone formation. It has been reported that OT may regulate maternal skeletal homeostasis during pregnancy and lactation. The fetal skeleton is unlikely to be mineralized effectively in the absence of calcium mobilized from the maternal skeleton [61]. It has been suggested that elevated OT levels during pregnancy and lactation not only enhance bone resorption by increasing the number of osteoclasts to make maternal calcium existing to the fetus, but also prevent unrestricted bone removal by inhibiting the activity of mature osteoclasts. Therefore, it was reported that recombinant OT or its analogs because of its skeletal anabolic action, might have potential utility in therapy for human osteoporosis [61].

Beta-blocker: Wiens et al found that beta-blocker use was associated with a significant decrease in fracture risk [62]. However, in 2008, Reid determinated that there was no any evidence to support the hypothesis that beta,-blockers reduce fracture numbers [63]. In 2012, Yang et al reported that beta-blockers are associated with reduced risk of fracture in older adults, but the effect size is likely to be modes [64]t. In summary, there was no an adequate evidence to support using beta-blockers in the treatment of osteoporosis.

Lithium: The mean (+/-SD) bone density in lithium treated patients was reported that 4.5% higher at the spine ($P<0.05$), 5.3% higher at the femoral neck ($P<0.05$) and 7.5% higher at the trochanter ($P<0.05$). In addition, lithium treated patients had lower serum total ALP ($P<0.005$), lower serum osteocalcin ($P<0.005$) and lower serum CTX ($P<0.05$) but the totalcalcium, PTH and urinary calcium excretion did not differ significantly between patients and controls. In conclusion, it was suggested that therapy with lithium carbonate may preserve or enhance bone mass [65].

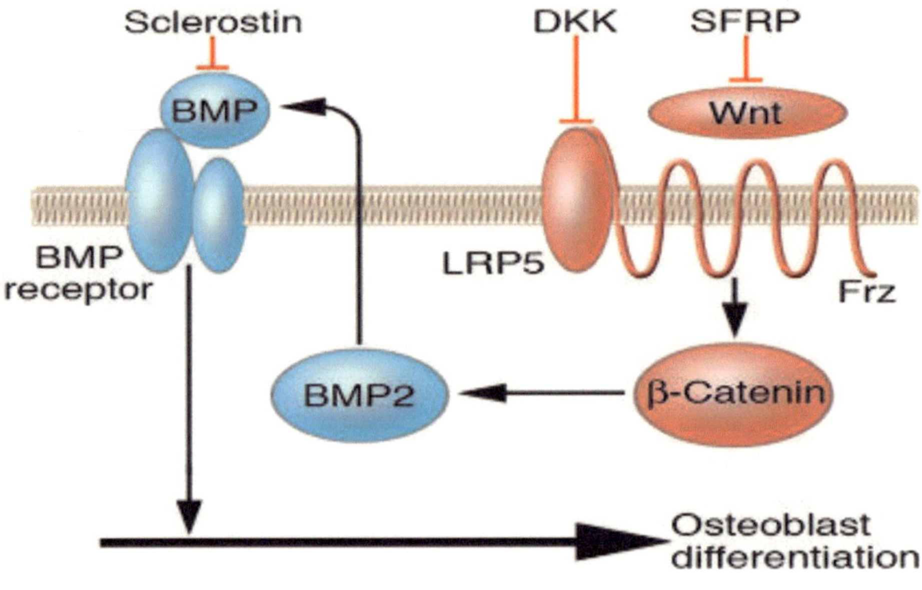

Figure 5. Modulation of Wnt signaling by sclerostin [73]

Anti-sclerostin monoclonal antibody: Sclerostin is a protein encoded by the SOST gene in osteocytes. It inhibits osteoblastic bone formation [66,67]. The binding of Wnt proteins to the LRP5/6-Frizzled co-receptor on the cell membrane of osteoblasts leads to stabilization of intracellular beta-catenin and regulation of gene transcription that promotes osteoblastic bone formation. Sclerostin is a modulator of osteoblast function. It antagonizes Wnt signaling and inhibits osteoblastic bone formation [68]. Recent studies reported that anti-sclerostin therapy enhances fracture healing and bone repair.[69-71]. AMG 785 is a humanized sclerostin monoclonal antibody, was first studied in humans. It enhances Wnt signaling and increase osteoblastic bone formation [72]. Figure 5

Treatment with AMG 785 has been well tolerated. In postmenopausal women with low bone mineral density (BMD) after 12 months of AMG 785 administration, increase in BMD is determined. Although there is no evidence that AMG 785 increases the risk of osteosarcoma, new studies are needed to modify this risk.

10. Conclusion

Aging is associated with impaired bone formation which is a principal pathogenetic cause mediating bone fragility in osteoporosis. Ideally, patients at high risk of fracture should be identified early and treated by a combination of lifestyle changes, correction of secondary causes of osteoporosis, and specific treatments to improve bone density and decrease fracture risk. By now, there were a limited number of therapeutic agent for activating bone formation and increasing bone mass and strength. More effective and better tolerated therapies will become available soon. We think that new treatments will be able to contribute to increase the currently low treatment rate of even severe osteoporosis by allowing approaches aimed at minimising fracture risk at the individual patient level.

Author details

Tulay Okman-Kilic[1] and Cengiz Sagiroglu[2]

*Address all correspondence to: ajlankilic@hotmail.com

1 Department of Obsterics and Gynecology, Trakya University, Medical Faculty, Edirne, Turkey

2 Tasyapi Health Group, Istanbul, Turkey

References

[1] World Health Organisation. Assessment of fracture risk and its application to screening for postmenopausal osteoporosis. World Health Organisation Technical Report Series. Geneva: WHO, 1994.

[2] Hock JM, Gera I. Effects of Continuous and Intermittent Administration and Inhibition of Resorption on The Anabolic Response of Bone to Parathyroid Hormone. J Bone Miner Res 1992;7:65–72.

[3] Schlüter KD. PTH and PTHrP: Similar Structures but Different Functions. News Physiol Sci. 1999;14:243-49.

[4] Marie PJ, Kassem M. Osteoblasts in Osteoporosis: Past, Emerging, and Future Anabolic Targets. Eur J Endocrinol. 2011;165 (1):1-10.

[5] Tam CS, Heersche JN, Murray TM, Parsons JA. Parathyroid Hormone Stimulates The Bone Apposition Rate Independently of Its Resorptive Action: Differential Effects of Intermittent and Continuous Administration. Endocrinology 1982;110:506-12.

[6] Uzawa T, Hori M, Ejiri S, Ozawa H. Comparison of The Effects of Intermittent and Continuous Administration of Human Parathyroid Hormone (1-34) on Rat Bone. Bone 1995;16:477-484.

[7] Neer RM, Arnaud CD, Zanchetta JR, Prince R, Gaich GA, Reginster JY, et al. Effect of Parathyroid Hormone (1-34) on Fractures and Bone Mineral Density in Postmenopausal Women with Osteoporosis. N Engl J Med 2001;344:1434-1441.

[8] Geusens P, Reid D. Newer drug treatments: their effects on fracture prevention. Best Practice and Clinical Rheumatology 2005;19(6):983-9.

[9] Subbiah V, Madsen VS, Raymond AK, Benjamin RS & Ludwig JA. Of Mice and Men: Divergent Risks of Teriparatide-Induced Osteosarcoma. Osteoporosis International 2010;21: 1041–1045.

[10] Manuele S, Sorbello N, Puglisi N, Grasso S, La Malfa L, Durbino G, et al. The teriparatide in the treatment of severe senile osteoporosis. Arch Gerontol Geriatr 2007;1:249-58.

[11] Reginster JY, Deroisy R, Jupsin I. Strontium ranelate: a new paradigm in the treatment of osteoporosis. Drugs of Today 2003;39(2):89-101.

[12] Nielsen SP. The biological role of strontium. Bone 2004;35:583-8.

[13] Marie PJ, Ammann P, Boivin G, Rey C. Mechanisms of action and therapeutic potential of strontium in bone. Carcified Tissue International 2001;69:121-9.

[14] Dahl SG, Allain P, Marie PJ, Mauras Y, Boivin G, Ammann P, et al. Incorporation and distribution of strontium in bone. Bone 2001;28:446-53.

[15] Baron R, Tsouderos Y. İn vitro effects of S12911-2 on osteoclast function and bone marrow macrophege differentiation. European Journal of Pharmocology 2002;450:11-7.

[16] Reginster JY, Lecart MP, Deroisy R, Lousberg C. Strontium ranelate: a new paradigm in the treatment of osteoporosis. Expert Opin Investig Drugs 2004;13(7):857-64.

[17] Marie PJ. Strontium ranelate: a physiological approach for optimizing bone formation and resorption. Bone 2006;38:10-4.

[18] Ammann P, Shen V, Robin B, Mauras Y, Bonjour J-P, Rizzoli R. Strontium ranelate improves bone resistnce by increasing bone mass and improving architecture in intact female rats. Journal of Bone and Mineral Research 2004;19(12):2012-20.

[19] Coulombe J, Faure H, Robin B, Ruat M. In vitro effects of strontium ranelate on the extracellular calcium-sensing receptor. BBRC 2004;323:1184-90.

[20] Reginster JY, Deroisy R, Dougados M, Jupsin I, Colette J, Roux C. Prevention or early postmenopausal bone loss by strontium ranelate: The randomized, two-year, double-masked, dose-ranging, placebo-controlled PREVOS trial. Osteoporos Int 2002;13:925-31.

[21] Reginster JY, Seeman E, De Vernejoul MC, Adami S, Compston J, Phenekos C, et al. Strontium ranelate reduces the risk of nonvertebral fractures in postmenopausal women with osteoporosis: treatment of peripheral osteoporosis (tropos) study. The Journal of Clinical Endocrinology and metabolism 2005;90(5):2816-22.

[22] Meunier JM, Roox C, Seeman E, Ortolani S, Budurski J, Spencor T, et al. The effects of strontium ranelate on the risk of vertebral fracture in women with postmenopausal osteoporosis. The New England Journal of Medicine 2004;350:459-68.

[23] Mycek MJ, Harvey R, Champe P (Çeviri: Ş. Oktay). Farmakoloji. İstanbul: Nobel Tıp Kitabevleri Ltd. Şti.; 1998:419-20.

[24] Raisz LG. Pathogenesis of osteoporosis: concepts, conflicts, and prospects. The Journal of Clinical Investigation 2005;115(12):3318-25.

[25] Watkins BA, Li Y, Seifert MF. Lipids as modulators of bone remodelling. Current Opinion in Clinical Nutrition and Metabolic Care 2001;4:105-10.

[26] Yoshida K, Oida H, Kobayashi T, Maruyama T, Tanaka M, Katayama T, et al. Stimulation of bone formation and prevention of bone loss by prostaglandin EP4 receptor activation. PNAS 2002;99(7):4580-5.

[27] Weinreb M, Suponitzky I, Keila S. Systemic administration of an anabolic dose of PGE2 in young rats increases the osteogenic capacity of bone marrow. Bone 1997;20(6):521-6.

[28] Yao W, Jee SSW, Zhou H, Lu J, Cui L, Setterberg R, et al. Anabolic effect of prostaglandin E2 on cortical bone of aged male rats comes mainly from modeling dependent bone gain. Bone 1999;25(6):697-702.

[29] Sonmez AS, Birincioglu M, Özer MK, Kutlu R, Chuong CJ. Effects of misoprostol on bone loss in ovariectomized rats. Prostaglandins and other Lipid Mediators 1999;57:113-8.

[30] Ahmet-Camcioglu N, Okman-Kilic T, Durmus-Altun G, Ekuklu G, Kucuk M. Effects of strontium ranelate, raloxifene and misoprostol on bone mineral density in ovariectomized rats. Eur J Obstet Gynecol Reprod Biol. 2009;147(2):192-4.

[31] Yasar L, Sönmez AS, Utku N, Özcan J, Çebi Z, Savan K, et al. Effect of misoprostol on bone mineral density in women with postmenopausal oateoporosis. Prostaglandins and Other Lipid Mediators 2006;79:199-205.

[32] Wanachewin O, Boonmaleerat K, Pothacharoen P, Reutrakul V, Kongtawelert P. Sesamin Stimulates Osteoblast Differentiation Through p38 and ERK1/2 MAPK Signaling Pathways. BMC Complement Altern Med 2012;12(1):71

[33] Boulbaroud S, Mesfioui A, Arfaoui A, Ouichou A, El-Hessni A. Preventive effects of flaxseed and sesame oil on bone loss in ovariectomized rats. Pak J Biol Sci 2008;11(13):1696–1701.

[34] Chang L, Karin M. Mammalian MAP kinase signalling cascades. Nature 2001;410:37–40.

[35] Suzanne M, Irie K, Glise B, Agnes F, Mori E, Matsumoto K, Noselli S. The Drosophila p38 MAPK pathway is required during oogenesis for egg asymmetric development. Genes Dev 1999;13:1464–1474.

[36] Hu Y, Chan E, Wang SX, Li B. Activation of p38 mitogen-activated protein kinase is required for osteoblast differentiation. Endocrinology. 2003;144(5):2068-74.

[37] LaRosa JC, He J, Vupputuri S. Effect of statins on risk of coronary disease: a meta-analysis of randomized controlled trials. JAMA 1999; 282 (24): 2340-6.

[38] Prevention of cardiovascular events and death with pravastatin in patients with coronary heart disease and a broad range of initial cholesterol levels. The Long-Term Intervention with Pravastatin in Ischaemic Disease (LIPID) Study Group. N Engl J Med 1998; 339 (19): 1349-57.

[39] Mundy G, Garrett R, Harris S, et al. Stimulation of bone formation in vitro and in rodents by statins. Science 1999; 286 (5446): 1946-9.

[40] Hamelin BA, Turgeon J. Hydrophilicity/lipophilicity: revelance for the pharmacology and clinical effects of HMG-CoA reductase inhibitors. Trends Pharmacol Sci 1998; 19: 26-37.

[41] Bauer DC. HMG CoA reductase inhibitors and the skeleton: a comprehensive review. Osteoporos Int 2003; 14 (4): 273-82.

[42] Maeda T, Kawane T, Horiuchi N. Statins Augment Vascular Endothelial Growth Factor Expression in Osteoblastic Cells via Inhibition of Protein Prenylation. Endocrinology 2003;144(2):681–692 doi: 10.1210/en.2002-220682.

[43] Pauly S, Luttosch F, Morawski M, Haas NP, Schmidmaier G, Wildemann B. Simvastatin locally applied from a biodegradable coating of osteosynthetic implants improves fracture healing comparable to BMP-2 application. Bone. 2009;45:505–511. doi: 10.1016/j.bone.2009.05.010.

[44] Fukui T, Ii M, Shoji T, Matsumoto T, Mifune Y, Kawakami Y, Akimaru H, Kawamoto A, Kuroda T, Saito T, Tabata Y, Kuroda R, Kurosaka M, Asahara T. Therapeutic effect of local administration of low-dose simvastatin-conjugated gelatin hydrogel for fracture healing. J Bone Miner Res. 2012 May;27(5):1118-31. doi: 10.1002/jbmr.1558.

[45] Ohlsson C, Bengtsson BA, Isaksson OGP, Andreassen TT, Slootweg M. Growth Hormone and Bone. Endocrine Reviews 1998; 19: (1) 55-79.

[46] Ransjö M, Lerner U, Ohlsson C. Growth hormone inhibits formation of osteoclast-like cells in mouse bone marrow cultures. J Bone Miner Res 1996;11 [Suppl]:T394

[47] Rosen CJ, Bilezikian JP. Clinical Review 123: Hot Topic Anabolic Therapy for Osteoporosis J Clin Endocrinol Metab 2001;86: 957–964.

[48] Donahue LR, Rosen CJ. IGFs and bone. The osteoporosis connection revisited. Proc Soc Exp Biol Med. 1998;219:1–7.

[49] Sugimoto T, Nishiyama K, Kuribayashi F, Chihara K. Serum levels of IGF-I, IGFBP-2, and IGFBP-3 in osteoporotic patients with and without spine fractures. J Bone Miner Res. 1997;12:1272–1279.

[50] Bauer DC, Rosen C, Cauley J, Cummings SR. Low serum IGF-I but not IGFBP-3 predicts hip and spine fracture: the study of osteoporotic fracture.J Bone Miner Res. 1998;23:S561.

[51] Rosen CJ, Pollak MF. IGF-I and aging: a new perspective for a new century. Trends Endocrinol Metab. 1999;10:136 –142.

[52] Ghiron L, Thompson J, Halloway L, Butterfield GE, Hoffman A, Marcus R. Effects of rhGH and IGF-I on bone turnover in elderly women. J Bone Miner Res.1995;10:1844 – 1852.

[53] Liu JM, Zhao HY, Ning G, Chen Y, Zhang LZ, Sun LH, Zhao YJ, Xu MY, Chen JL IGF-1 as an early marker for low bone mass or osteoporosis in premenopausal and postmenopausal women. J Bone Miner Metab (2008) 26:159–164

[54] Pak CYC, Sakhaee K, Zerwekh JE, Parcel C, Peterson R, Johnson K. Safe and effective treatment of osteoporosis with intermittent slow release NaF: augmentation of vertebral bone mass and inhibition of fractures. J Clin Endocrinol Metab.1989; 68:150 –159.

[55] Pak CYC, SakhaeeK, Adams Huet B, Piziak V, Petersen RD, Poindexter JR. Treatment of postmenopausal osteoporosis with slow-release NaF. Ann Intern Med. 1995;123:401– 408.

[56] Pak CYC, Zerwekh JE, Antich PP, Bell NH, Singer FR. Slow-release sodium fluoride in osteoporosis. J Bone Miner Res. 1996;5:561–564.

[57] Ringe JD, Kipshoven C, Coster A, Umbach R. Therapy of established postmenopausal osteoporosis with monofluorophosphate plus calcium: dose related effects on bone density and fracture rate. Osteop Int.1999; 9:171–178.

[58] Reginster JY, Meurmans L, Zegels B, et al. The effect of sodium monfluorophosphate plus calcium on vertebral fracture rate in postmenopausal women with moderate osteoporosis.Arandomized controlled trial. Ann Intern Med. 1998;129:1– 8.

[59] Ringe JD, dorst A, Kipshoven C, Rovati LC, Setnikar I. Avoidance of vertebral fractures in men with idiopathic osteoporosis by a three-year therapy with calcium and low-dose intermittent monofluorophosphate. Osteop Int. 1998;8:47–52.

[60] Shimazaki C, Uchida R, Nakano S, Namura K, Fuchida SI, Okano A, Okamoto M and InabaT. High serum bone-specific alkaline phosphatase level after bortezomib-combined therapy in refractory multiple myeloma: possible role of bortezomib on osteoblast differentiation. Leukemia 2005;19, 1102–1103.

[61] Tamma R, Colaianni G, Zhu LL, DiBenedetto A, Greco G, Montemurro G, Patano N, Strippoli M, Vergari R, Mancini L, Colucci S, Grano M, Faccio R, Liu X, Li J, Usmani S, Bachar M, Bab I, Nishimori K, Young LJ, Buettner C, Iqbal J, Sun L, Zaidi M, Zallone A. Oxytocin is an anabolic bone hormone. Proc Natl Acad Sci U S A. 2009;106(17):7149-54

[62] Wiens M, Etminan M, Gill SS, Takkouche B. Effects of anti-hypertensive drug treatments on fracture outcomes: a meta-analysis of observational studies. J Intern Med 2006;260:350-62

[63] Reid IR. Effects of beta-blockers on fracture risk. J Musculoskelet Neuronal Interact. 2008 Apr-Jun;8(2):105-10. Review.

[64] Yang S, Nguyen ND, Eisman JA, Nguyen TV. Association between beta-blockers and fracture risk: A Bayesian meta-analysis. Bone. 2012;51(5):969-974.

[65] Zamani A, Omrani GR, Nasah MM. Lithium's effect on bone mineral density. Bone. 2009 Feb;44(2):331-4

[66] Poole KE, van Bezooijen RL, Loveridge N, Hamersma H, Papapoulos SE, Lowik CW, Reeve J. Sclerostin is a delayed secreted product of osteocytes that inhibits bone formation. FASEB J 2005;19(13):1842-1844.

[67] van Bezooijen RL, Roelen BA, Visser A, van der Wee-Pals L, de Wilt E, Karperien M, Hamersma H, Papapoulos SE, ten Dijke P, Löwik CW. Sclerostin is an osteocyte-expressed negative regulator of bone formation, but not a classical BMP antagonist. J Exp Med 2004;199(6):805-814.

[68] Lewiecki EM. Sclerostin: a novel target for intervention in the treatment of osteoporosis. Discov Med. 2011;12(65):263-73. Review.

[69] Li X, Ominsky MS, Niu QT, Sun N, Daugherty B, D'Agostin D, Kurahara C, Gao Y, Cao J, Gong J, Asuncion F, Barrero M, Warmington K, Dwyer D, Stolina M, Morony

http://dx.doi.org/10.5772/54452

S, Sarosi I, Kostenuik PJ, Lacey DL, Simonet WS, et al. Targeted deletion of the sclerostin gene in mice results in increased bone formation and bone strength. J Bone Miner Res 2008; 23(6):860-869.

[70] Li X, Ominsky MS, Warmington KS, Morony S, Gong J, Cao J, Gao Y, Shalhoub V, Tipton B, Haldankar R, Chen Q, Winters A, Boone T, Geng Z, Niu QT, Ke HZ, Kostenuik PJ, Simonet WS, Lacey DL, Paszty C. Sclerostin antibody treatment increases bone formation, bone mass, and bone strength in a rat model of postmenopausal osteoporosis. J Bone Miner Res 2009b;24(4):578-588.

[71] Ominsky MS, Vlasseros F, Jolette J, Smith SY, Stouch B, Doellgast G, Gong J, Gao Y, Cao J, Graham K, Tipton B, Cai J, Deshpande R, Zhou L, Hale MD,Lightwood DJ, Henry AJ, Popplewell AG, Moore AR, Robinson MK, Lacey DL, Simonet WS, Paszty C. Two doses of sclerostin antibody in cynomolgus monkeys increases bone formation, bone mineral density, and bone strength. J Bone Miner Res.2010;25(5):948-59.

[72] Padhi D, Jang G, Stouch B, Fang L, Posvar E. Single-dose, placebo-controlled, randomized study of AMG 785, a sclerostin monoclonal antibody. J Bone Miner Res 2011;26(1):19-26.

[73] Lawrence G. Raisz. Pathogenesis of osteoporosis: concepts, conflicts, and prospects. J Clin Invest .2005;115(12):3318-25.

[74] Amgen and UCB. Amgen and UCB announce positive phase 2 results of AMG 785/ CDP7851 in patients with postmenopausal osteoporosis (PMO). http://www.amgen.com/media_pr_detail.jsp?releaseID=1553039. (accessed 1 Jun 2011).

Chapter 12

Osteoporosis in Spaceflight

Satoshi Iwase, Naoki Nishimura and Tadaaki Mano

Additional information is available at the end of the chapter

http://dx.doi.org/10.5772/54708

1. Introduction

1.1. Renal stones during spaceflight

No major medical diffifulties were experienced during spaceflight in the era of Russian Vostok/ Voshot or spaceflight programs of Mercury and Gemini, however, when prolonged stays in space stations began in the 1980's, astronauts or Russian cosmonauts had an increased risk of suffering from renal stones, and resultant bone loss. The detailed mechanism behind this phenomenon is still unknown, but one explanation is that unloading of the skeleton that would normally bear the bodyweight led to calcium (Ca) leaving the bones for the bloodstream. The Ca entered the kidneys, filtered into the urine, causing hypercalciuria, and increased the risk of kidney stone formation. Such stones formed in the kidney break down and travel into the ureter, causing flank pain. Thus astronauts continually subjected to risks of bone and Ca loss while in microgravity [Buckey, 2006].

Factors that seem to affect the bone and Ca loss while in microgravity are as follows; low light levels, high environmental CO_2 levels, and minimal skeletal loading. It is reported that urinary Ca excretion increases by 60-70 % within a few days of entering the microgravity. Data from the Skylab program in 1973-74, when nine astronauts stayed in the space station for 28 to 84 days, showed that the estimated rate of Ca loss from the bone per month was 0.3% of the total body Ca [Whedon et al. 1974].Data from the Mir program indicated that the bone losing the most Ca losing bone is the coxal bone estimated to lose 1.5% of the total body Ca per month [Le Blanc et al. 2000]. Skylab was a space station launched and operated by NASA (National Aeronautics and Space Administration of the USA) and was the America's first space station, which orbited the Earth from 1973 to 79, and included a workshop, a solar observatory, and other systems with the weight of 77 tons. Mir (мир, peace/world) was a space station that operated in low Earth orbit from 1986 to 2001, at first by Soviet Union and then by Russia. Assembled in orbit from 1986 to 96, Mir was the first modular space station and had a greater mass than that of any previous spacecraft until its deorbit on March 21, 2001. Many experiments including biomedical sciences.

In spite of rapid bone loss under conditions of weightlessness, a slow recovery rate is reported. Data from the Mir program showed that approximately 12% of bone was lost during 4.5 months in space while only 6% recovered in a year on the Earth [Linenger 2000]. Follow-up study of the Skylab crew members after 28-84 days of the microgravity exposure suggested that not all the bone lost on the station had been recovered [Tilton et al. 1980]. These findings indicate the seriousness of bone loss under conditions of microgravity, which could present significant problems, and may progress to osteoporosis, in long-duration spaceflight. Bone loss under conditions of weightlessness should be strictly monitored and controlled.

2. Calcium metabolism during spaceflight

During spaceflight, several factors influence the Ca metabolism, including alterations in diet intake, low lighting, increased ambient CO_2, and the most important factor is unloading of the bodyweight when considering the long duration spaceflight.

The recommended Ca^{2+} intake is 1,000 mg/day, and nutritionists prepare the space food to satisfy this criterion.

In spacecraft, where no sunlight or ultraviolet light exposure is occurs, vitamin D deficiency may develop without sufficient Ca intake, which causes poor mineralization of bone, diminished intestinal Ca absorption, decreased serum Ca^{2+} levels. These situations may cause an increase in parathormone, but actually, sufficient Ca intake protects the bone loss, and serum Ca^{2+} level has been proved to be increased, and parathormone level is suppressed..

Compared with the low CO_2 level on the Earth, which is 0.03% of the atmosphere, confined and isolated circumstances such as in spacecraft or a space station have increased CO_2 levels of 0.7-1%, which affects the acid-base balance, and consequently the bone metabolism. Increased CO_2 levels in inhaled air cause acidosis, and carbonates and phosphates in the bone play important roles in neutralizing the acidosis, which leads to bone resorption [Bushinsky et al., 1997]. Although CO_2 levels >1% were reported to have some effects on urinary bone absorption markers [Drummer et al. 1998], respiratory acidosis may decrease the urinary pH, and increase the risk of kidney stone formation [Coe et al. 1992].

Bone remodeling and the remodeling changes during spaceflight are profoundly dependent on genetic factors in terms of the baseline level [Boyden et al. 2002, Judex et al. 2002]

3. Bone formation factors

3.1. Mechanical loading

The mechanism by which bone senses and responds to loading has yet to be fully clarified yet. Frost [1987] postulated that bone has a mechanostat that senses strain and maintains bone mass

http://dx.doi.org/10.5772/54708

at an appropriate level to keep the strain within an appropriate range, showing that exceeding the setpoint of bone strain bone modeling intiates reduction of the strain back to the setpoint had been carried out. Surveys on athletes indicated that high weight bearing, which is observed in weightlifters and significant impact loading in gymnasts resulted in significantly high bone mass [Nilsson & Westlin, 1971, Uusi-Rasi et al. 1971, Taaffe et al. 1997, Huddleston et al., 1980].

As for the gravity-induced high bone mass density, evidence has shown that heavy-weight people exhibited higher bone density, and spinal injury patients with a wheelchair lose significantly bone mass at lower extremity while not in the lumbar spine [Biering-Sorensen et al., 1988, 1990]. The impact of contact with the ground on the bones of the coxa and the lower extremities is an important factor to maintain the bone mass density [Kreb et al., 1998].

Not only impacts or weight bearing on the bone, but also muscular contractions also play a role in strain bearing on the bone at 1 G [Kreb et al., 1998, Schulthesis et al., 1991]. However, 0 G conditions may influence the skeletal loading both through a loss of ground reaction forces and through marked reduction in the forces needed to move the weightless limbs.

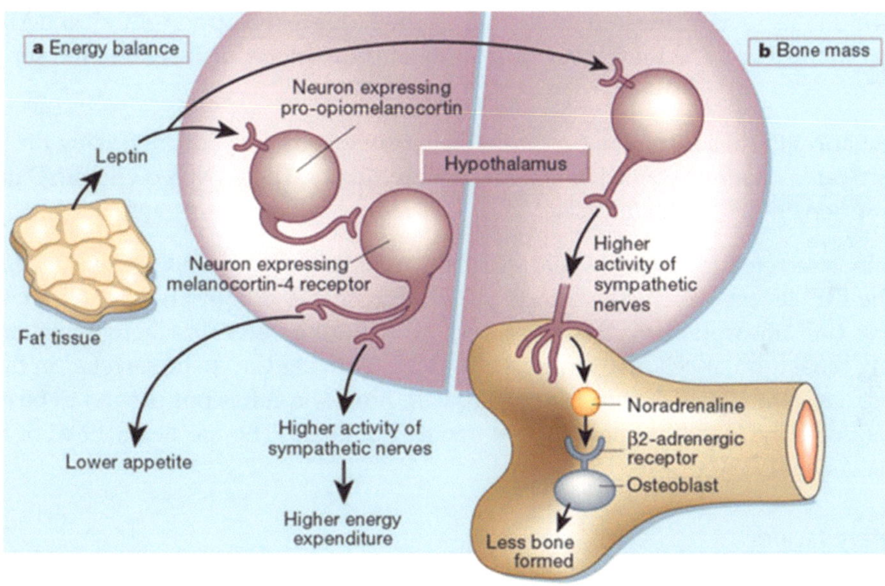

Adapted with permission from Flier JS: Nature 420(6916): 619, 621-622(2002)

Figure 1. Regulation of energy balance and bone mass Leptin suppresses appetite and enhances sympathetic nerve activity through the hypothalamus elevating energy expenditure. At the same time higher activity of the sympathetic nervous system inhibits bone formation of osteoblasts, inducing bone loss.

3.2. Hormones

Sex hormones, estrogens and androgens are associated with bone mass density; however, there seems to be no significant changes in sex hormones during spaceflight. Growth hormone increases the bone mass, but it does not seem to have a relationship with spaceflight. Insulin-like growth factor (IGF-1) has also been shown to be an agent that can increase bone mass, and in animal experiments performed during the Space Shuttle experiment, administration of IGF-1 to rats during the 10 days of the Shuttle flight increased bone formation in the humerus.

Parathormone has a complex effect on the bone. Its ultimate goal is to increase the serum Ca^{2+} level, so that without enough Ca^{2+} intake or vitamin D deficiency, it acts on bone resorption and reduces the bone mass. The action sites of parathormone are the bone, the kidney, and the intestine.

The mechanism of parathormone action on the bone is indirect since osteoclasts have no receptor of parathormone, rather parathormone binds to osteoblasts to increase their expression of RANKL (receptor activator of nuclear factor kappa-B ligand, osteoclast differentiation factor) and inhibits their expression of osteoprotegrin. Osteoprotegerin binds to RANKL and inhibits it from interacting with RANK (receptor activator of nuclear factor kappa-B, receptor of osteoclast differentiation factor). The binding of RANKL to RANK is facilitated by the decreased amount of osteoprotegerin, and stimulates osteoclast precursors to fuse. It resulted to form new osteoclasts, which ultimately enhances bone resorption.

Parathormone also acts on the kidney to enhance the active reabsorption of Ca^{2+} and Mg^{2+} from the distal tubules and the thick ascending limb, and maintains or increases the serum Ca^{2+} levels.

It also enhances the absorption of Ca^{2+} from the intestine indirectly, by increasing the production of activated vitamin D, which is activated in the kidney. The activated vitamin D increases the absorption of Ca^{2+} by the intestine.

Calcitonin is secreted from the thyroid gland by an increase in serum Ca^{2+} levels, and acts to lower the Ca^{2+} levels, which counteracts parathormone. Calcitonin lowers Ca^{2+} levels by 1) inhibiting Ca^{2+} absorption by the intestines, 2) inhibiting osteoclast activity in bones, 3) inhibiting renal tubular cell reabsorption of Ca^{2+} by allowing Ca^{2+} to be secreted in the urine. Therefore, calcitonin protects bone from Ca^{2+} loss, however, it has not proved to be effective in preventing bone loss in immobilization in either animals [Thomas et al., 1995] or humans [Hantman et al., 1973].

3.3. Dietary factors

Ca, vitamin D, and vitamin K are the essential factors for bone formation, and their oral intake is recommended during spaceflight.

3.4. Electric fields and vibration

Studies have shown exposure of marrow culture to low-frequency, low-intensity electric fields inhibited the recruitment of osteoclasts [Rubin et al., 1996]. Low magnitude (0.25 G) and high frequency (30-90 Hz) vibration has been proved to be effective in inhibiting bone loss and increasing bone formation in humans [Bosco et al., 1999, Rubin et al. 2004]. This vibration constitues a promising countermeasure against bone loss in spaceflight, and studies are now being conducted to clarify the optimal magnitude and frequency.

http://dx.doi.org/10.5772/54708

4. Bone resorption factors

4.1. Immobilization

The unloading of weight bearing on bone on Earth is associated with prolonged bed rest, immobilization, or paralysis. Studies of patients with spinal cord injury have demonstrated that approximately 30–50% of lower extremity bone mass can be lost before reaching a plateau, which occurs an average of approximately 16 months after admission [Biering-Sorensen et al. 1990, Garland et al. 1992].

4.2. Hormones

Chronic increase in parathormone levels enhances resorption, which causes osteoporosis. This increase in parathormone is sometimes produced by lower serum Ca^{2+} and vitamin D; however, intermittent administration of parathormone with enough Ca^{2+} levels with vitamin D can also be anabolic. Thyroid hormones and glucocorticoid can be a cause of osteoporosis, but it is unlikely to occur in space.

4.3. Dietary factors

High Na^+ intake enhances Na^+ excretion as well as urinary Ca^{2+} excretion. A high level of dietary protein also provides an acid load, which causes bone loss mediated by skeletal buffering. Therefore, it is favorable for space food to contain low salt as well as low protein.

5. Bone loss and osteoporosis in spaceflight

Skylab missions were the first opportunity to study the Ca metabolism in space [Whendon et al., 1974]. These included the unmanned Skylab 1, Skylab 2 with 3 crew members staying 29 days of stay, Skylab 3 also with 3 crew members staying 59 days, and Skylab 4 again with 3 crew members staying 84 days. Thereafter, various Space Shuttle Programs have been conducted to examine the effects of space flights on Ca metabolism in humans.

Urinary excretion of Ca^{2+} is enhanced promptly just after microgravity exposure, and remains elevated for several months throughout weightlessness exposure or eventually returns to normal depending on individual. The mechanism behind individual differences has not benn well clarified. Data from two Russian cosmonauts demonstrated no Ca^{2+} excretion increases were observed after 218 days of microgravity exposure [Grigoriev et al., 1994]. The reason for this lack of an increase in Ca^{2+} might be the effectiveness of countermeasure program.

5.1. Bone loss markers during spaceflight

Frozen urine samples from the Skylab mission were subsequently examined; the data showed that N-telopeptide was increased throughout the flight [Smith et al., 1998], and C-telopeptide also remained elevated throughout on a-180 day Mir flight [Caillot-Augusseau et al., 1998].

Elevation of these two markers demonstrated that the increased urinary Ca^{2+} was due to an increase in bone resorption. Osteocalcin, a bone formation marker, measured during a 180-day Mir flight showed a decrease.

5.2. Bone loss location

Bone mineral density was measured before and after flights on the Mir program. The changes per month were as follows; +0.6% in the skull, +0.1% in the arm, −1.07% in the spine, −1.35% in the pelvis, −1.16% in the femoral neck, −1.58% in the trochanter major, −1.25% in the tibia, and −1.50% in the calcaneus, all per month, with comparable results obtained from the International Space Station [Lang et al., 2004].

The bones that are most affected during spaceflight seems to be weight bearing bones, such as the pelvis (os coxae), the trochanter major of the femur, the femoral neck, the tibia, and the calcaneus.

5.3. Parathormone and Vitamin D

Data from the Skylab program exhibited a slight increase in serum Ca^{2+} levels and decrease in parathormone. Spacelab Life Sciences 1 (9 days), and 2(14 days) flights and a 180-day Mir flight showed decreased serum parathormone levels in crew members, and active vitamin D levels were also decreased, which in turn reduced Ca absorption [Caillot-Augusseau et al., 1998].

5.4. Summary

In summary, bone resorption is increased, bone formation is decreased, bone loss occurs in weight-bearing areas, and parathormone is suppressed during space flight, which are comparable to the data from immobilization under conditions of bedrest or spinal cord injury.

6. Sympathetic modulation of bone metabolism during spaceflight

It has been reported that sympathetic neural traffic to bone inhibits the function of osteoblasts and enhances that of osteoclasts thus facilitating bone loss. Possible roles of the sympathetic nervous system in the mechanisms of bone loss in humans exposed to long-term space flight will be discussed [Mano et al., 2010].

6.1. Alterations in sympathetic neural traffic under microgravity

Sympathetic neural traffic indirectly measured by plasma noradrenaline level has been reported to increase during spaceflight compared with the pre-flight control level [Christensen & Norsk, 1998, Ertl et al., 2002], and vagal activity estimated by power spectral analysis of heart rate variability has been shown to be reduced after long-term spaceflight [Cooke et al., 2000, Mano, 2005].

http://dx.doi.org/10.5772/54708

Microneurographically, on the other hand, recorded neural traffic in humans is known to reflect muscle and skin sympathetic nerve activity (MSNA and SSNA), and MSNA controls the vasomotor function of the muscular bed, responding to blood pressure changes against gravitational stress [Iwase et al., 1987, Mano 1990, Mano et al., 2009]. MSNA was found to be suppressed during an exposure to short-term microgravity induced by parabolic flight [Iwase et al., 1999], to mild lower body positive pressure (10-20 mmHg LBPP) [Fu et al., 1998], and to thermoneutral head-out water immersion [Miwa et al., 1996] responding to the loading or unloading of cardiopulmonary receptor stimulated by cephalad fluid shift. Contrarily, MSNA was enhanced after an exposure to long-term microgravity in spaceflight and its simulation induced by dry immersion (Iwase et al., 2000), and 6°head-down bed rest (Kamiya et al., 2000), caused by various mechanisms including plasma volume loss, changes in baroreflex, and vascular compliance after the human body has acclimated to microgravity situation..

As for the sympathetic influence on bone metabolism, sympathetic stimulation facilitated bone resorption, while it inhibited ossification by osteoblasts mediated by hypothalamus and leptin in mouse. Loading of weak chronic stress in mouse reduced the osteoblastic activity with elevated noradrenaline, which was prevented by β-blocker [Kondo et al., 2005]. The beneficial effects of β-adrenergic blocker on bone mass and metabolism were reported in mice and rats [Minkowitz et al., 1991, Pierroz, et al., 2006]. Other studies were controversial, however, recent studies have indicated that there are two systems that regulate bone metabolism; one through β_2 receptors in bone which facilitates osteolysis and inhibits osteogenesis, and the other that facililtates osteogenesis through a kind of neuropeptide called CART (cocaine amphetamine regulated transcript) [Elefteriou et al., 2005].

From human studies, there have been reports that administration of β-blockers may reduce the risk of bone fracture as well as higher bone density (Graham et al., 2008, Levasseur et al., 2005, Pasco et al., 2004, 2005, Reid et al., 2005a, b, Reinmark et al., 2004, 2006, Schlienger et al., 2004, Turker et al., 2006)

6.2. Space flight-related changes in sympathetic regulation on bone metabolism

Prolonged exposure to microgravity in space for 14 days enhanced the sympathetic neural traffic in humans as evidenced by the Neurolab mission[Cox et al., 2002, Fu et al., 2002, Levine et al., 2002, Ertl et al., 2002], with comparable results in elevated noradrenaline spillover and clearance in space [Ertl et al., 2002]. Corresponding results were obtained from simulated microgravity including dry immersion [Iwase et al., 2000] or head-down bed rest [Kamiya et al., 2000]. Elderly people generally have low bone mass and density and high sympathetic neural traffic to muscles although response to gravitational stress becomes lowered (Iwase et al. 1991). Our preliminary data show that changes in sympathetic neural traffic to muscles after long-term bedrest of 20 days had a significant correlation with changes in the urinary secretion level of deoxypyridinoline (Mano et al., 2009, Nishimura et al., 2010) (Fig.2), which a specific marker for bone resorption (Robbins et al., 1994). On the basis of these findings, it is postulated that an exposure to prolonged microgravity enhances the sympathetic neural traffic to bone, which increases the noradrenaline level, inhibits osteogenesis and facilitates osteolysis through β-receptors to induce bone mineral loss; however, it is no better than hypothesis.

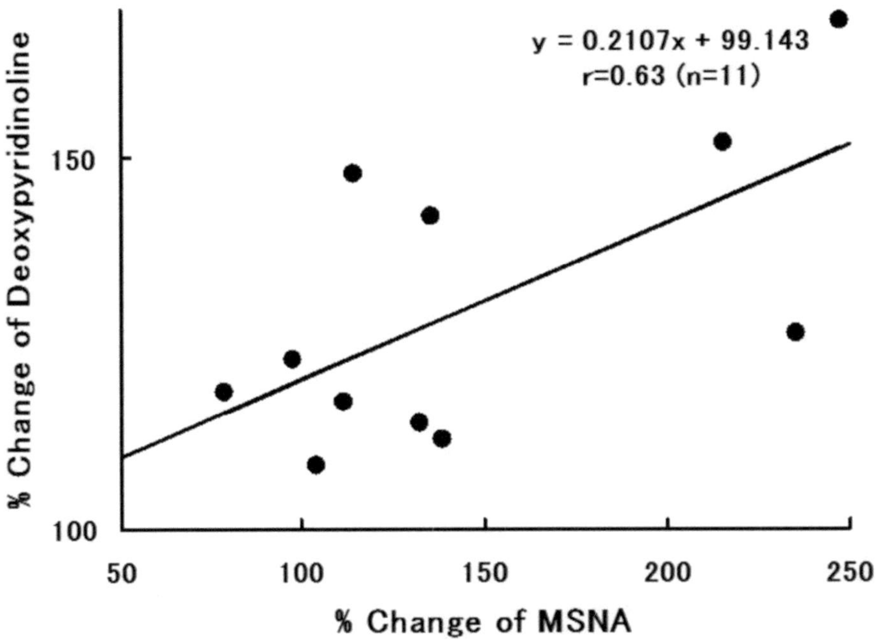

Adapted with permission from Nishimura N et al: Space Utiliz Res. 26: 122-124 (2010)

Figure 2. Correlation between muscle sympathetic nerve activity (MSNA) and urinary secretion of deoxypyridinoline in healthy humans exposed to long-term bed rest. A significant correlation was found between percent changes in burst numbers per minute of MSNA recorded microneurographically from the tibial nerve (abscissa) and percent changes in urinary secretion of deoxypyridinoline (ordinate) in 11 young healthy male subjects (24±5 years old) exposed to long-term head-down bed rest (20 days).

7. Countermeasures for space-related osteoporosis

The bone has difficulty regaining its density and once it is lost, as shown by the studies of bed rest and spinal cord injury patients. Data from spaceflight suggest that this slow recovery is also exhibited by astronauts as well [Linenger, 2000, Tilton et al., 1980]. Bone can be recovered, but it takes a longer time to recover it than to lose it. This means that the prevention of bone loss is a more preferable than its recovery by aggressive rehabilitation. The strategy of "less loss to regain fast" might be an effective way to minimize the necessary amount of postflight rehabilitation needed and to extend the time people can remain in microgravity.

7.1. Vitamin D and calcium intake

The low light levels in the spacecraft necessitate sufficient oral intake of vitamin D and Ca since parathormone levels are suppressed during spaceflight. Oral intake of 600–800 IU/day vitamin D is recommended in the absence of sunlight although 400 IU/day is usually adequate to maintain bone mass density [Holick, 1996].

The Ca intake necessary to minimize a negative Ca balance is approximately 1,000 mg of elemental Ca (~40% of $CaCO_3$), which is currently recommended for space station flights up to 360 days [Weaver, 2000]. Howver, excessive oral intake of Ca is associated with a risk of hypercalciuria due to skeletal unloading, which may lead to high risk of kidney stones. However, kidney stones may not develop because orally administered Ca may bind to oxalate in the intestine and reduce the oxalate absorption [Heller 1999]. Therefore, Ca intake during spaceflight should be taken orally [Martini & Wood, 2000].

7.2. Physical factors

Exercise upon exposure to weightlessness has been incorporated into some countermeasure programs, however, exercise alone cannot prevent the bone loss. The current exercise program for the ISS is a combination of aerobic and resistive exercises for 2.5 hrs, 6 days/week. Data from the space flight demonstrate that bone loss occurs mainly in the femur, tibia, calcaneus, and vertebrae. Therefore, exercise should be concentrated on these bones, and impact loading should primarily be provided rather than static loading [Taaffe et al., 1997].

Hip joint: Some of the larger bone losses observed in the space program have been concentrated in the hips (os coxae mainly) [Le Blanc et al., 1999]. A study using hip joint pressure sensors has demonstrated that peak joint forces can range from 3–4 times when walking, 5.5 times with jogging, and as high as 8.7 times bodyweight with stumbling [Hall, 1995], which are do not seem to be generated during the exercise in microgravity. The peak pressure in the articulatio coxae (hip joint) during supine isometric abduction was 3.78 mPa, which was as high as those during walking of 3.64 mPa [Strickland et al., 1992], and that during rising from a seated position, was 7.14 mPa [Hodge et al., 1986]. These data suggest that running on a treadmill generates an insufficient load to generate enough loads, but short periods of high loading using abduction, adduction and squatting would be necessary to load sufficient pressures on the hip joint.

Lumbar spine: The bodyweight is loaded on the L_3 vertebra when standing under conditions of 1 G state, but unloaded vertebrae would lose their bone mass density under microgravity. The concern is the minimum period of standing position required to maintain the bone mass, which has not been clarified. Moreover, the even if this duration is clarified; weight loading under weightlessness is difficult. Whether a shorter duration of a higher load can provide the same bone protection as a longer duration of a lower load has also yet to be solved.

Femur: The femoral neck and the trochanter major are the principal sites of weight bearing under the condition of 1 G, and are site at which significant bone mass is lost during the spaceflight. The femoral shaft mainly consists of cortical bone and the loss of bone mass from the femoral shaft were −1.6% on average after 4–6 months of spaceflight [Oganov, 1996]. The kind of exercise that be most effective to prevent bone loss from the femur is not known.

Tibia: The proximal tibia consists of trabecular and cortical bone, and its loss of bone mass was reported to be −1.25% per month. The most effective exercise to prevent the bone loss from this area seemed to be squatting exercise.

Calcaneus: The calcaneus receives a reaction force from the ground of 2–3 times of body weight to the foot while running under 1 G. The fact that the calcaneus of gymnasts exhibits increased bone density suggests that not only the number of loading cycles but also peak loading is significant in increasing bone mass density in the calcaneus [Taaffe et al., 1999].

7.3. Pharmacological factors

Since bone mass is adequate at the onset of spaceflight, the optimal strategy for pharmacotherapy against bone loss is the prevention of bone loss, not the acceleration of bone formation, when the loading is removed during spaceflight. Several drugs have been proposed for the prevention of bone loss under microgravity.

7.3.1. Bisphosphonates

Bisphosphonates have two phosphonate (PO_3) groups and have a similar structure to pyrophosphate. They bind to hydroxyapatite in the bone matrix, and prevent the bone loss by inhibiting the osteoclastic bone resorption. Bisphosphonates have been demonstrated to be effective in preventing bone loss during bed rest studies [Grigoriev et al., 1992, Rodan & Fleisch, 1996, Thompson et al., 1990, LeBlanc et al., 1998]. Among several kinds of bisphosphonate, pamidronate has been proved to suppress bone mineral loss and to prevent the formation of renal stones during bedrest study (Watanabe et al., 2004).

In 2010, LeBlanc and Matsumoto proposed an experiment on the effectiveness of bisphosphonate as a countermeasure to spaceflight-induced bone loss. The astronauts chose either oral administration of alendronate at 70 mg once per week or intravenous administration of zoledronate at 4 mg before flight, and were examined their bone density by DEXA (dual energy x-ray absorptiometry), QCT (quantitative computed tomography), and pQCT (peripheral qualitative computed tomography), bone metabolism markers including bone formation and resorption markers, and renal stone formation. One of the co-investigators, Ohshima reported successful results in suppressing the space flight-induced bone loss and renal stone formation [Ohshima, personal communication].

The disadvantages of bisphosphonates are local irritation of the upper gastrointestinal (GI) tract, and poor absorption from the GI tract. Therefore, the oral administration of bisphosphonates requires the intake with 200 mL of water and for the subject to remain upright posture for at least 30 min, and until after consumption of the first food of the day to facilitate delivery to the stomach. The problem is that an upright posture cannot be achieved in space under conditions of microgravity. Another problem is the possibility of osteonecrosis of the maxilla and the mandible occurring although the incidence of this is low [Durie et al., 2005]. Since these osteonecroric or osteolytic phenomena are always accompanied by physiological stress (mastication), iatrogenic trauma (tooth extraction/denture injury), or tooth infection [Ruggiero et al. 2004, 2008], it is preferable to prevent such phenomena.

Bisphosphonates are hardly metabolized, and high concentrations of them are maintained in the bones for long periods. Because bone formation is closely coupled to bone turnover, long-term use of these compounds with the resultant suppression of bone turnover can compromise

http://dx.doi.org/10.5772/54708

the healing of even physiological microinjuries within bone. Osteonecrosis of the maxilla and the mandible likely results from the inability of hypodynamic and hypovascular bone to meet an increased demand for repair and remodeling because several kinds of manipulation are associated with this necrosis.

7.3.2. *Thiazide diuretics and potassium citrate*

Thiazide diuretics and potassium citrate are not usually considered drugs for bone loss prevention, but are usually used for kidney stone prevention; they act by markedly reducing the urinary Ca level.

7.3.3. *Selective estrogen receptor modulators*

Estrogen is effective for bone mass preservation in both men and women, but it has a side effect of thrombophlebitis, which would be a very significant for bedrest subjects or astronauts in the space.

7.3.4. *Statins*

There is some evidence suggesting that statins might be effective to increase bone mass, in addition to their main role; however, no data from bedrest or immobilization studies have shown the effectiveness of their use. Therefore it might be too early to apply it to astronauts in spaceflight.

7.3.5. *Parathormone*

Parathormone has anabolic effects on bone, and also acts on the kidney to stimulate the resorption of Ca^{2+} and enhance the synthesis of vitamin D. In this sense, parathormone may stimulate the bone formation, increase vitamin D synthesis, and stimulate Ca^{2+} resorption. Since the suppression of bone resorption is favorable for stimulating bone formation during spaceflight, the administration of parathormone appears strategically unfavorable.

7.4. Artificial gravity

For human space voyages of several years duration, such as those envisioned for the exploration of Mars, astronauts would be at risk of catastrophic consequences should any of the systems that provide adequate air, water, food, or thermal protection fail. Beyond that, astronauts will face serious health and/or safety risks resulting from severe physiologic deconditioning associated with prolonged weightlessness [Buckey 1999]. The principal physiologic deconditioning risks are related to physical and functional deterioration of the loss of regulation of several systems including blood circulation, decreased aerobic capacity, musculo-skeletal systems, and altered sensory-motor system performance. These physiologic effects of weightlessness are generally adaptive to spaceflight and present a hazard only following G-transitions upon return to Earth or landing on another planet [Young 1999]. Among them, bone mineral metabolism would be greatly affected during prolonged spaceflight.

7.4.1. Why artificial gravity?

Space biomedical researchers have been working for many years to develop "countermeasures" to reduce or eliminate the deconditioning associated with prolonged weightlessness. Intensive and sustained aerobic exercise on a treadmill, bicycle, or rowing machine coupled with intensive resistive exercise has been used on U.S. and Russian spacecraft to minimize these problems. The procedures were uncomfortable and excessively time-consuming for many astronauts, and their effectiveness for maintaining bone, muscle, and aerobic fitness has not been demonstrated, owing, at least in part to the low reliability of the devices used to date. Furthermore, they have had inconsistent effects on postflight orthostatic hypotension or sensory-motor adaptive changes. With the exception of fluid loading before reentry, other kinds of countermeasures (e.g., diet, lower body negative pressure, or wearing a "penguin suit" to force joint extension against a resistive force) have been either marginally effective or present an inconvenience or hazard.

To succeed in the near-term goal of a human mission to Mars during the second quarter of this century, the human risks associated with prolonged weightlessness must be mitigated well beyond our current capabilities. Indeed, during nearly 45 years of human spaceflight experience, including numerous long-duration missions, research has not produced any single countermeasure or combination of countermeasures that is completely effective. Current operational countermeasures have not been rigorously validated and have not fully protected any long-duration (>3 months) astronauts in low-Earth orbit. Thus, it seems unlikely that they will adequately protect astronauts journeying to Mars and back over a three-year period.

Although improvements in exercise protocols, changes in diet, or pharmaceutical treatments of individual systems may be of value, they are unlikely to eliminate the full range of physiologic deconditioning. Therefore, a complete research and development program aimed at substituting for the missing gravitational cues and loading in space is warranted.

The urgency for exploration-class countermeasures is compounded by the limited availability of flight resources for vallidating a large number of system-specific countermeasure approaches. Furthermore, recent evidence of rapid degradation of pharmaceuticals flown aboard long-duration missions, putatively because of radiation effects, raises concerns regarding the viability of some promising countermeasure development research. Although the rotation of a Mars-bound spacecraft will not be a panacea for all the human risks of spaceflight (artificial gravity cannot solve the critical problems associated with radiation exposure, isolation, confinement, and environmental homeostasis), artificial gravity does offer significant promise as an effective, efficient, multi-system countermeasure against the physiologic deconditioning associated with prolonged weightlessness. Virtually all of the identified risks associated with cardiovascular deconditioning, myatrophy, bone loss, and neurovestibular disturbances, space anemia, immune compromise, neurovegetative might be alleviated by the appropriate application of artificial gravity.

7.4.2. Why artificial gravity with exercise?

While short radius centrifuge has been proposed several times, only the loading of artificial gravity has not so effective to prevent spaceflight deconditioning. Also human-powered short-arm centrifuge is effective to load exercise to the astronaut. Considering the size of the International Space Station, it is appropriate to employ the short-radius centrifuge

In 1999, Iwase proposed the manufacture of the facility of artificial gravity with ergometric exercise, and it was subsequently installed at Nagoya University [Iwase 2005]. Several studies were performed using this short-radius centrifuge with an ergometer. In 2002, bedrest study was carried out to validate the effectiveness of artificial gravity with ergometric exercise. In 2005, the facility was moved to Aichi Medical University, and bedrest studies were performed to finalize the protocol. In 2006, this daily AG-EX step-up protocol (1.4 G of artificial gravity load with 60W of ergometric exercise, and the load was stepped up by 0.2 G and 15 W respectively) has been shown to be effective to prevent cardiovascular, musculoskeletal, and bone metabolism deconditioning, while an alternate-day protocol failed to prevent this. In this experiment, bone metabolism was moderately ameliorated by this protocol, but not completely.

The authors proposed installing a short-radius centrifuge facility at the International Space Station, and using it to prevent this spaceflight deconditioning including bone loss. This project, Artificial GRavity with Ergometric Exercise (AGREE project) is promising for the prevention of bone loss in spaceflight (Fig. 3).

8. Bone loss monitoring in space

Most of the space medicine studies on bone metabolism have utilized the blood/urine samples collected before, during, and after spaceflight, and analyzed them in laboratories on Earth. However, during prolonged spaceflight now and in the future, the astronauts or spaceflight surgeons will necessitate to collect samples by themselves and to analyze them in the space station or spacecraft to assess the effects of any countermeasures. Although dual X-ray absorptiometry (DEXA) is effective to measure the bone mass, it cannot detect small changes in bone metabolism so may not provide timely information on the effects of countermeasures..

At least, serum/urinary Ca levels and blood/urinary markers of bone resorption should be determined and monitored, and additional information on bone mass (and/or density) and bone formation/resorption markers in blood and urine is desirable.

Guidelines for bed rest standardization [2012] suggest the use of osteocalcin, bone-specific alkaline phosphatase (BSAP), N-terminal propeptide of type I procollagen (P1NP) as bone formation markers, and N-telopeptide, C-telopeptide, and deoxypyridinoline as bone resorption markers.

Further measurements for bone loss using miniature mass spectrometers and ultrasound may be possible. In particular, ultrasound echography of the bone would be helpful to measure the

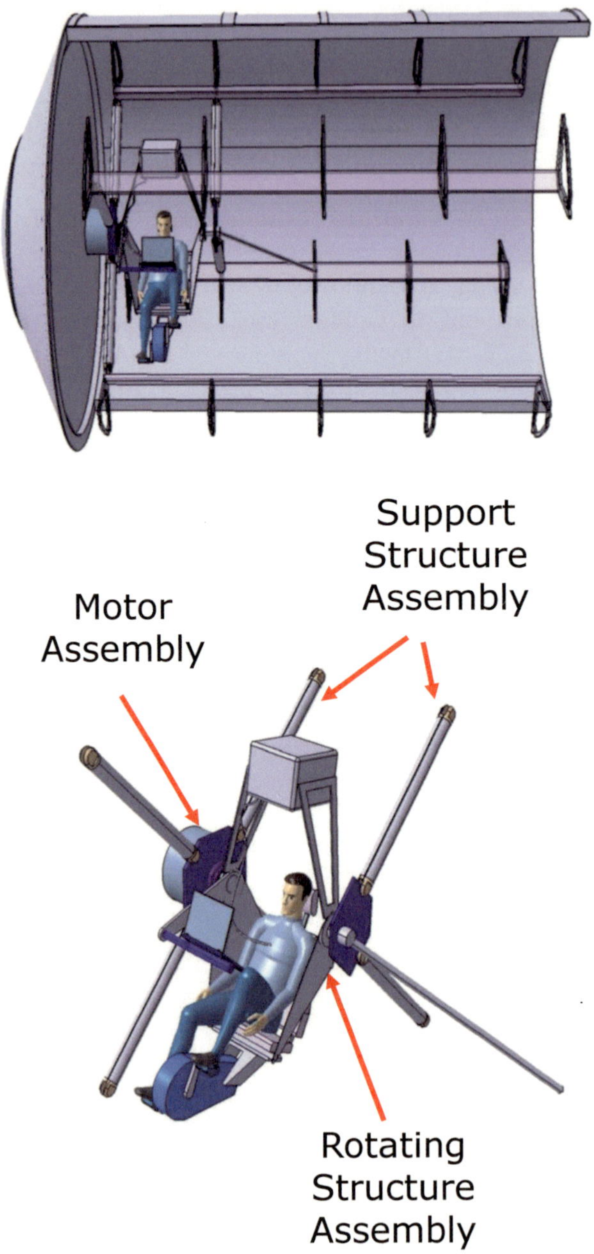

Figure 3. Short arm centrifuge to be installed in the International Space Station.

bone mass/density. Determination of bone mass/density at the hip joint or the calcaneus is helpful to assess the bone status and to validate the countermeasure programs in space [National Osteoporosis Society].

http://dx.doi.org/10.5772/54708

9. Conclusion and summary

In conclusion, it is favorable to administer bisphosphonate orally with artificial gravity with exercise in order to prevent the osteoporosis in space. Monitoring of the blood and urine samples in a space station or spacecraft by a simple method is necessary to assess the effectiveness of any countermeasure program against bone loss..

Author details

Satoshi Iwase[1*], Naoki Nishimura[1] and Tadaaki Mano[2]

*Address all correspondence to: s_iwase@nifty.com

1 Department of Physiology, Aichi Medical University, Yazako-Karimata, Nagakute, Japan

2 Gifu University of Medical Sciences, Seki, Gifu, Japan

References

[1] Biering-sørensen, F, Bohr, H. H, & Schaadt, O. P. Bone mineral content of the lumbar spine and lower extremities years after spinal cord lesion. Paraplegia. (1988). , 26, 293-301.

[2] Biering-sørensen, F, & Bohr, H. H. Schaadt OP Longitudinal study of bone mineral content in the lumbar spine, the forearm and the lower extremities after spinal cord injury. Eur J Clin Invest. (1990). , 20, 330-335.

[3] Bosco, C, Colli, R, Introini, E, Cardinale, M, Tsarpela, O, Madella, A, Tihanyi, J, & Viru, A. Adaptive responses of human skeletal muscle to vibration exposure. Clin Physiol.(1999). , 19, 183-187.

[4] Boyden, L. M, Mao, J, Belsky, J, Mitzner, L, Farhi, A, Mitnick, M. A, Wu, D, Insogna, K, & Lifton, R. P. High bone density due to a mutation in LDL-receptor-related protein 5. N Engl J Med. (2002). , 346, 1513-1521.

[5] Buckey JC JrPreparing for Mars: the physiologic and medical challenges. Eur J Med Res (1999). , 4, 353-356.

[6] BuckeyJC Jr. Bone Loss, In: Space Physiology, by Buckey, JC Jr., (2006). Oxford University Press, New York, NY, , 1-31.

[7] Bushinsky, D. A, Riordon, D. R, Chan, J. S, & Krieger, N. S. Decreased potassium stimulates bone resorption. Am J Physiol. 272: FF780, (1997). , 774.

[8] Caillot-augusseau, A, Lafage-proust, M. H, Soler, C, Pernod, J, Dubois, F, & Alexandre, C. Bone formation and resorption biological markers in cosmonauts during and after a 180-day space flight (Euromir 95). Clin Chem. (1998)., 44, 578-585.

[9] Christensen, N. J. Norsk P: Sympathoadrenal activity is increased in humans during spaceflight. J Gravit Physiol. 5, (1998)., 13-P14.

[10] Coe, F. L, Parks, J. H, & Asplin, J. R. The pathogenesis and treatment of kidney stones. N Engl J Med. (1992)., 327, 1141-1152.

[11] Cooke, W. H, Ames, I. V J. E, Crossman, A. A, Cox, J. F, & Kuusela, T. A. Tahvanaine KUO, Moon LB, Drescher J, Baisch FJ, Mano T, Levine BD, Blomqvist GC, Eckber DL : Nine months in space: effects on human autonomic cardiovascular regulation. J Appl Physiol. (2000)., 89, 1039-1045.

[12] Durie BGMKatz M, Crowley J. Osteonecrosis of the jaw and bisphosphonates. N Engl J Med (2005)., 353, 99-102.

[13] Elefteriou, F, Ahn, J. D, Takeda, S, Starbuck, M, Yang, X, Liu, X, Kondo, H, Richards, W. G, Bannon, T. W, Noda, M, Clement, K, & Vaisse, C. Karsenty G: Leptin regulation of bone resorption by the sympathetic nervous system and CART. Nature. (2005)., 434(7032), 514-520.

[14] Ertl, A. C, Diedrich, A, Biaggioni, I, Levine, B. D, Robertson, R. M, Cox, J. F, Zuckerman, J. H, Pawelczyk, J. A, & Ray, C. A. Buckey JC Jr, Lane LD, Shiavi R, Gaffney FA, Costa F, Holt C, Blomqvist CG, Eckberg DL, Baisch FJ, Robertson D: Human muscle sympathetic nerve activity and plasma noradrenaline kinetics in space. J Physiol. (2002)., 538, 321-329.

[15] Frost, H. M. Bone "mass" and the "mechanostat": a proposal. Anat Rec. (1987)., 219, 1-9.

[16] Fu, Q, Sugiyama, Y, & Kamiya, A. Shamsuzzaman ASM, Mano T: Responses of muscle sympathetic nerve activity to lower body positive pressure. Am J Physiol. 275: HH1259, (1998)., 1254.

[17] Gill, S. B, & Valencia, M. P. Sabino MLC, Heideman GM, Michel MA. Bisphosphonate-related osteonecrosis of the mandible and maxilla: clinical and imaging features. J Comp Assist Tomogr (2009)., 33, 449-454.

[18] Graham, S, Hammond-jones, D, Gamie, Z, Polyzois, I, & Tsiridis, E. Tsiridis E: The effect of β-blockers on bone metabolism as potential drugs under investigation for osteoporosis and fracture healing. Expert Opin Investig Drugs. (2008)., 17, 1281-1299.

[19] Grigoriev, A. I, Morukov, B. V, Oganov, V. S, Rakhmanov, A. S, & Buravkova, L. B. Effect of exercise and bisphosphonate on mineral balance and bone density during 360 day antiorthostatic hypokinesia.. J Bone Miner Res. 7 Suppl 2: SS455, (1992)., 449.

[20] Grigoriev, A. I, Morukov, B. V, & Vorobiev, D. V. Water and electrolyte studies during long-term missions onboard the space stations SALYUT and MIR. Clin Investig. (1994). , 72, 169-189.

[21] Hall, S. J. The biomechanics of the human lower extremity. In: Basic Biomechanics, edited by Hall SJ, (1995). Mosby, New York, , 208-242.

[22] Hantman, D. A, Vogel, J. M, Donaldson, C. L, Friedman, R, Goldsmith, R. S, & Hulley, S. B. Attempts to prevent disuse osteoporosis by treatment with calcitonin, longitudinal compression and supplementary calcium and phosphate. J Clin Endocrinol Metab. (1973). , 36, 845-858.

[23] Heller, H. J, Stewart, A, Haynes, S, & Pak, C. Y. Pharmacokinetics of calcium absorption from two commercial calcium supplements. J Clin Pharmacol. (1999). , 39, 1151-1154.

[24] Hodge, W. A, Fijan, R. S, Carlson, K. L, Burgess, R. G, Harris, W. H, & Mann, R. W. Contact pressures in the human hip joint measured in vivo. Proc Natl Acad Sci U S A. (1986). , 83, 2879-83.

[25] Holick, M. F, & Vitamin, D. and bone health. J Nutr. 126(4-Suppl):1159S-1164S, (1996).

[26] International Academy of Astronautics Study GroupBone standard measures. In: International Academy of Astronautics Study Group eds, Guidelines for standardization of bed rest studies in the spaceflight context, (2012). , 44-46.

[27] Iwase, S, & Mano, T. Saito M: Effects of graded head-up tilting on muscle sympathetic nerve activities in man. Physiologist: 30, SS63, (1987). , 62.

[28] Iwase, S, Mano, T, Watanabe, T, & Saito, M. Kobayashi F: Age-related changes of sympathetic outflow to muscles in humans. J Gerontol. 46: MM5, (1991). , 1.

[29] Iwase, S, Mano, T, Cui, J, Kitazawa, A, Kamiya, A, Miyazaki, S, Sugiyama, Y, & Mukai, C. Nagaoka S: Sympathetic outflow to muscle in humans during short periods of microgravity produced by parabolic flight. Am J Physiol. 46: RR426, (1999). , 419.

[30] Iwase, S, Sugiyama, Y, Miwa, C, Kamiya, A, Mano, T, Ohira, Y, Shenkman, B, & Egorav, A. Kozlovskaya IB: Effects of three days of dry immersion on muscle sympathetic nerve activity and artrial blood pressure in Human. J Auron Nerv Sys. (2000). , 79, 156-163.

[31] Iwase, S. Effectiveness of centrifuge-induced artificial gravity with ergometric exercise as a countermeasure during simulated microgravity exposure in humans. Acta Astronaut (2005). , 57, 75-80.

[32] Judex, S, Donahue, L. R, & Rubin, C. Genetic predisposition to low bone mass is paralleled by an enhanced sensitivity to signals anabolic to the skeleton. FASEB J. (2002). , 16, 1280-1282.

[33] Kamiya, A, Iwase, S, Kitazawa, H, Mano, T, & Vinogradova, O. L. Kharchenko IB: Baroreflex control of muscle sympathetic nerve activity after 120 days of 6 degrees head-down bed rest. Am J Physiol Regul Integr Comp Physiol. 278: RR452, (2000). , 445.

[34] Kondo, H, Nifuji, A, Takeda, S, Ezura, Y, Rittling, S. R, Denhardt, D. T, Nakashima, K, & Karsenty, G. Noda M: Unloading induces osteoblastic cell suppression and osteoclastic cell activation to lead to bone loss via sympathetic nervous system. J Biol Chem. (2005). , 280(34), 30192-30200.

[35] Krebs, D. E, Robbins, C. E, Lavine, L, & Mann, R. W. Hip biomechanics during gait. J Orthop Sports Phys Ther. (1998). , 28, 51-59.

[36] Lang, T. LeBlanc A, Evans H, Lu Y, Genant H, Yu A. Cortical and trabecular bone mineral loss from the spine and hip in long-duration spaceflight. J Bone Miner Res. (2004). , 19, 1006-1012.

[37] LeBlanc ASchneider V, Shackelford L, West S, Oganov V, Bakulin A, Voronin L. Bone mineral and lean tissue loss after long duration space flight. J Musculoskelet Neuronal Interact. (2000). , 1, 157-60.

[38] LeBlanc ADDriscol TB, Shackelford LC, Evans HJ, Rianon NJ, Smith SM, Feeback DL, Lai D. Alendronate as an effective countermeasure to disuse induced bone loss. J Musculoskelet Neuronal Interact. (2002). , 2, 335-343.

[39] LeBlanc AMatsumoto T, Jones J, Shapiro J, Lang T, Smith SM, Shackelford L, Sibonga J, Evans H, Spector E, Nakamura T, Kohri K, Ohshima H. Bisphosphonate as a countermeasure to space flight-induced bone loss., http://www.dsls.usra.edu/meetings/hrp(2010). pdf/Bone/1094LeBlanc.pdf

[40] Levasseur, R, Dargent-molina, P, Sabatier, J. P, & Marcelli, C. Breart G: Beta-blocker use, bone mineral density, and fracture risk in older women: results from the Epidemiologie de l'Osteoporose prospective study. J Am Geriatr Soc. (2005). , 53, 550-552.

[41] Linenger, J. M. OFF the planet, (2000). McGraw-Hill, New York.

[42] Mano T: Sympathetic nerve mechanisms of human adaptation to environments-Findings obtained by recent microneurographic studies- EnvironMed. (1990). , 34, 1-35.

[43] Mano, T. Autonomic neural functions in space. Curr Pharm Biotechnol. (2005). , 6, 319-324.

[44] Mano, T, Iwase, S, Nishimura, N, Fu, Q, Cui, J, & Shamsuzzaman, A. S. Kamiya A: Gravitational stress on the sympathetic nervous system in humans. Invasive and non-invasive studies of the human autonomic nervous system. A Satellite Meeting of ISAN2009, September 5-6, 2009, Sydney, (2009). , 22-23.

[45] Mano, T, Nishimura, N, & Iwase, S. Sympathetic neural influence on bone metabolism in microgravity. Acta Physiol Hung. (2010). , 97, 1354-1361.

[46] Martini, L. A, & Wood, R. J. Should dietary calcium and protein be restricted in patients with nephrolithiasis? Nutr Rev. (2000). , 58, 111-117.

[47] Minkowitz, B, Boskey, A. L, Lane, J. M, & Pearlman, H. S. Vigorita VJ: Effects of propranolol on bone metabolism in the rat. J Orthop Res. (1991). , 9, 869-875.

[48] Miwa, C, Mano, T, Saito, M, Iwase, S, Matsukawa, T, & Sugiyams, Y. Koga K: Ageing reduces symptaho-suppressive response to head-out water immersion in humans. Acta Physiol Scand. (1996). , 158, 15-20.

[49] National Osteoporosis SocietyPosition statement on the use of quantitative ultrasound in the management of osteoporosis. National Osteoporosis Society, Camerton, Bath, UK, (2001).

[50] Nilsson, B. E, & Westlin, N. E. Bone density in athletes. Clin Orthop Relat Res. (1971). , 77, 179-182.

[51] Nishimura, N, Iwase, S, Shiozawa, T, Sugenoya, J, Shimizu, Y, Takada, M, Inukai, Y, Sato, M, Kanikowska, D, Suzuki, S, Ishida, K, Akima, H, Katayama, K, & Masuo, Y. Mano T: Effectiveness of countermeasure to bone metabolic deconditioning induced by simulated microgravity exposure (in Japanese). Space Utiliz Res. (2010). , 26, 122-124.

[52] Oganov, V. S, & Schneider, V. S. Skeletal system. In: Space Biology and Medicine, edited by Nicogossian AE, Gazenko OG. (1996). American Institute of Aeronautics and Astronautics, Reston, VA, , 247-266.

[53] Pasco, J. A, Henry, M. J, Sanders, K. M, Kotowicz, M. A, & Seeman, E. Nicholson GC: Beta-adrenergic blockers reduce the risk of fracture partly by increasing bone mineral density: Geelong osteoporosis study. J Bone Miner Res. (2004). , 19, 19-24.

[54] Pasco, J. A, Henry, M. J, Nicholson, G. C, & Schneider, H. G. Kotowicz MA: Beta-blockers reduce bone resorption marker in early postmenopausal women. Ann Hum Biol. (2005). , 32, 738-745.

[55] Pierroz, D. D, Bouxsein, M. L, & Rizzoli, R. Ferrari SL: Combined treatment with beta-blocker and intermittent PTH improves bone mass and microarchitecture in ovariectomized mice. Bone. (2006). , 39, 260-267.

[56] Reid, I. R, Gamble, G. D, Grey, A. B, Black, D. M, Ensrud, K. E, & Browner, W. S. Bauer DC: beta-Blocker use, BMD, and fractures in the study of osteoporotic fractures. J Bone Miner Res. (2005a). , 20, 613-618.

[57] Reid, I. R, Lucas, J, Wattie, D, Horne, A, Bolland, M, Gamble, G. D, & Davidson, J. S. Grey AB: Effects of a beta-blocker on bone turnover in normal postmenopausal

women: a randomized controlled trial. J Clin Endocrinol Metab. (2005b). , 90, 5212-5216.

[58] Rejnmark, L, Vestergaard, P, Kassem, M, Christoffersen, B. R, Kolthofff, N, & Brixen, K. Mosekilde L: Fracture risk in perimenopausal women treated with beta-blockers. Calcif Tissue Int. 75: 365-372, (2004).

[59] Rejnmark, L, & Vestergaard, P. Mosekilde L: Treatment with beta-blockers, ACE inhibitors, and calcium-channel blockers is associated with a reduced fracture risk: a nationalwide case-control study. J Hypertens. (2006). , 24, 581-589.

[60] Robins, S. P, Woitge, H, Hesley, R, Ju, J, & Seyedin, S. Seibel MJ: Direct, enzyme-linked immunoassay for urinary deoxypyridinoline as a specific marker for measuring bone resorption. J Bone Miner Res. (1994). , 10, 1643-1649.

[61] Rodan, G. A, & Fleisch, H. A. Bisphosphonates: mechanisms of action. J Clin Invest. 97: 2692-2696, (1996).

[62] Rubin, J, Mcleod, K. J, Titus, L, Nanes, M. S, Catherwood, B. D, & Rubin, C. T. Formation of osteoclast-like cells is suppressed by low frequency, low intensity electric fields. J Orthop Res. (1996). , 14, 7-15.

[63] Rubin, C, Recker, R, Cullen, D, Ryaby, J, Mccabe, J, & Mcleod, K. Prevention of postmenopausal bone loss by a low-magnitude, high-frequency mechanical stimuli: a clinical trial assessing compliance, efficacy, and safety. J Bone Miner Res. (2004). , 19, 343-351.

[64] Ruggiero, S. L, Mehrotra, B, Rosenberg, T. J, & Engroff, S. L. Osteonecrosis of the jaws associated with the use of bisphosphonates: a review of 63 cases. J Oral Maxillofac Surg. (2004). , 62, 527-534.

[65] Ruggiero, S. L, & Woo, S. B. Biophosphonate-related osteonecrosis of the jaws. Dent Clin North Am. (2008). , 52, 111-128.

[66] Schlienger, R. G, Kraenzlin, M. E, & Jick, S. S. Meier CR: Use of beta-blockers and risk of fractures. JAMA. (2004). , 292, 1326-1332.

[67] Schultheis, L. The mechanical control system of bone in weightless spaceflight and in aging. Exp Gerontol. (1991). , 26, 203-214.

[68] Smith, S. M, Nillen, J. L, Leblanc, A, Lipton, A, Demers, L. M, Lane, H. W, & Leach, C. S. Collagen cross-link excretion during space flight and bed rest. J Clin Endocrinol Metab. (1998). , 83, 3584-3591.

[69] Strickland, E. M, Fares, M, Krebs, D. E, Riley, P. O, Givens-heiss, D. L, Hodge, W. A, & Mann, R. W. In vivo acetabular contact pressures during rehabilitation, Part I: Acute phase. Phys Ther. (1992). , 72, 691-699.

[70] Taaffe, D. R, Robinson, T. L, Snow, C. M, & Marcus, R. High-impact exercise promotes bone gain in well-trained female athletes. J Bone Miner Res. (1997). , 12, 255-260.

[71] Taaffe, D. R, Duret, C, Cooper, C. S, & Marcus, R. Comparison of calcaneal ultrasound and DXA in young women. Med Sci Sports Exerc. (1999). , 31, 1484-1489.

[72] Thomas, T, Skerry, T. M, Vico, L, Caulin, F, Lanyon, L. E, & Alexandre, C. Ineffectiveness of calcitonin on a local-disuse osteoporosis in the sheep: a histomorphometric study. Calcif Tissue Int. (1995). , 57, 224-228.

[73] Thompson, D. D, Seedor, J. G, Weinreb, M, Rosini, S, & Rodan, G. A. Aminohydroxybutane bisphosphonate inhibits bone loss due to immobilization in rats. J Bone Miner Res. (1990). , 5, 279-286.

[74] Tilton, F. E, Degioanni, J. J, & Schneider, V. S. Long-term follow-up of Skylab bone demineralization. Aviat Space Environ Med. (1980). , 51, 1209-1213.

[75] Turker, S, & Karatosun, V. Gunal I: Beta-blockers increase bone mineral density. Clin Orthop Relat Res. (2006). , 443, 73-74.

[76] Uusi-rasi, K, Sievänen, H, Vuori, I, Heinonen, A, Kannus, P, Pasanen, M, Rinne, M, & Oja, P. Long-term recreational gymnastics, estrogen use, and selected risk factors for osteoporotic fractures. J Bone Miner Res. (1999). , 14, 1231-1238.

[77] Watanabe, Y, Ohshima, H, Mizuno, K, Sekiguchi, C, Fukunaga, M, Kohri, K, Rittweger, J, Felsenberg, D, & Matsumoto, T. Nakamura T: Intravenous pamidronate prevents femoral bone loss and renal stone formation during 90-day bed rest. J Bone Miner Res (2004). , 19, 1771-1778.

[78] Weaver, C. M. LeBlanc A, Smith SM. Calcium and related nutrients in bone metabolism. In: Nutrition in Spaceflight and Weightlessness Models, edited by Lane HW, Schoeller DA, (2000). CRC Press, Boca Raton, FL., , 179-196.

[79] Whedon, G. D, Lutwak, L, Reid, J, Rambaut, P, Whittle, M, Smith, M, & Leach, C. Mineral and nitrogen metabolic studies on Skylab orbital space flights. Trans Assoc Am Physicians. (1974). , 87, 95-110.

[80] Young, L. R. Artificial gravity considerations for a mars exploration mission. Ann N Y Acad Sci (1999). , 871, 367-378.